FOUNDATIONAL STRENGTH

The Basics for Starting Training

John Flagg

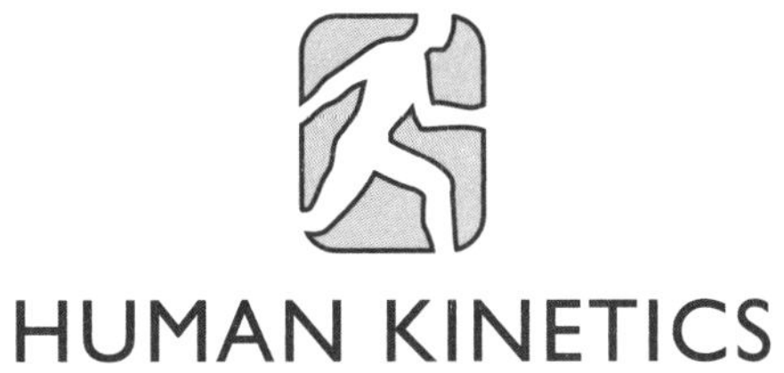

Library of Congress Cataloging-in-Publication Data

Names: Flagg, John, 1983- author.
Title: Foundational strength : the basics for starting training / John Flagg.
Description: Champaign, IL : Human Kinetics, 2026. | Includes bibliographical references and index.
Identifiers: LCCN 2024038950 (print) | LCCN 2024038951 (ebook) | ISBN 9781718216013 (paperback) | ISBN 9781718216020 (epub) | ISBN 9781718216037 (pdf)
Subjects: LCSH: Weight training. | Muscle strength.
Classification: LCC GV546 .F53 2026 (print) | LCC GV546 (ebook) | DDC 613.7/13--dc23/eng/20241113
LC record available at https://lccn.loc.gov/2024038950
LC ebook record available at https://lccn.loc.gov/2024038951ISBN: 978-1-7182-1601-3 (print)

Acquisitions Editor: Korey van Wyk; **Senior Developmental Editor:** Laura Pulliam; **Managing Editor:** Kim Kaufman; **Copyeditor:** Kirsten Aldrich; **Indexer:** Andrea Hepner; **Permissions Manager:** Laurel Mitchell; **Graphic Designer:** Denise Lowry; **Cover Designer:** Keri Evans; **Cover Design Specialist:** Susan Rothermel Allen; **Photograph (cover):** miodrag ignjatovic/E+/Getty Images; **Photographs (interior):** © Human Kinetics; **Photo Production Specialist:** Amy M. Rose; **Photo Production Manager:** Jason Allen; **Senior Art Manager:** Kelly Hendren; **Illustrations:** © Human Kinetics; **Printer:** Sheridan Books

We thank The Bear Cave in Salisbury, Maryland, for assistance in providing the location for the photo shoot for this book.

Human Kinetics books are available at special discounts for bulk purchase. Special editions or book excerpts can also be created to specification. For details, contact the Special Sales Manager at Human Kinetics.

Printed in the United States of America   10 9 8 7 6 5 4 3 2 1

The paper in this book is certified under a sustainable forestry program.

Human Kinetics
1607 N. Market Street
Champaign, IL 61820
USA

United States and International
Website: **US.HumanKinetics.com**
Email: info@hkusa.com
Phone: 1-800-747-4457

Canada
Website: **Canada.HumanKinetics.com**
Email: info@hkcanada.com

E8808

To my wife, Nikki, and my two girls, Joleen and Maddox,
Thank you for always being all-in on me
and my eccentric dreams with weights and barbells
while also tolerating my terrible Dad jokes
and laughing at them
(because you actually find them hilarious).

CONTENTS

FOREWORD

In 2015, we created a community of coaches and health care providers who were ready to break the status quo and set a new standard of care for athletes—and who actually trained hard themselves. This community of professionals understood athletes because they *were* athletes. We called this new community Clinical Athlete. This is where I first met John Flagg.

John was the perfect representation of the mission—strong as hell and a top-tier clinician and coach. Something that stuck out to me right from the beginning was how voracious he was about learning and improving his craft—be it professionally or athletically—with an intense, competitive drive to get better.

Over time, I got to know John on a deeper level, and within a few years, he became a Clinical Athlete subject matter expert for barbell training because (1) it was obvious that there was nobody whose knowledge we trusted more, (2) he applies his knowledge by coaching lifters on a daily basis, and (3) he trains as hard as anyone I've seen and puts up ridiculous numbers in the gym. He's the true embodiment of "walking the walk."

We've sent him all over the country to teach coaches, clinicians, and athletes who wanted to learn from the best. These are people who want to understand the essential barbell lifts, inside and out. I've personally witnessed the magic: John leading multiday courses, with people absolutely getting after it. This way of teaching and learning is great, but there's just one problem: There's only so much content that can be packed into a course that lasts just a few days.

Imagine having a comprehensive manual from a leading expert on barbell training—a place where *all* of the details can be shared. That's what you're getting with this book. No stone is left unturned; you will understand the four essential lifts in a way that transforms your professional and athletic skill set. It's a step-by-step guide and is especially great for new lifters and coaches.

John has broken down the lifts in great detail and with clear photos to help you learn the basics—the phases, the mechanics, the technique—but does so in a way that is digestible, that busts myths, and that helps you understand what matters and what doesn't when implementing the lift in the real world. Then there are the bigger-picture principles, like how athletes learn to move and how skillful exercise selection can drive the movement skill that you're looking for. And, of course, programming: the topic that fuels many Internet wars these days. This book will help you rise above all of that, providing you with a deeper understanding of programming principles that can be applied in any athletic context.

I'm really proud of John for bringing this project to life and am equally excited for it to bring you all the training gains. Here's to future PRs.

—Quinn Henoch, PT, DPT, Clinical Athlete Cofounder

PREFACE

Lifting weights has changed my life, and not just in the sense that most people think. It's literally changed everything about me. It's changed my body, as you'd expect. I've squatted over 900 pounds (408 kg) and bench pressed over 500 pounds (227 kg) in competition. It has undoubtedly changed the way my body looks and feels, and by that, I don't mean that I feel beat up all the time. I feel great, and I look like a guy that can squat 900 pounds (408 kg) and still run around the yard at full speed with his kids. It's incredible. Those are the changes people expect though. I'm not talking about those.

It's changed the way I think. If you had told me years ago what my body was capable of, I would have called you a liar. Just eight years before I squatted that 900 pounds (408 kg), I had 700 pounds (318 kg) on my back for a photography project a friend of mine was doing, and it felt like the weight was sucking my soul right out of my body. I racked it after he took the shot and immediately turned around and told him, "There's no way I will ever actually be able to squat that." Years of work later, and it's a warm-up set. Lifting weights has broken down countless mental barriers for me and for the athletes and clients who I have worked with. It's freed me of beliefs that were limiting me and stopping me from progressing not just in the gym but in my life and my career. I've experienced firsthand how the simplest change can lead to the biggest shift in a person's life. You just need to swap out the phrase "I can't" for "I can."

It's changed my relationships. I am proud to say that my wife and I have a very strong bond and that our relationship has grown through some tough times. Much of that strength stems from lessons learned in the gym while under a barbell, learning to fail and struggling just to add a few more pounds to the bar. Progress takes time and effort, and the pursuit of progress is not a short sprint but a long marathon. That mentality has taught me a kind of patience and an enjoyment of the process that has spilled over into the rest of my life. My relationship with my wife and family is the biggest reflection of this. With sustained effort, we have been able to grow, just like muscles in the gym. In my professional life, I have coached at every level—from Division 1 athletes and national- and international-level powerlifters all the way down to youth sports teams. I'm currently running the strength-and-conditioning program for my daughters' cheer organization. It's dozens of girls, ranging from 5 to 20 years old and with little or no experience with what I'm teaching them. For some people, that may sound like a nightmare. For me, it's a blast. We crank up the music, and everyone has a big smile on their face the whole time because it's fun—and we make it even more fun together by focusing on the discomfort of it. I find discomfort to be a positive because growth comes from discomfort. Those girls figured out early that the work they are doing, no matter how hard it is, will lead them to where they want to be and that the only way to get there is through that discomfort. So they might as well embrace it.

Lifting weights changed my career. It's true; lifting heavy round circles connected to a metal bar literally changed the trajectory of my entire career. Officially,

I'm an athletic trainer. That's what the piece of paper I went to school for says. I decided early on, however, that I wanted to be proactive with my athletes. Why wait until they suffer an injury to help them? Why not make them bigger, faster, and stronger than everyone else so that they can do the damage instead? I had been training (if you could call it that) since I was 15 years old. I knew that the solution to so many of the issues that I was seeing in athletes wasn't in the treatment of injury but in the prevention—or at least the decreased risk—of injury. That became the ethos behind my clinical practice as an athletic trainer working extensively in Physical Therapy offices ,and it dictated all the education and experience I gained moving forward. That was nearly 20 years ago, and I've taken that knowledge and used it to create a coaching course for Physical Therapists, the *Clinical Athlete Powerlifting Coaching Certification*, and to build a business that works with more than 100 athletes—ranging from beginners to world-champion lifters—while helping thousands of other clients and coaches learn how to use a barbell to get the results they want.

I wrote this book because I want all of this for you.

If you are someone who is wondering how best to get started at the gym for the first time, this book is for you. This book contains the basics of what is tried-and-true when it comes to strength training. You can use this to get started and to keep going for years to come. You can build strength and the body you want while also learning the lessons from training that can help you to build a better life and mind.

If you are a coach, or even a student in college who is taking their first exercise-science class, this book is for you. This isn't a cookbook or a compilation of "how tos" that you can copy and paste from. This is a way of thinking about the barbell and about training that can serve as the foundation of your coaching practice. It is a framework to help you serve anyone that steps in front of you with the confidence and assurance that what you do with them will work, and that they will enjoy it.

If you are a health care provider and wondering just how to make a bigger difference in your practice, welcome to the family. The following pages will help you create an accessible and sustainable training program and a pathway for your patients to not only get back to their baseline health, but exceed it.

I wrote this book because lifting changed my life, and I want all of that for you. Welcome to *Foundational Strength.* I hope you enjoy the ride.

ACKNOWLEDGMENTS

Writing a book is something that I never thought I would do. I'm a big meathead, after all, and I figured that my ideas and everything that I've learned from lifting weights for the last 20-plus years and from coaching thousands of clients would live in my brain until I was gone. That, or that my daughters would fall in love with weightlifting and carry it on. That was until my good friend and colleague, Korey VanWyk, emailed me one day and asked if I wanted to write a book. I was floored. I was honored, but I was also as nervous as I could be. Thankfully, he knew me well, and he guided me through, explaining what the process would look like and what kind of impact the book could make. It was that impact that got us on the same page and that inspired this work. If it weren't for him and his faith in me, these pages wouldn't exist. I'm forever grateful for you, Korey, for sending me that email and for always thinking of me when it comes to knowledge about strength.

The next person I want to thank is Laura Pulliam, my editor for this project. To say that she is blessed with the greatest level of patience of anyone who has ever lived would be an understatement. This process took longer than expected; I had a few run-ins with writer's block, and there were some life events (like a move) that came up, resulting in numerous delays. Laura was there the whole time, gently guiding me along the path and answering my questions. Her edits and her advice drove me to think outside the box, leading to an even better book in the end. She found a way to pull so much out of my brain, and this book wouldn't be nearly what it is without her.

I can't forget my parents, Mary Beth and Rod Flagg. I am who I am because of them. They introduced me to the culture of physical fitness, and they still exercise on a regular basis to this day. They taught me the basics. They taught me how to lean in to the learning process of failure. They taught me how to persevere and never quit. (Hell, my mom wrote a textbook on computer programming, which showed me that anything was possible if you worked hard at it.) Without them I would have never picked up a barbell, become the athlete and the coach I am, or gained the knowledge to fill these pages. Love you, Mom and Dad.

Lastly, my wonderful wife, Nikki, and my two girls, Joleen and Maddox. They are my rocks. They laughed with me when I couldn't figure out how to end a chapter. They cried with me when I thought that I wasn't the guy for the job. They celebrated with me at the end of every milestone. They understood every late night and every weekend when Daddy had to write, and they stuck with me the whole time. And since my wife is the one person brave enough to spot me while I lift, she literally kept me alive during the whole process. I love you, lots and lots, forever and ever.

Chapter 1

The Foundation

Walking into the gym for the first time can bring on a lot of different feelings: excitement, joy, anticipation, and—let's be totally honest here—fear, uncertainty, and intimidation. All of these feelings are completely normal and to be expected. Those feelings of fear and uncertainty are just your brain telling you that you may not have it all figured out. Spoiler: No one does. The important part is that you're here now, and it's time to learn.

I distinctly remember my first time walking into a weight room. *I was terrified*. It was in middle school, before the start of my eighth-grade football season. I didn't even know what a barbell was, let alone any of the other stuff in the gym. I did nothing that day other than watch everyone else. I was too afraid to mess something up and have everyone laugh at me.

I didn't actually start lifting weights until high school, and that was only with some dumbbells that my dad had gotten me (supplemented by the occasional trip to the local Powerhouse Gym). Still having zero clue what I was doing, I would go in and use every single machine there until I could barely move my legs. Then I'd struggle to drive home as my legs shook whenever I tried try to use the gas or the brakes. It was all trial and error until I found some real mentors and coaches to help me along the way.

I've worked in weight rooms at all levels for over 25 years—in high schools, in college programs from D3 to D1, with professional teams, and at elite powerlifting facilities. I've met some of the best coaches in the world, and I have picked their brains over. The one big lesson I've learned from all of them is this: Never underestimate the importance of the basics. The basics build the foundation needed to achieve success. The gym is the ultimate place for transformation. You will get stronger here. You will look better. You will gain confidence and discipline. To do all those things though, you need to lay a strong foundation. So we're going to start with the absolute foundation of lifting. But first, let me introduce you to the main tool we will be using to build that foundation: the barbell.

Why the Barbell?

This is a barbell book, and I'm not shy about saying that. I want to make it clear that there are many tools out there to get stronger. Most of this book is going to focus on one tool: the barbell. Kettlebells, dumbbells, rubber bands, and Atlas stones are great (shout-out to my Strongman people out there), but not one of these measures up to the barbell. Why?

No tool is perfect, and the bar is no exception. With that said, the barbell is an easy tool to learn. Most people can snag a bar and learn how to squat, bench, deadlift, row, and press safely in under an hour. Will they be experts? No. They will be able to do it again tomorrow though. And the next day, and the next, and the next, and so on. That ease of learning makes it great for getting started, and we all know the hardest part is just getting started.

The barbell is also incredibly accessible and versatile. If you walk into most gyms in the country, you can find a barbell in a rack that can be used any number of ways. It is balanced, so you can do hundreds of movements with it safely ranging from the most basic, like a squat, all the way to some of the most complex movements, like a snatch. You can put one end of it on the ground and do single-arm work. It can be loaded with far more weight than other implements, making progress easier to measure. The options are fairly limitless.

Lastly, you can load it up. Using a squat as an example, there is a limit to how much weight you can hold in front of you with a kettlebell or a dumbbell. They make 135-pound kettlebells (61 kilograms), but handling them in a position to squat is cumbersome and difficult for most trainees. Even for those who can get that kind of weight into position, the barbell would still be a better option to overload that kind of movement. You could use the heaviest kettlebell or dumbbell you can find and just do more reps, but there is a limit to how long you can hold that weight in that position. With a barbell, you can increase the weight far beyond those other tools and hold the bar in a better position to get the most out of it. That gives you more options to progress by increasing weight in a manageable way. Figure 1.1 shows three different examples that highlight the versatility of the barbell.

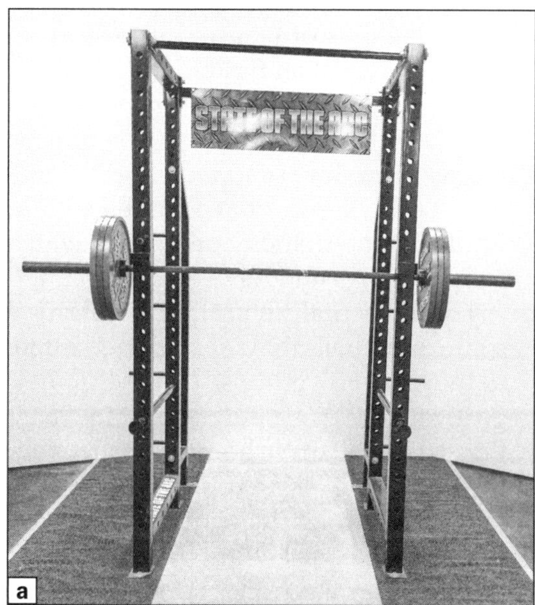

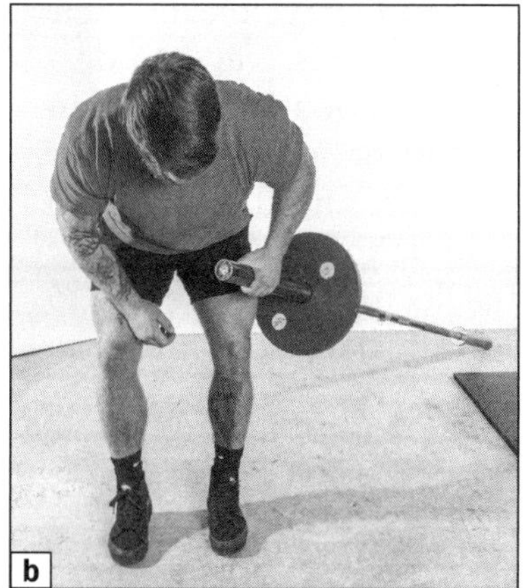

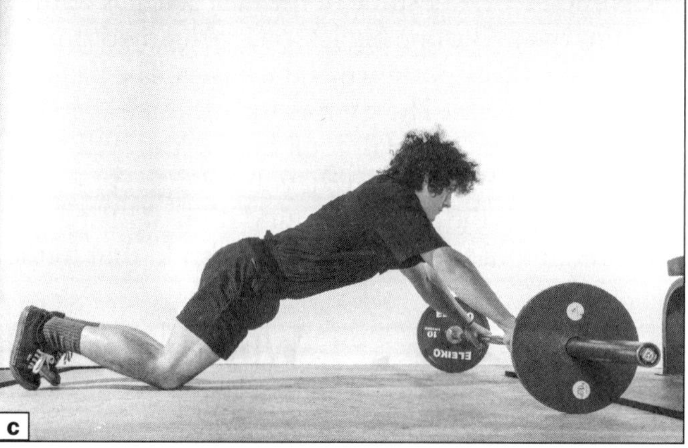

FIGURE 1.1 The versatility of the barbell: *(a)* a fully-loaded barbell on a squat rack, *(b)* a barbell in a landmine setup for use as a single-sided implement, and *(c)* the barbell as a rolling implement for core exercise.

Benefits of Lifting Weights

Now let's look at the benefits of lifting weights. This is not going to be an exhaustive list—that would go on for way too long—but let's hit the highlights.

Enhanced Athletic Performance and Physique

Let's face it, many people start lifting because they want to look like they lift. There is another benefit to increased muscle: It's functional weight. Your muscles are what move your body. The stronger they are, the more capacity you have to move the way you want to. Have you ever seen a sprinter who wasn't jacked? Even marathon runners have begun to focus on strength training to supplement their running, leading to faster times, more muscular physiques, and healthier seasons. The key is that strength training puts stress on the body that it will adapt to, and those same adaptations carry over on the field, on the court, and even in everyday life.

Decreased Risk of Chronic Disease

Strength training can decrease your risk of chronic disease. It can also lead to decreased mortality and morbidity, increased bone density, decreased resting heart rate, and decreased blood pressure.

It is estimated that falls will cost the health care system 101 *billion* dollars by 2030 (NCOA 2023). How are falls relevant here? Falls result in bone fractures. As we age, bone density naturally decreases. The best way to slow down that process is to put stress on the bone, and it's going to take more than going for a walk. An even better idea here is prevention; start lifting weights earlier in life and get ahead of that aging process. On top of that, resting heart rate and blood pressure have been shown to benefit from all forms of exercise, not just cardiovascular exercise. There is evidence that strength training alone can have a positive impact on heart health. Heart disease remains the number one killer in the United States, and strength training is another tool to combat that.

Increased Emotional Well-Being

It feels really cool when you can jump up from the couch really quickly and easily, or carry in all the groceries on your own. It's great when you no longer worry about being able to do something because you know that you can based on what you do in the gym. These are some of the tangible and measurable benefits of strength training. The intangible emotional and psychological benefits are even more far-reaching.

Some of these benefits may be more important to you than others. Except for being more badass—everyone wants that. Either way, only you can determine the risk–reward ratio that you are happy with. The more you push the limits, the higher the risk but even then, the risk remains low. You can experience the benefits simply by starting and then staying consistent. Throughout this book, we will go over multiple ways to reduce risk further by making smart decisions and by having a solid foundation to build from.

Let's flip the script for a moment. Outside of performance in the gym, lifting can change your life for the better. It can help you reduce injuries in other aspects of your life. Being stronger and having denser bones means you will be more capable. People will start asking you to help them move their couch, so there are some drawbacks. The fact is that your enhanced capabilities will give you the ability to live a fuller and richer life with fewer limitations.

Anatomy of a Barbell

Learning the anatomy of the barbell is our next step. It's a simple tool, but if you are using it for the first time or haven't used it regularly, these frames of reference will be important moving forward.

Size and Weight

Barbells are standardized when it comes to their basic measurements (see figure 1.2). They weigh 45 pounds (20 kg), give or take a few ounces. They are a little longer than 86 inches (218 cm), and most of them are 28.5 millimeters in diameter. Bars may vary slightly, but these measurements are standard at this point, so you can trust this will be the size and the weight of most of the bars that you use.

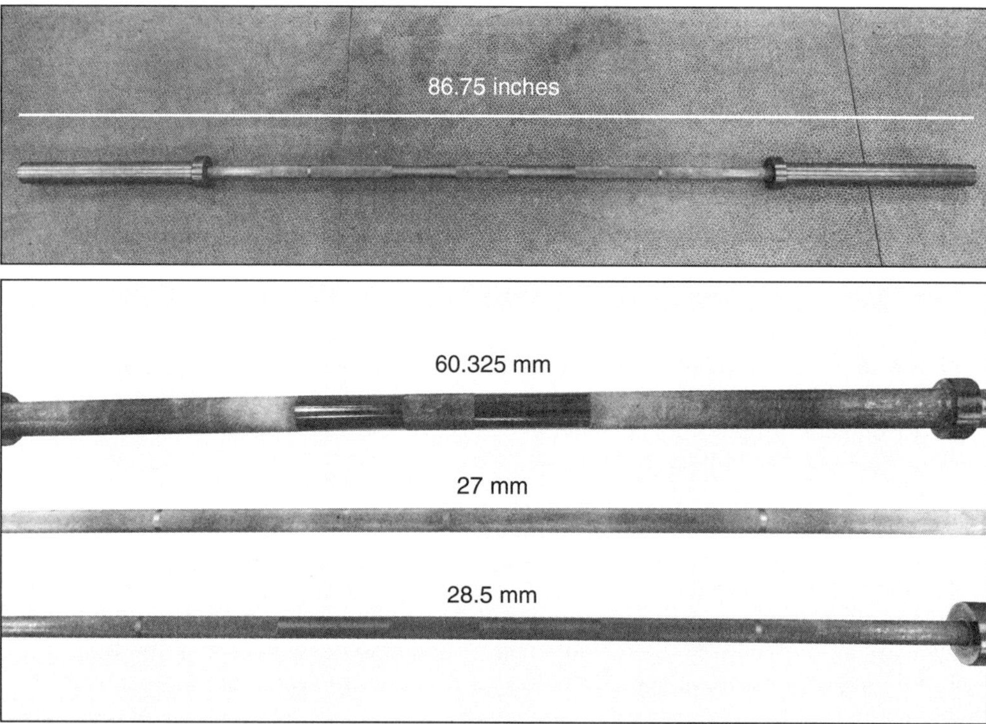

FIGURE 1.2 The barbell is a standardized piece of equipment. You can expect it to meet the measurements shown in the figure with only slight variations.

Sleeve and Collar

The first parts of the bar to know are the sleeves and collars (see figure 1.3). The sleeves are where you slide the plates on, and the collars are what stop the plates. When you put plates on, they should be tight against the collar. Additionally, the collars indicate the maximum width of your grip. I'm not a big advocate of draping the hands over the collars or sleeves, so the insides of the collars are a good frame of reference. Not many people need to go that wide, but it's good to know that reference point.

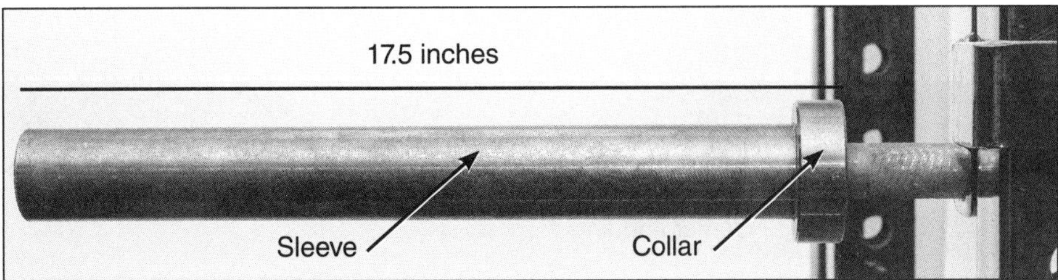

FIGURE 1.3 The sleeve and collar of the barbell serve two purposes: the sleeve is the correct diameter for holding plates securely on the bar, and the collar serves as a barrier and prevents you from setting hands too far apart.

Knurling

The next part to know is the knurling. This is the textured pattern on the bar that helps you grip it. Knurling can vary from bar to bar and is typically described as being either more or less *aggressive* (see figure 1.4 for three examples of knurling ranging from more aggressive to less aggressive). The most aggressive knurling maximizes grip and is used often in high-end powerlifting bars. While it maximizes grip, it also maximizes discomfort until your hands get used to it. Smoother, or less aggressive bars are more comfortable, but the grip can be more difficult. In most commercial gyms, the bar knurling will be moderate. At certain points in the book, I will mention the start of the knurling as a reference point. This is where the smooth middle section of the bar meets the start of the knurling. Of special note here are bars with a center knurl. This is important for squatting because it helps to keep the bar in a better position on your back. Not all bars have this, and it's not required to have a center knurl to squat (see figure 1.5), but boy is it helpful.

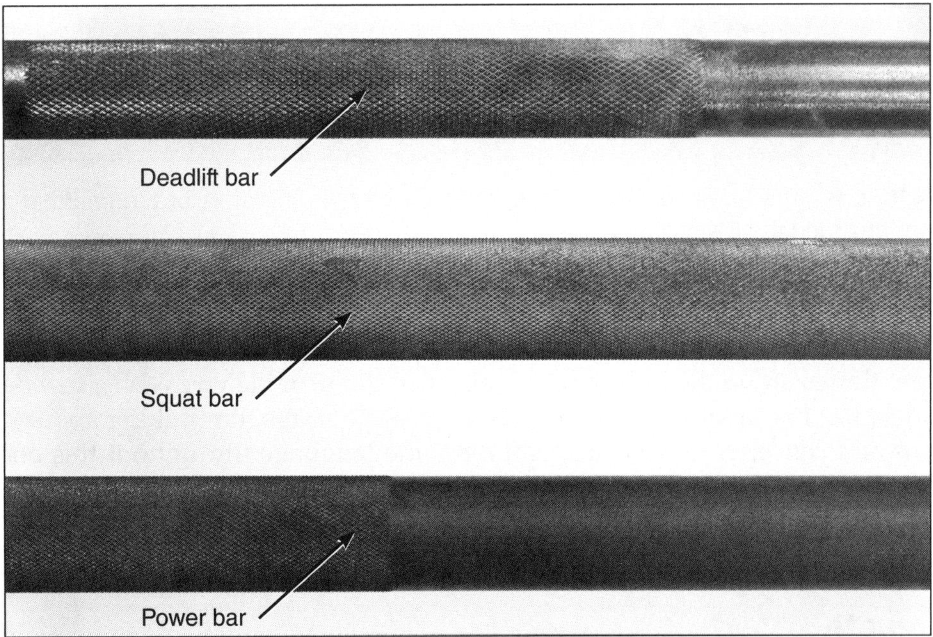

FIGURE 1.4 Knurling: the deadlift bar has the most aggressive knurling, while the squat bar is slightly less aggressive than a deadlift bar but more aggressive than the power bar.

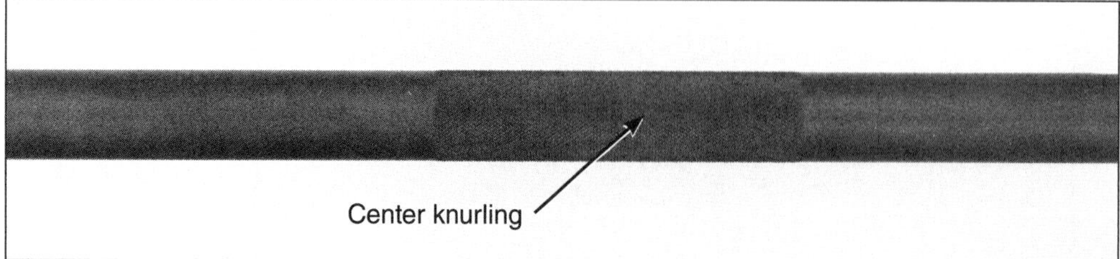

FIGURE 1.5 A bar with a center knurl is ideal for helping secure the bar on the shoulders for a back squat.

Rings

This last landmark also has to do with the knurling. On most bars you will see two rings on each side that look like a break in the knurling. Only specific bars used for powerlifting or for Olympic weightlifting have only one ring on each side. As shown in figure 1.6, for the bars that have two rings, the inside ring is known as the *power ring* and is the reference point for the maximum allowable grip width for bench pressing in powerlifting competitions. The outside ring is known as the *Olympic ring* and relates to the grip position for the snatch, the clean, and the jerk in Olympic weightlifting. In this book, we will use the same ring (the power ring) every time to help standardize your own setup to the bar and where to put your hands.

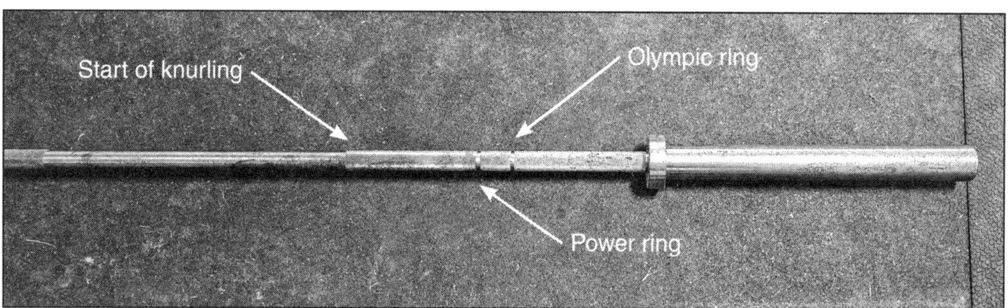

FIGURE 1.6 The three common landmarks on a barbell: the start of the knurling, the power ring, and the Olympic ring.

Key Foundational Terms and Concepts

To get things off on the right foot, we also need to provide you with a few definitions. I'm not talking about the definition of your abs. I'm talking about key terms and concepts so we can speak the same language throughout this book. If we aren't on the same page now, it's going to be hard to move forward. Not only that, but these are universal definitions in strength training that will help you navigate other books and articles on the subject.

Strength

Strength is defined as the quality or state of being physically strong. That definition makes "strength" more of a relative term with its actual definition being more individually based.

It could mean an 800-pound (363 kg) squat, or a bigger tackle on the football field. It could mean higher jumps and more body control in gymnastics, or a stronger base in cheer. It could mean picking up and carrying your kids without pain or discomfort. In this book, there will be many ways to develop the quality of strength, but that strength—and your journey toward it—is yours to define.

Program

A program is the plan, devised by you or a coach, for your training. The duration and difficulty of a program depends on the desired outcome. It outlines which days of the week you train, the exercises you need to complete each session, and the details of how much work you need do with each exercise. A good program should be compatible with your life and your available time commitment, and it should adjust as you approach and surpass your goals. It allows you to track and measure progress over time as well as to compare and contrast methods used in your training so you can learn what you respond best to. That's how to develop more individualized programs that will continue to drive progress. You can't win at something you aren't measuring and tracking, and the program is the framework for that.

To be clear, there is no magic program. There is no perfect program. It is typically easy to tell the difference between a good one and a bad one (you will absolutely learn that from this book), but there are no secrets in any of them. From this point forward, avoid any program that claims to be "secret" like the plague. You will find everything you need to know about programming and how to create your own in chapter 9.

Session

A session is a single day of prescribed training within the program. It consists of everything you do in the gym: your warm-up, your main workout, and your cool-down. It can last anywhere from 30 minutes to three hours depending on your goals and experience level. Sessions fill out a week of training in your program.

Block

A block is a cluster of weeks in a row within your program. Most commonly, they are 8 to 12 weeks. During this time, your training builds to a particular goal such as muscle growth or maximum strength. A block helps to organize training by focusing on one or two goals at a time while also allowing for proper recovery. A common mistake is when new lifters try to do too much with their training. Getting stronger, losing weight, and gaining muscle all at the same time sounds great, but losing weight and gaining muscle tend to compete with each other as goals. Picking one or the other in combination with getting stronger is a smarter path. How to better select goals will be covered in chapter 9.

Repetitions and Sets

A repetition, or a rep, is when an exercise has been performed from its starting point to its end point once. Sets are the number of times you will complete a certain number or repetitions. Sets and reps are written together in a program like this: sets × reps. For example, if you have to do three sets of eight reps for a particular exercise, it is written in the program as "3 × 8." Nearly every coach, trainer, or program you find will express it this way. However, if the program you find was originally Russian, then you can expect these numbers to be inverted: reps × sets. As downloading strength programs from the Internet becomes more common, this is an important point to note.

Exercise, or Main Movement

The terms *exercise* and *main movement* are often used interchangeably. The main movement, or exercise, is the focus exercise for the day as identified in your program. This is the exercise that is most important to the session. For example, if you compete in powerlifting, it's common for the back squat to be your main movement for the day since that is a lift that is used in competition.

Variation

A variation is a movement that is similar to the main movement that you are doing that session. For example, you may have the back squat as the main movement in your program on a particular day, with a front squat programmed in on the same day as a variation. The variation exercise is still a squat, so it will count toward your squat volume (more on that later), but it's not identical to your main movement.

Accessories

Accessories are movements, or exercises, that complement the rest of the program. Typically, they are single-joint exercises like triceps extensions or leg curls. They help to build strength where there is weakness and to create more muscle mass in specific areas. They can also help reduce injury.

Frequency

Frequency is the number of times you train each week or how many times you train a movement in a week. For example, if your frequency is four, you are training four days per week. If you train four days a week and squat two of those days, you have a training frequency of four and a squat frequency of two.

Volume

Volume is the number of sets and reps you do for a particular movement. There are many ways to look at volume. You can look at exercise volume, session volume, weekly volume, or block volume. So let's take a second to break this down using the back squat as an example. Let's say you train the back squat two days a week and do three sets of eight reps each session. Your exercise volume would be 24 (or 3 × 8). Your weekly volume would be double that, or 48, since you squat two times a week. If the block is eight weeks long with the weekly volume staying the same, that would be 384 (or 48 × 8). Now let's say that on one of those days, you have a back squat for three sets of eight reps and a front squat for three sets of five reps. The exercise volume for the back squat would be 24 (or 3 × 8), and the exercise volume for the front squat would be 15 (or 3 × 5), making the session volume for squats 39 (or 24 + 15). Just like your math teacher told you in the ninth grade: Math is important! Why? Knowing your total volume can help you track how much work you are doing over time and help inform you about how well you are recovering. There is a science to this. Just randomly adding sets or an additional 5 pounds (2 kg) every single week won't cut it. Learn to do the math so that when the time comes to use it, you can.

Intensity

Intensity is what everyone thinks about. It's the weight on the bar. The most accurate way to measure intensity is to have a known one-repetition maximum (1RM), or the most weight you can lift once. Your 1RM is equal to 100 percent intensity. You can then use that number to prescribe the weights for each session. The closer the weight is to your one-repetition maximum, the higher the intensity of the exercise. As an absolute beginner, or even as someone returning to the gym after a bit of a hiatus, testing your maximum to find out where you are is poor practice. Do not hop into the car to go find your 1RM. Instead, you can use an estimated one-rep maximum or another metric, which we will define next.

A Note on Intensity and Volume

Intensity is often misunderstood as being about how tired or fatigued training makes you. "I am so tired and sore from that intense workout," is a normal thing to say in conversation, but it is inaccurate in terms of what intensity means in the context of strength training. Intensity is strictly relative to your 1RM. Calculating your total volume and knowing what your intensity is at that volume can help you better understand fatigue in a session or through your training program.

As time goes on, volume and intensity in a program will rise, creating more fatigue. This is when most trainees start to feel more tired after a session and between sessions. It's important to pay attention to this. As your fitness and strength increases, so will your capacity to handle intensity and volume. However, we all have our limits, and volume and intensity can't just continue to go up without having a negative impact on your recovery and performance. Scheduling downtime and adjusting the volume and intensity during program blocks can help manage this. We will cover that in more detail in chapter 9.

Rating of Perceived Exertion

Rating of perceived exertion, or RPE, is how hard something feels on a scale of 1 to 10, with a 10 being maximum difficulty and 1 being no challenge at all. This is important to learn when first starting out so you can intelligently guide yourself and appropriately manage your volume and intensity. We aren't robots, so performance can change as a result of many factors. Using your RPE can help you make good decisions in the gym (like when to push harder and when not to).

Specificity

Specificity is based on the principle that your body adapts to the challenges you present it with. It's important that the training you do be specific enough to make your body adapt in order to achieve your goal. If you want to bench more, you have to do the bench press or some close variation of it. Doing more squats isn't going to blow up your bench. Your goals dictate your training, so train specifically for them.

Equipment and Safety Recommendations

Now let's talk about equipment and what you need in order to train and stay safe while doing so. If the gym you go to has a barbell, it more than likely will have a squat rack and a bench press too. When it comes to large pieces of equipment, those three are literally all you need to get started with what you will find in this book. In fact, they're really all you will ever need. The world is your oyster with those three simple things. If you are looking to set up a home gym, the same applies. You could operate in a ten-foot-by-ten-foot space the following things.

- *A full squat rack.* I suggest a cage type, such as the Rogue R-3 or the Titan T-3.
- *A flat bench.* You'll use this for presses.
- *A barbell.* I suggest the Rogue Ohio Power Bar.
- *Plate weights.* For most, the common 300-pound (136 kg) sets are a good starting point. The base for my athletes is four 45-pound (20 kg) plates, two 25-pound (11 kg) plates, four 10-pound (5 kg) plates, and two 5-pound (2 kg) plates.

When it comes to personal equipment, my biggest suggestion is to get a pair of shoes appropriate for lifting. What does this mean? Your shoes should be flat-bottomed and have limited cushioning. Running shoes and most cross-trainers do not fit the bill here. The cushioning in these types of shoes has a tendency to compress under weight, which can create an unstable base by putting the foot in inconsistent positions during a lift. There is a reason Converse Chuck Taylors are popular in the lifting world. They are simple, cheap, and effective. Their firm, flat soles aid in creating stability between your foot and the floor. Personally, I find that the sole on the Adidas Sambas has better grip, but either option is easy to find and affordable.

Clips, as shown in figure 1.7, are essential to have on each end of the bar at any weight. Clips go on the sleeves of the barbell and hold the weight plates in position, preventing them from sliding off. Nothing is worse, or potentially more dangerous, than having a plate slide off mid-set. Once you put a plate on the bar, slide the clip on. Safety catches, such as pins or struts, also need to be in place (see figure 1.8). These will catch the bar and prevent it from coming down on you if you fail a lift. A bar crashing on you during a failed lift can lead to injury or worse, but it's completely preventable with the proper use of safety equipment. Don't take the safety of yourself and those around you for granted.

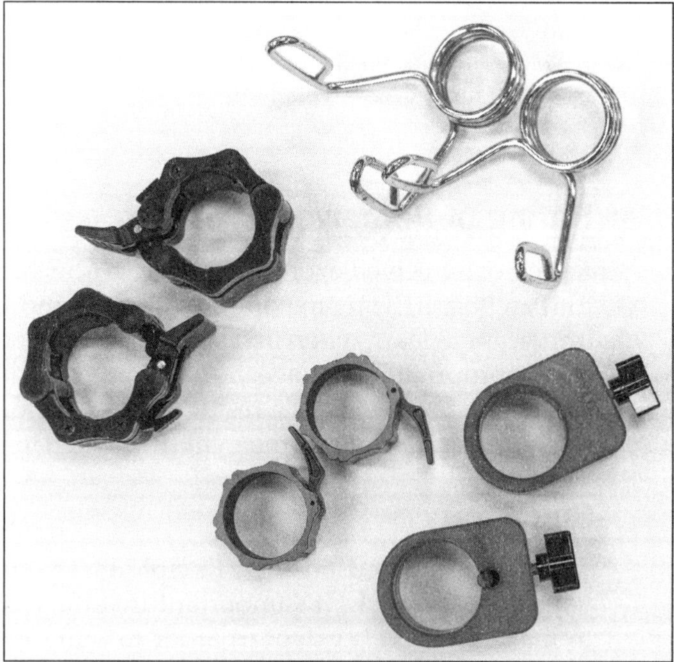

FIGURE 1.7 As soon as a plate goes on the bar, use clips to prevent it from moving or falling off.

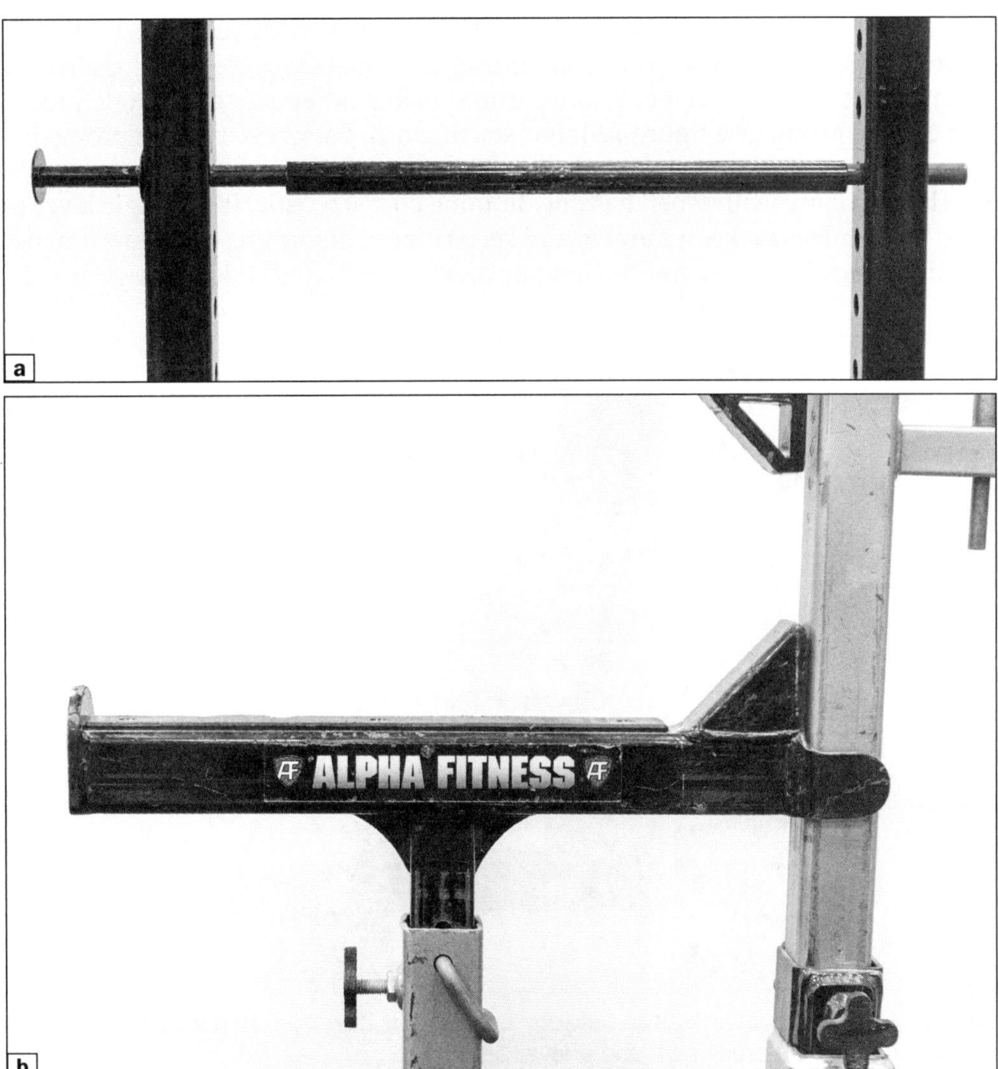

FIGURE 1.8 Common safety catches: *(a)* safety pins and *(b)* struts.

While not essential when starting out, a good belt is something to add to your holiday wish list. I'm partial to the Inzer Forever Belt. This is something you can hand down to your kids, and it costs around $100. A belt will help you create more intra-abdominal pressure, which helps to stabilize your lumbar spine while lifting. It does this by creating more tactile feedback to your core musculature and to the surrounding areas. We will discuss bracing later on in the book, but a belt is a great tool to help learn proper bracing, and it's been shown to increase lifting performance by 5 to 10 percent.

Finding and selecting a good belt can be overwhelming. Belts are made of either cloth or leather. Cloth belts are more flexible and are secured on the lifter with Velcro straps. These can be a great starting point for many because they are less expensive. However, as you learn to brace harder and lift heavier the Velcro on these belts often pops open mid-lift.

Leather belts are the standard, in my opinion. There are different sizes in terms of the thickness: The two most common sizes are 13 millimeters and 10 millimeters. If you are a smaller lifter with a waist between 22 and 29 inches (56 to 74 cm), I suggest a 10-millimeter belt. This size is slightly less stiff, making it more functional for those with smaller frames. For everyone else, I suggest the 13-millimeter size. Leather belts are secured using either a lever, a single prong, or a double prong (see figure 1.9). For starting out, I suggest a single prong; it's the easiest to adjust, to get on and off, and to grow into.

A high-quality leather belt has one defining characteristic: It's a single layer of solid leather. This makes it durable and keeps it from deforming over time. I'm not kidding when I say that you can get one of these and hand it down to your kids.

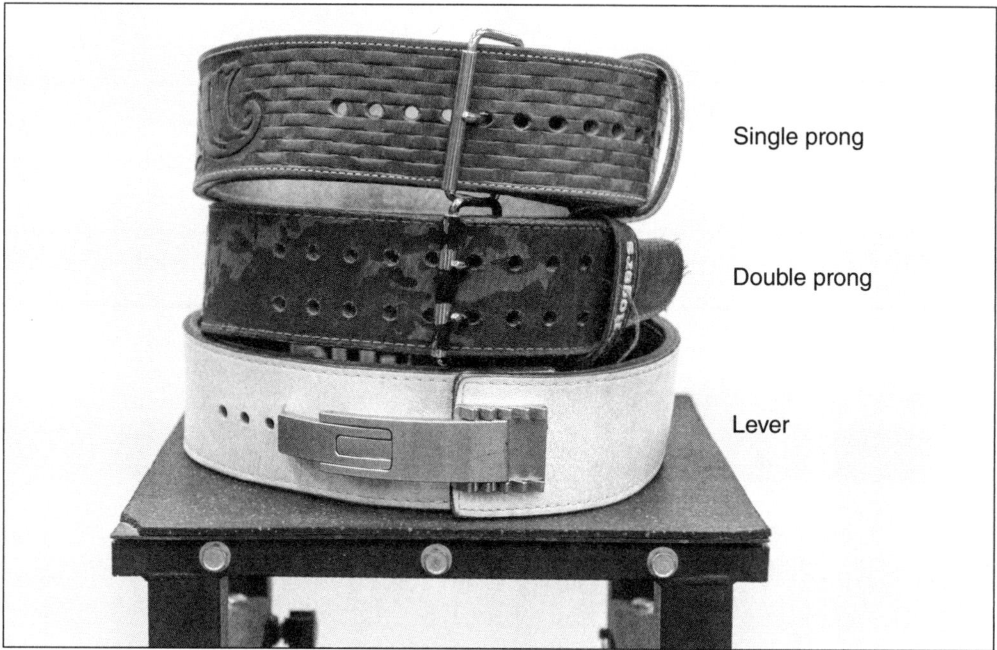

FIGURE 1.9 The main difference between belt types is how they latch together: a single-prong belt, a double-prong belt, and a lever belt.

How Likely Am I to Get Injured?

There is a stigma around lifting because many believe that it can lead to injury. I'm here to tell you that that is true. The reality is that you can get hurt doing literally anything. The fact that it *can* happen isn't what we need to focus on. We need to focus on the *rate* at which it happens and measure that against the benefits of the activity.

The *British Journal of Sports Medicine* estimates the rate of injury for weightlifting to be 2.4 to 3.3 injuries per 1,000 hours of training (Aasa et al. 2017). They defined "injury" as having to cease competition or training for a period of time. In other words, for every 1,000 hours that you train, you can expect to have two to three injuries that may interrupt your training. One thousand hours is a lot of time in the gym. Compare that to 7.2 injuries per 1,000 hours for soccer and even 4.8 injuries per 1,000 hours for basketball (Prieto-González 2021). So weightlifting has a really low rate of injury. Even at elite levels, the rate is around five injuries per 1,000 hours.

The Science of Strength Gains

This subject could fill an entire book, but for our purposes, I will keep this brief. To get stronger and grow, muscle needs to have a stimulus. When it comes to weight training, this stimulus is the weight you use. That stimulus causes damage to the muscles—not so much that it creates injury, but enough to cause micro tears in the muscle. These heal through recovery and stimulate the muscle to grow back bigger and stronger. This is the basis of the principle of specific adaptations to imposed demands, or SAID. In other words, your body will adapt and change in response to what you train, how you lift, and what you lift with. This book will give you the fundamentals to control and guide this process.

You can't just do the same thing over and over. If the body adapts, which it is very good at doing, then doing the same sets, reps, and weights all the time will lead to progress at first and then nothing. Progression is only created through change. That could mean more volume, more intensity, or even different exercises (more on that later). There are many methods you can use, but the basic SAID principle remains the same. The fundamental science of strength and muscle growth is based on applying stimulus on the muscle itself, and the barbell is perfect for that.

That wraps up the first chapter of this book. The definitions and concepts here will continue to pop up as we move forward, so if you need to read through this chapter again or bookmark it for future reference, then go ahead and do that. Let's move on to the next phase: the warm-up.

Chapter 2

The Warm-Up

Before we begin talking about lifting, we must have a discussion about warm-ups—what they do for you, why you do them, and how to put them together to not only be effective but to also save you time. Your warm-up is everything you do prior to your big working sets for the day. It's done before you load the bar with whatever amount of weight you're going to lift. Over the years, warm-ups have taken many forms—light running or jumping rope, long periods of static stretching, dynamic warm-ups with jumping and skipping movements, and more. What we cover here will give you the tools to create the best and most efficient warm-up possible that will be specific to what you are about to do.

Understanding the Importance of the Warm-Up

There are multiple reasons to start each training day with a solid warm-up:

- To increase blood flow and raise the temperature in tissues.
- To increase tissue pliability for more range of motion.
- To increase nervous system involvement, which increases performance.

Increased Blood Flow

Do you remember when you were a kid and your gym teacher made you do laps at the start of each class because it was "good for you"? They were right; but there is more to it.

Increased blood flow has a lot of benefits when it comes to your performance. First: It helps transport oxygen and glucose to working muscles where they are then converted into the energy needed to fuel exercise and muscle contractions. Second: It helps transport carbon dioxide and other waste products away, which is vital because otherwise, glucose and oxygen can't get to the muscles efficiently and they will fatigue more quickly. These waste products also contribute to muscle soreness. This explains why we are particularly sore when we are just starting out or returning to the gym after long break: We aren't as efficient at clearing out these waste products when our fitness level is lower.

Additionally, increased blood flow improves muscle tissue's ability to contract efficiently. What does this mean exactly? Muscle tissue is unique in that it can contract and relax at a very fast rate. Much of this is controlled in the muscle by *motor units*. Think of a motor unit as a computer chip that receives the signal from the brain or from a load on the muscle. When that signal is strong enough, the muscle contracts. There are hundreds of motor units in each muscle that help determine how quickly and how hard a muscle contracts. The stronger the signal, the more of these units come to the party. This activates larger and more powerful muscle fibers, creating a fast and powerful contraction. It has been shown that when blood flow to the muscle is increased, these motor units and the surrounding structures are more efficient (Hammer et al., 2020). That's going to lead to faster contractions that are less fatiguing, which will increase performance.

This isn't a small detail. This can make a difference when you add five pounds (2 kg) to the bar, and it can affect how hard a set feels. We talked about volume in the first chapter; being able to add five pounds (2 kg) to a workout or having the workout feel easier are measurable aspects of progress. These small progressions over time can make a huge impact on your training. Give yourself every advantage possible.

Do I Go Hard or Go Home?

Starting off with a specific warm-up for the lift you are about to do in the gym is a great way to shake off the rust from the day and get yourself psychologically ready. If you're crunched for time, you can shorten the warm-up. Skipping the warm-up, however, is a bad idea. Anyone who tells you otherwise is just flat-out wrong.

Even if you need to shorten your warm-up for time, it shouldn't be easy or even worse, lazy. The warm-up should be done at a brisk pace and should be approached with intent. It's the time to get physically and mentally ready for the workout. At the same time, this shouldn't turn into an all-out effort before the workout even starts. Save that for the big lifts. What I like to shoot for here is simple: You should start to get that first appearance of sweat on your forehead, and you should feel your body temperature and heart rate increase. Get past the early part where you feel short of breath and a little out of shape (everyone feels this way during the warm-up, even elite athletes), and start to control your breathing. By the time you reach this point, everything should feel loose and ready to go. That's the sign of a good warm-up.

Increased Tissue Pliability

Another benefit of the warm-up is increased tissue pliability and capacity to tolerate stretch. For effective weight training, you need to be able to go through your full available range of motion. You don't want to start your workout feeling like you just got out of bed—stiff from lying down for eight hours. The increase in blood flow from a proper warm-up will decrease that stiffness and increase your available range of motion. When enough blood is present in the muscle and its temperature is increased, the muscle becomes more pliable, allowing it to stretch and return to normal length more efficiently. This also leads to a higher tolerance for stretch. Let's go back to the example of getting out of bed. When you get out of bed and try to touch your toes, you may not be able to because of how tight it feels or how painful it is. However, if you stand up and repeat trying to touch your toes a few times, you can do it (or at least get closer). Two things are happening here: The act of going through that range of motion increases blood flow, which enhances the pliability of the muscles involved and allows you to reach farther and farther. Additionally, the parts of your muscles that communicate the feeling of the stretch to your brain start to downregulate that message. In other words, they go from screaming, "Stop it!" to saying, "Hey, this isn't so bad." This response is crucial to performing your lifts at a high level and continuing to see progress.

Increased Nervous-System Involvement

That big soft squishy thing in your skull is the gatekeeper to your progress in the gym. You won't be able to trick it, confuse it, or find a way around it. Your brain follows rules; those rules are based on threat, prediction, and automation.

Let's talk about threat first. Your brain is still wired to keep an eye out for saber-toothed tigers. Even now—long after the last saber-toothed tiger disappeared—the remains of that wiring are still deeply embedded in your hardware. A potential threat is something the brain sniffs out quickly and then responds to. The feeling of stiffness, of a stretch, of a pin prick, or of pain are all sensations brought about by threat sensors in your brain. We touched on this in the last section with the example of the sensation of stretch being downregulated with a good warm-up. The same concept applies when it comes to your brain. If you go into the gym, load your maximum weight on the bar, and try to squat that thing cold, you are more than likely going to get smushed. At best, you might grind through one rep, but it will be an ugly one. Even with weights at 70 percent of your maximum, it's going to feel rough. This is because the brain perceives what you are about to do as a threat. It tells your entire body that it's in danger and downregulates your performance. Downregulation is a response by the brain to reduce the body's response to a stimulus. So in this example, because that maximal attempt wasn't prepared for, or upregulated for, the brain interpreted the weight as something that was trying to kill you. In response, it sent a weaker signal to your muscles to contract. That weaker signal got picked up by the motor units we talked about before, and fewer of them show up to the party. The result was a slower and less powerful contraction.

So what does all this mean for your warm-up? Your warm-up gradually introduces your brain to what is about to happen. It decreases the threat response in the brain through gradual exposure. Your brain has to know that you are going to be okay, and then it will upregulate performance to meet the demands you are putting on it. You can't trick your brain, but you can ease it into cooperation.

Now let's talk about prediction and automation. When was the last time you thought about how you brush your teeth? I mean each and every step: How are you going to put the toothpaste on the brush? Are you going to start brushing on the top row of teeth? The bottom row? Will you brush up and down first? Or side to side? You probably think I'm ridiculous for asking these questions, but I have a three-year-old at the time of this writing and let me tell you, she thinks *hard* about how to brush her teeth. It's a task. It takes a lot of energy for her to brush her teeth. For you, it doesn't. Let's explore why and how it applies to building foundational strength.

Because you have been brushing your teeth for a lot longer than my daughter has, your brain has automated this process. Through repetition, it's been predicted, mapped out in the brain, and outsourced, so it takes very little energy to perform. Your brain is amazing at figuring out how to automate tasks so that they take as little energy as possible.

The same process will happen with your lifting. Each workout, each exercise, and each repetition is a learning opportunity for your brain. When you first start out, you may feel like a baby giraffe. Each rep will feel a little different, a little off-balance, and maybe a little random. As time goes on, your brain will learn the bigger details of the lifts and make them more automatic. Every single rep won't be the same, but they will get better and better over time. That's going to take more reps to do though.

This is where your warm-up comes into play. I've mentioned a few times that it needs to be specific. If you are going to warm up to squat, squats need to be part of the warm-up. This will add specific learning opportunities for your brain to get better at squatting while making your warm-up more fun and effective.

This explains why people see such immense progress when they first start. The increase in skill as a result of the brain automating some of these processes makes the entire movement more efficient. If you use less energy with each rep, then you can either add weight or add reps while maintaining the same level of fatigue. Are you getting stronger? You are, because the weight on the bar is going up, but the big difference is your improved level of skill. This is a recipe for success and the foundation of the rest of the progress that you will make. I like to think of each training session as practice for each movement. The warm-up is a part of each session. If you skip it, you'll miss out on reps, miss out on learning, and miss out on progress.

Should I Use a Foam Roller or Similar Tool in My Warm-Up?

Here's the deal: I'm not going to tell you that you should or should not use a foam roller or one of those cool jackhammer massage drills that your best friend just bought on Amazon. I will, however, tell you what these tools do and don't do compared to what they claim to do. Let's start with what they don't do.

Foam rollers and other similar tools claim to change tissue structure, increasing the pliability of tissue. In other words, they claim to make you more mobile by lengthening muscles, breaking up adhesions that decrease range of motion, and increasing local blood flow. Unfortunately, these claims don't look to be true based on current research. In reality, it would take a tremendous amount of force—similar to the force of being run over by a road paver—to create these kinds of tissue changes. I'm pretty sure that's not a great health decision.

However, we do see that when people use implements like a foam roller, they experience an increase in their range of motion for a short time (roughly five minutes.) This is more than likely due to the discomfort that these tools produce. Weirdly, it's the actual pain and discomfort of using these tools that result in that benefit. The theory is that the pain increases the body's tolerance to stretch within that specific tissue. In essence, the pain you feel when you use a foam roller on your hamstrings is why you can then stretch them more before the pain of the stretch comes on. It creates a small window that can be used to get some movement in. So what's the difference between warming up with something like a foam roller and using the more active approach of movements clustered together the way it's been presented in this chapter? It is this: While you can get the same increased range of motion from foam rolling that you get with specific warm-up movements, you completely miss out on the skill acquisition from the exercises.

The choice is still yours. If foam rollers and similar modalities make you feel better and you are willing to spend your time doing it, then go for it. Just stay clear on what it's actually doing, and don't fall victim to some of the false claims.

Creating an Effective Warm-Up

Putting together an effective warm-up doesn't have to be complicated. Simpler is better, especially when it comes to time management. That's why the initial framework that I like to use for a warm-up is called *clustering*. Clustering is performing your specific warm-up exercises while also completing your warm-up sets for the main movement of the session. Clustering combines the traditional warm-up exercises that are relevant to the main movement with the actual main-movement warm-up. This gets you the most bang for your buck in a short time. It also allows you to feel how the other exercises are affecting the main movement in the moment, giving you better feedback on their usefulness and a better read on your level of performance that day. For example, if your main movement is a bench press and your general warm-up exercises are banded pull-aparts, pec flies, and shoulder dislocates, then warming up for a 135-pound (61 kg) working set for the bench press would look like this:

Shoulder dislocates × 10

Banded pull-aparts × 10

Pec flies × 10

Bench press with bar × 10

Shoulder dislocates × 10

Banded pull-aparts × 10

Pec flies × 10

Bench press with 95 pounds (43 kg) × 10

Shoulder dislocates ×10

Banded pull-aparts × 10

Pec flies × 10

First working set of bench press at 135 pounds (61 kg)

In this example, you have three general warm-up exercises to help increase blood flow to relevant upper-body musculature in the bench press. I suggest sticking to light sets of 10 to 15 reps for two to three rounds of each exercise to make sure you are thoroughly warmed up. At the end of each round, you have a set of the main movement in order to get that skill practice in for your brain as you work up to the weight that you are going to use for the day. You can find a list of general, nonspecific warm-up exercises for each lift in chapter 9.

There's no need to do more than three sets of the nonspecific, lower-load exercises. For example, let's say you were working up to 315 pounds (143 kg) for the squat, and the warm-up progression on the bar looks like this:

Bar

135 pounds (61 kg)

185 pounds (84 kg)

225 pounds (102 kg)

275 pounds (125 kg)

315 pounds (143 kg)

You could stop doing the other warm-up exercises after the set with either 185 pounds (84 kg) or 225 pounds (102 kg) depending on how you feel.

There is a lot of flexibility here to make this your own. Are you working around an injury and have specific rehab exercises given to you by a physical therapist? Slide them in here instead, and cluster them close to the main movement. Is the main movement feeling a bit off while you roll through your cluster? Adjust one of the other exercises in the warm-up to see if there is a change and if there isn't, modify the main exercise for the day based on that information. It really can be that simple. You don't need gimmicks or fancy tools. This gives you total control and freedom over your session with the ability to make informed decisions based on your warm-up. That is smart training that can keep you lifting for a lifetime.

Before we wrap up this chapter, I want to cover an important concept regarding warm-ups and exercise selection. If something during those first sets of the main movement feels funky, the solution is to spend time in that specific position. It doesn't have to be a heavy-loading or a specialized exercise. It can be as simple as adding a pause during the main lift as part of your warm-up, right at the spot where you feel less comfortable. Your first instinct might be to avoid those positions, but that would fly in the face of everything that we have learned about the warm-up thus far. Instead, spend some time in those positions and get comfortable there. Don't force them—ease into them. You'll soon find yourself getting more comfortable than ever.

Here's a specific example: One of the lifters I work with was dealing with some lower-back pain in the squat. He felt some pain about halfway down in the squat, and he always felt a little tight in the front of their hips. We selected a half-kneeling stretch for the front of the hips and a rack-assisted pause squat right where the pain typically started. Then it was straight into the first set of squats. The cluster looked like this:

Half-kneeling stretch for 30 seconds on each side

Pause squat while holding the rack for five deep breaths

Squat with bar 10 times

We capped the weight for the pause squats at 225 pounds (102 kg), to ensure a pain-free transition to the working sets, and did three rounds of this cluster. The guidelines for this were simple: Pause in the squat where the discomfort starts, breathe and relax through it, and don't push into any pain that you can't tolerate. This was really effective. When there was no more back pain in the squat, we changed up the warm-up. The key factor here is that we selected an exercise specifically for spending time where there was a problem and gradually increased the range as the warm-ups went along. To this day, this athlete still has no pain with squatting and has continued to see massive strength improvements.

All in all, those are the absolute basics of constructing and utilizing a warm-up. Here are a few key things to remember:

- Don't overcomplicate this. Keep it simple and relevant to the main movement you are doing in the workout, and adjust based on how you are feeling.
- It shouldn't take 45 minutes just to get ready. Ten to 15 minutes is plenty of time to get going and set yourself up for a great workout.
- Cluster the warm-up exercises together with your main-movement warm-up sets to stay efficient and to help gauge how the workout is going to go.

Chapter 3

The Squat

While playing favorites isn't my thing, I have to say that the squat is my favorite lift. It's simple, is effective at building muscle and strength, and can be the cornerstone for a weight-loss program. Plus, everyone has some level of experience with it if they have ever sat in a chair! That's the good stuff that makes me love it. There are also hard parts that make me love it too. The squat takes discipline, perseverance, and dedication. It's the lift that takes the longest to master, is typically the most intimidating, and is surrounded by so much myth and dogma (but don't worry—that's what this chapter is here for). Being a great squatter sets you apart from everyone else at the gym. I can still remember looking like a baby giraffe the first time I squatted at the gym, but I made massive improvements in the first few months. I also remember a three-year-long plateau when I couldn't get past 644 pounds (292 kg). Now well into the 800s (360 kg), I can say the squat is the lift that I have enjoyed most on my journey.

The barbell back squat is also the lift that took me the longest to incorporate when I first started lifting. It wasn't until I started pursuing powerlifting that I dedicated myself to it and started squatting regularly, and even then it was the most intimidating lift for me. Many thoughts would run through my head, including, "Am I even doing this right?"; "How many people are looking at me?"; and "Don't fall over; don't fall over; don't fall over. . ." The point of this chapter is to eliminate those thoughts and have you confident that you can walk into any gym in the country, grab a bar, and start squatting.

Reasons Why You Should Squat

The squat is the lift that has the most practical benefit for your life, followed closely by the deadlift. So why should you squat? Put simply, a squat is a sit-to-stand lift. Activities like getting in and out of chairs, in and out of bed, on and off the couch, and on and off the toilet all include the basic movements of the squat. Having the strength to reliably sit to stand is important for long-term health because it decreases the risk of falls. While this may not be a concern for you right now, squatting regularly as part of a program can ensure that it never will be (Lui-Ambrose et al. 2004).

Squats are also the foundation of athletic development. Period. The way you squat is going to depend on your sport, but the squat needs to be included in your program. Why? The first reason has to do with your strength-to-body weight ratio. The stronger you are in relation to your body weight, the greater your capacity for athletic performance. The squat strengthens more than just the legs; it hits the whole posterior chain (hips, lower back, middle back, glutes, hamstrings, calves, and upper back), and all of these muscles are vital in athletic performance and power development. Will the squat alone make you run faster or jump higher? No, but it will enhance the rest of your training to help you get the best results possible.

I know that different people find different things rewarding. With that said, you are reading a book about barbell training, so more than likely you are someone who finds lifting weights rewarding. In my experience, no lift has carried over to peoples' everyday lives as much as squat has. No other lift has led to as many stories of increased quality of life and confidence due to improved performance of that lift. My absolute favorite example involves an older client I worked with. She had just gotten into the 100-pound (45 kg) club squatting the week before, and when she came into the gym on Monday she was beaming—smiling from ear to ear and with a story to tell. Was it about that squat specifically? Nope. This is what she said:

> John, you won't believe what happened this weekend. I went out to see my family, and my daughter had just gotten a puppy. Because of its energy, she was keeping it crated for a little while before letting it out. In the past, I would have had to strategize about what I was going to do when that puppy was let out. Where should I sit? How should I sit? Who will bring the puppy over to me and set it on my lap? How long will I be able to actually hold it before I get tired? So here is the bizarre part: None of those thoughts came. It wasn't until I stood up from the ground that I realized I had never even started those thoughts in my head. What I actually did was I got down on the ground, opened that crate, pulled that puppy right out, and sat on the floor to play with it—*without even thinking about it*. Isn't that weird? I've gotten so confident over the last few weeks that I'm walking around just living life.

Are Squats Bad for Your Knees?

You will often hear that squats are bad for your knees and that you will pay for the wear and tear on your body. This is a myth that needs to die and die hard, just like my favorite Christmas movie.

Here are the facts: The specific adaptations to imposed demand (SAID) principle indicates that your body will adapt to the stimulus you apply to it. The training you do and the stimulus that you put on your body will cause you to get better at that exact thing. What this means is that your tissues will adapt to squatting over time. Muscle tissue is the fastest to adapt, with ligaments, cartilage, and bone following suit. This makes lifts like squats protective from injury, especially when executed properly and with mindful progression, as outlined in this book. The real culprit when it comes to wear and tear on the body is time. Time is not kind to any of us, and none of us can escape the degenerative processes of the body. That process is accelerated not by exercise but by a lack of it. Squatting, and squatting well, will increase your strength and joint health in the long term. So the next time someone tells you squats are bad for your knees, let them know otherwise.

I often hear these kinds of stories in connection with the squat. So many people—people just like you—don't think they can do it. But you can, and it's a massive confidence builder for everyone.

Elements of the Squat

It's time to cover the basic elements of the squat: everything you need to understand to be ready to get under the barbell and start learning this movement. We will go over each position: the start, the descent, the bottom of the squat, and the ascent. Every squat has these elements, and at the end of this chapter you will know them well.

But before we begin, let me say this: There is no perfect squat. Let me repeat that. There is no perfect squat. There are guidelines, but each person's squat will look a little different based on how they are built, as shown in figure 3.1. This is normal, and I want to set that expectation for you right now. Your squat is going to be your squat. It may not look like the pictures in this book or like the squats of people on the Internet or like your best friend's. That's why this section is important; it will give you the tools to evaluate your particular squat and make it better. Training is an extended process that takes time, and cookie-cutter approaches don't work here. So let's take a deeper look into what the back squat is and how to perform it.

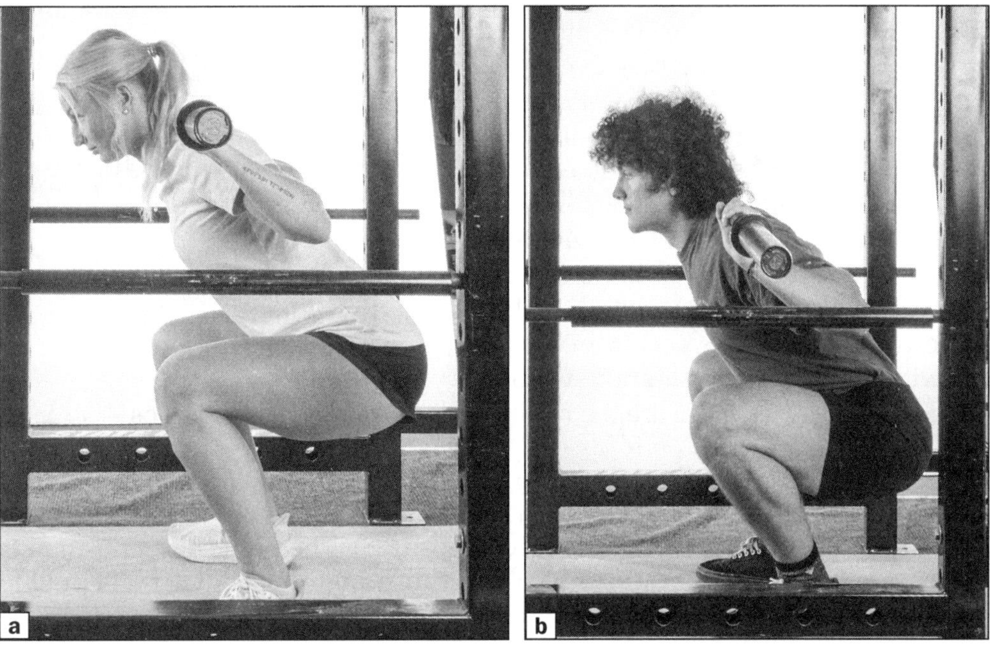

FIGURE 3.1 Comparison of two squats where the athletes have different body types, resulting in visibly different body positions.

Bar-Lifter Unit

The first aspect of the squat that we are going to cover is the bar-lifter unit, which is created once you have the bar on your back and are ready to lift. The combined mass, or weight, of both you and the bar creates a new center of gravity (see figure 3.2). This is important, because that center of gravity will dictate the position of the bar and your body while you lift, creating something we can actually track called a *bar path*. Let's break it down.

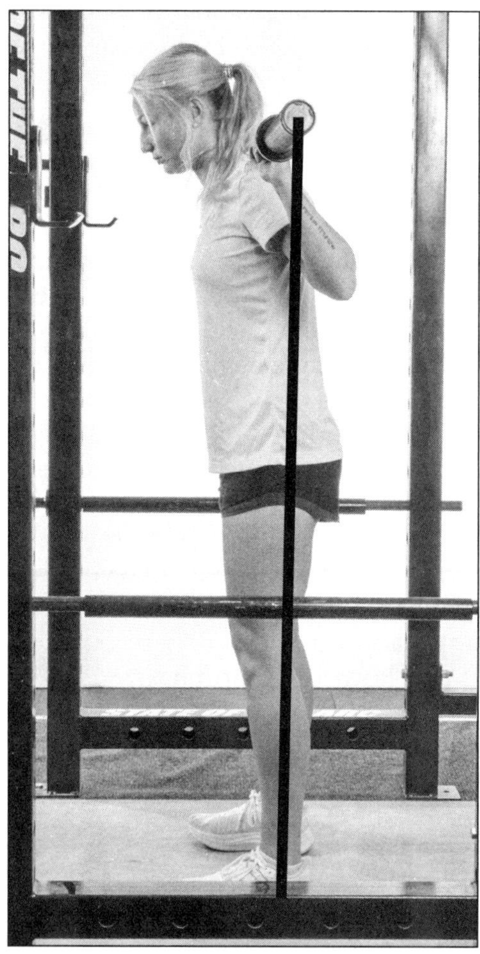

FIGURE 3.2 The barbell combines with the lifter to create the bar-lifter unit. Notice that the line for the center of gravity passes through the midfoot.

Bar Positioning

There is more to squatting with a barbell than just putting it anywhere on your back. Where you put the bar will affect the bar-lifter unit as well as your body position during the movement itself. There is no right or wrong position for the bar, and I like to look at bar position as existing on a spectrum. The highest position possible is known as the *high-bar position*, and the lowest is known as the *low-bar position*. Every point in between these two positions is also a viable option, and through your lifting career you will more than likely use all of them. It is important to understand how each position affects the lift though, so you know what to expect from each. We will cover the high-bar and low-bar positions here since those are the most commonly used bar positions.

High-Bar Position

The high-bar position is just underneath that large bony knot at the base of your neck, also known as the *C7 vertebra* (see figure 3.3). The highest bar position is always going to be under this bony spot, because anything above it will put too much pressure on the neck and not provide enough contact to keep the bar stable. The high-bar position also places the bar right across your upper traps, helping you to stabilize and better distribute the total weight of the bar.

In this high-bar position, the bar-lifter unit has a center of gravity right over the midfoot, without any change in torso angle (see figure 3.4). The high-bar position also allows you to stay much more upright during the entire movement, most notably in the start position, where it will look like you are standing up straight, and in the bottom of the lift where you will remain relatively upright. Also, the knees will travel farther forward during the lift with the higher bar position, something we will cover later.

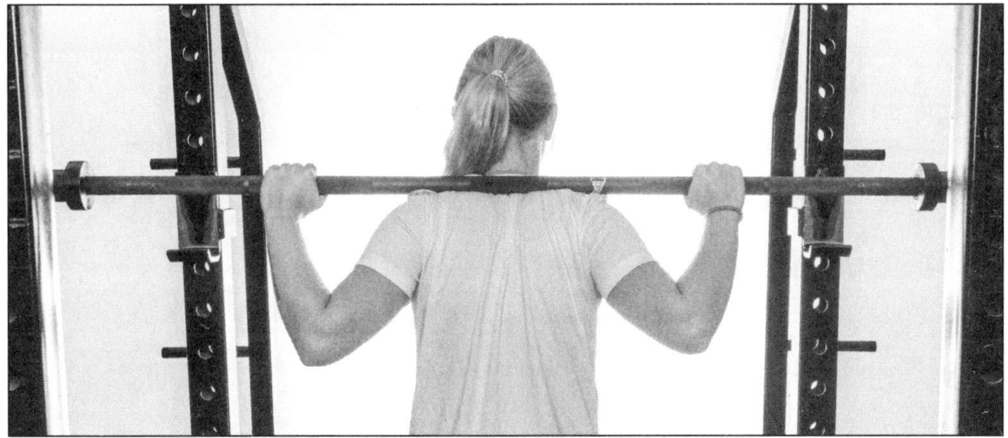

FIGURE 3.3 High-bar position of the barbell, just below the C7 vertebra of the cervical spine.

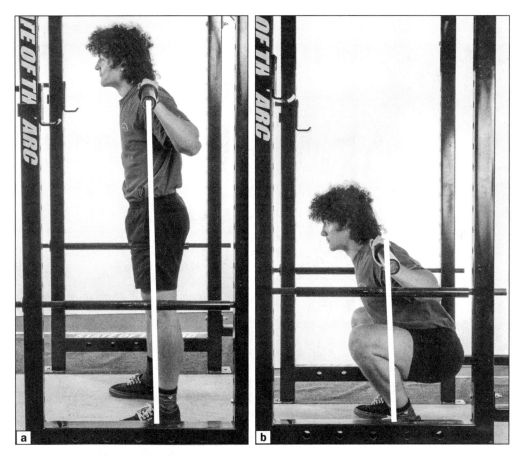

FIGURE 3.4 In the high-bar position, notice that the center of gravity remains over the midfoot *(a)* at the start position and *(b)* all the way at the bottom of the squat.

Low-Bar Position

The low-bar position is when the bar is locked on the rear delts and mid traps (see figure 3.5). I have seen a handful of lifters bring the bar lower than this, but I don't suggest positioning it any lower than the rear delts. This position starts with the bar behind the midfoot. In order to create a balanced center of gravity, the torso leans forward throughout the lift to bring the bar back over the midfoot (see figure 3.6). The degree of this lean is going to depend on the height and limb length of the lifter and can range from 10 to 30 degrees.

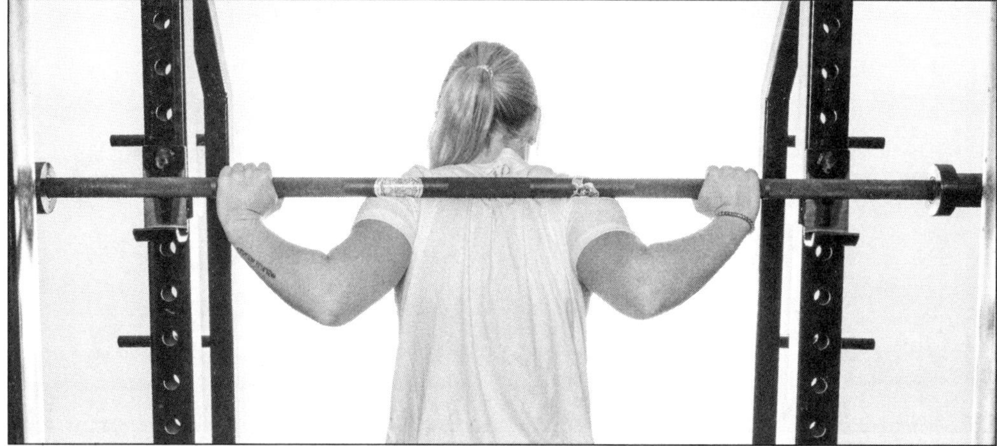

FIGURE 3.5 Low-bar position just above the rear deltoids, locking the bar in and preventing it from sliding lower.

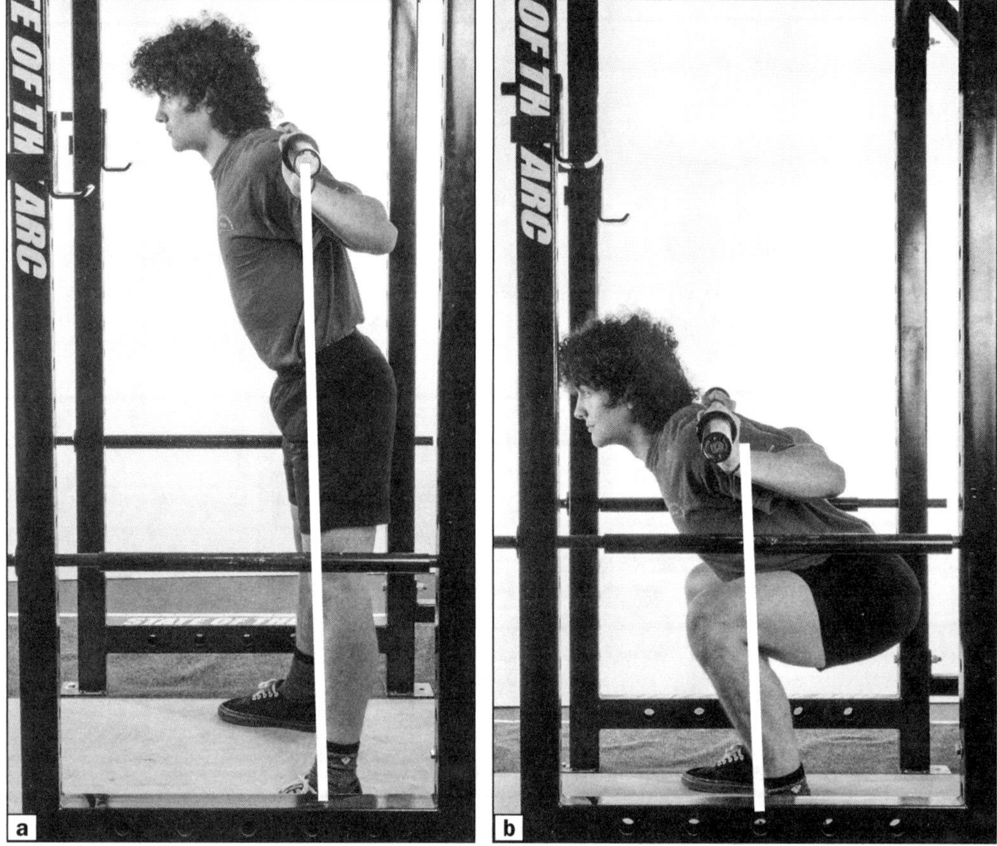

FIGURE 3.6 In the low-bar position, notice that the center of gravity remains over the midfoot *(a)* at the start position and *(b)* all the way at the bottom of the squat.

So what bar position is the best? High-bar and low-bar each have their pros and cons. High-bar requires less upper-body mobility to get into position and tends to be an easier position to start with. But you can't move as much weight compared to the low-bar because it's not as leveraged a movement. What exactly do I mean by *leveraged*? The low-bar position sets the hips back slightly more compared to the high-bar position. This puts the hips in a position where they contribute to the lift earlier and more directly. With this increased contribution, more total muscle mass is used to lift the weight. Most people observe that they lift about 10 percent less with the high-bar position. On the flip side, the low-bar position is harder to achieve because it requires greater range of motion in the shoulders and is notably less comfortable (Glassbrook et al. 2017).

One important thing to note about both bar positions: When you are first starting out, neither is going to be comfortable. The bar is going to dig into skin that hasn't really had anything like that on it before. It's going to feel heavy and awkward. If max strength is your goal, the feeling of it being heavy never really goes away, even as you get stronger. What will go away is the discomfort of the pressure on your upper back and the awkwardness of the movement. It takes time and reps, but it's completely worth it.

Bar Path

For both high-bar and low-bar positions, the bar path should be as straight of a line as possible throughout the lift. To achieve this, keep the bar-lifter unit center of gravity right over your midfoot. Not the ball of your foot. Not the heel. Right in the middle of your foot. Typically, this is where you would see the strap of a weightlifting shoe come across your foot or where the knot would be when you tie your low-top shoes. There are ways to position yourself and the bar to keep the bar path in the right spot, which we will cover shortly, but basically, the bar-lifter unit stays over the midfoot through the whole movement. This will create a straight bar path (see figure 3.7).

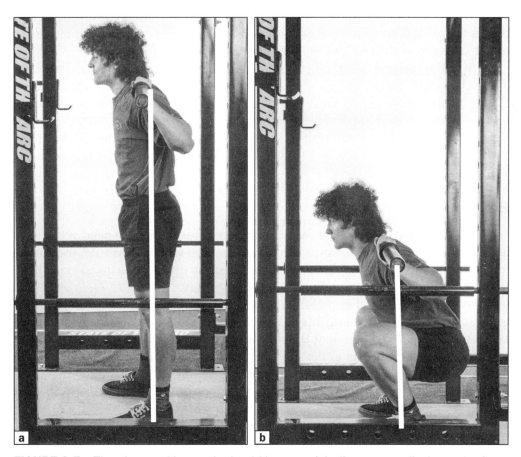

FIGURE 3.7 The observed bar path should be a straight line, perpendicular to the floor.

Why is that straight bar path important? It's because adding a horizontal vector (forces that push you forward or backward) would make moving the weight that much harder. You know what this means: It's biomechanics time. The objective of the back squat is to move the weight down to depth and then stand back up. The most efficient way to do this is to go straight down and straight up. That straight line is the path of least resistance, so to speak. It takes the least amount of energy to complete, so you will be able to do more weight or more reps. If we add side-to-side or front-to-back movement of the weight into the equation, the energy expenditure becomes less efficient. You use more energy to move the weight, making reps harder and the weight feel heavier, which in turn makes progress slower and can create an artificial ceiling to your performance. The body is incredible at adapting to what you ask it to do, but it has its limits. Being efficient with the bar path will be a determining factor in your progress in terms of lifting more weight and doing more reps.

A note on injury here: Injury tends to happen when you either drastically change your position during a lift (to a position you aren't used to) or when you attempt to do something you aren't prepared for (like lifting maximally without training properly leading up to it). The content in this book will help you avoid both of those situations.

This helps explain why you might see that one lifter in the gym move with what looks like terrible technique and yet have no problems. That lifter's body has adapted to that movement and is prepared to perform in that manner, and because that lifter has regularly done the movement that way, we can't say it increases their risk for injury. Does it limit progress in regard to weight on the bar, strength and hypertrophy improvements, and sustainable volume? All data points to yes. You have to work on technique and make it more efficient in order to get stronger over time, and that should always be the priority.

With both positions, there is one constant that you should look for: The torso angle should remain relatively the same as you do the movement. With some lifters, if you were to cut off the lower-body portion of a video of them squatting, you wouldn't be able to tell if they were at the top or bottom of the movement. That is how well they maintain the same torso angle through the entire squat. Being aware of this will create a very straight and efficient bar path, and that's what you want.

Bar Speed

I want to cover two topics here: what to expect in terms of bar speed when you are lifting, based on research on bar path and barbell velocity through the movement; and the general guidelines about bar speed to answer the question of how fast you should move during the squat.

There is a common belief that the bar speed in the squat, or how fast the lifter is moving, should be the same throughout the entire movement. This ends up not being the case when we look at the data on velocity and force in squats. We've found very distinct points in the lift where we can anticipate the lifter slowing down or speeding up. You can see this in figure 3.8. As the squat progresses, there are distinct spikes in force in the short periods of time that correspond with typical sticking points in the lift. These changes in force and velocity at these very distinct points of the lift mean that it is expected to see different speeds throughout. Understanding this can help you know when something is normal and when it is not, so you don't have to chase ghosts in your training.

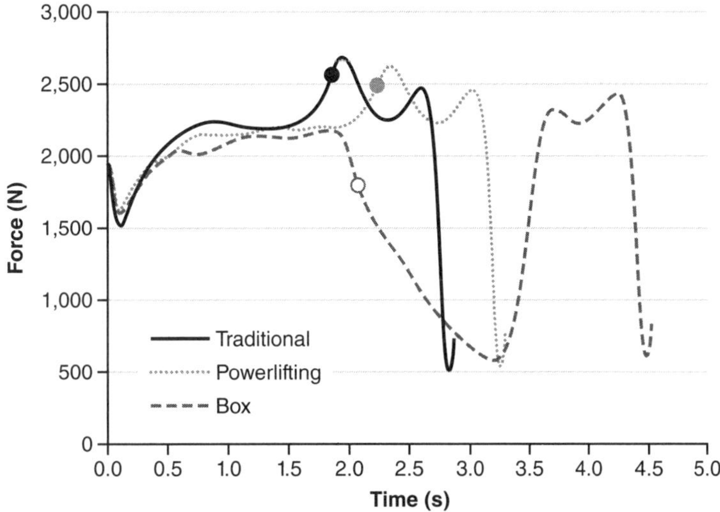

FIGURE 3.8 Force over time in three executions.

Reprinted by permission from P.A. Swinton, R. Lloyd, J.W. Keogh, et al., "A Biomechanical Comparison of the Traditional Squat, Powerlifting Squat, and Box Squat," *Journal of Strength Conditioning & Research 26*, no. 7 (2012):1805-16.

The speed of descent will vary based on the lifter, and we will cover that in a second. What I want to focus on now is what happens once the lifter comes out of the bottom, or out of the hole, which is indicated on the chart by the first gray dot on the dotted line representing the powerlifting squat. As you can see in figure 3.8, there are two peak velocities and two overcoming phases. These look like small hills with two distinct peaks on the dotted line for the powerlifting squat. Everyone expects the first difficult point of the lift to be coming out of the bottom as you reverse the direction of the weight and have to create the overcoming force to get the bar moving upward. Once the bar starts moving from there, you hit your first peak force. This is where people think they are just going to keep going at that speed. Wrong. There is a second phase between that first peak force and the top of the movement. Around half to three-quarters of the way up, the bar will start to slow down during a transition phase. At this time, you create a secondary overcoming force and hit a second peak force until you get to lock-out, when your body naturally taps the brakes to slow you down so you don't throw the bar off your back. This is important to recognize. I've seen many intermediate and advanced lifters chase ways to make this middle phase faster when, in reality, it is the naturally slow and hard portion of the lift (after getting out of the hole). The type of squat doesn't matter. A traditional high-bar squat, a powerlifting squat, and a box squat all have this presentation of two peak velocities.

An important thing to recognize here is that the speed at which you move completely depends on your ability to maintain your position through the lift. This is especially true in the descent of the squat because that sets up your position for the way up. So only move as fast as you can while maintaining your position. If you go too fast and lose position, you are less efficient with your strength and won't reap the benefits of that increased speed (Miletello et al. 2009). I've seen so many new lifters ask on social media, "Should I be moving faster at this point of the lift?" A few months later, they're still frustrated and trying everything to move faster, but their technique has diminished because of it, and with it their gains. Ultimately, maintaining position is what's most important.

My favorite example of maintaining position in the lift regardless of the speed is an absolute legend in barbell sport and bodybuilding. Stan Efferding has squatted over 800 pounds (363 kg) on numerous occasions while in his 40s. His descent in the squat is mega slow—so slow that the first time you watch it, you may think YouTube is broken. I assure you it is not. Stan moves that slowly so that he can maintain position with the extreme amount of weight he is moving and set himself up for success on the way up. He has been quoted many times as saying that he's tried to move faster, and it just flat out wasn't as effective. The key is to move as fast as you can, with position being the number one priority. Your squat will thank you for it.

The Phases of the Squat

The squat is broken down into four distinct phases: the start position, the descent, the hole, and the ascent. I don't include the finishing position here because it is identical to the start position. We are going to explain what each position should look like, how to get into each position and execute it, and things to think about during each one of them. It's good to think of these positions as building blocks. Each one sets up and leads to the success of the next one. Loss of position in one will affect the entire remainder of the lift. The degree of detail that we will cover may seem excessive, but I look at this like building a house. Would you live in one that was a rushed construction? Let's begin at the top with the start position.

Start Position

The entire lift begins here. A bad start position makes the rest of the lift harder. First things first: You want to make it so that your setup and approach to the bar becomes a routine, and here we will explain how to do that.

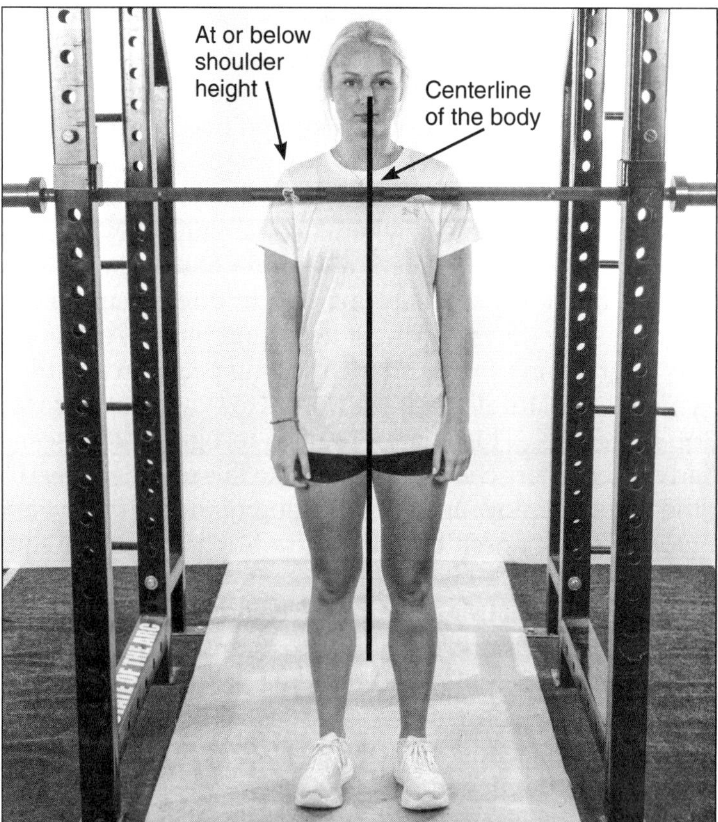

FIGURE 3.9 The bar should be between these two reference points on the rack. Remember that it's better to have it too low than to have it too high if there isn't an option in between.

Set Up the Bar

Make sure the bar is set up in the rack at just about shoulder height. If the hooks holding the bar are weird or off for your height, be conservative and set them one notch lower. It's better to be a little low here than to have the bar too high, forcing you onto your tiptoes to get it off the rack. Check out figure 3.9 for a great example of where the bar should be set up in relation to your height.

Position the Hands

Your hands are the first thing you should get set on the bar. A great starting place is just outside shoulder width, and make sure you are using the rings as landmarks, as we discussed earlier in the book. That way you are even on each side of the bar. Grasp the bar, and squeeze it with your whole hand (see figure 3.10). A firm grip on the bar helps you start creating tension right from the start.

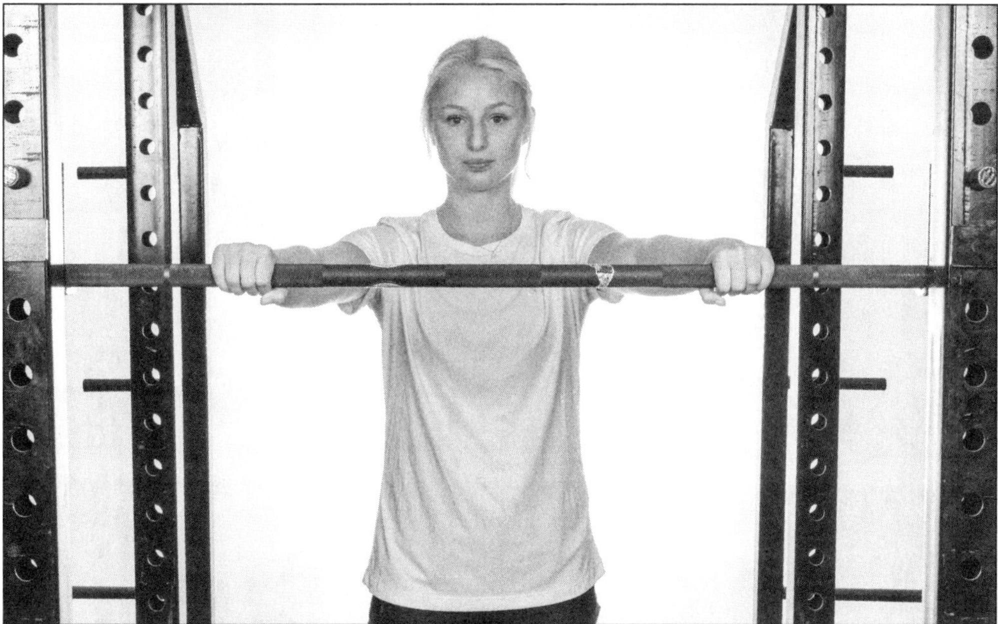

FIGURE 3.10 Take a firm grip of the bar just outside shoulder width.

Get Under the Bar

The next step is to get under the bar, but that doesn't mean you just jump under it and unrack it. Start by ducking your head under the bar and stepping underneath it. At the same time, use your arms to help pull yourself under the barbell. As you do this, try to keep your wrists neutral or in a straight line. This neutral wrist position helps control the bar better by limiting its ability to roll and is more stable than a wrist that is bent back. This will start ramping up that tension in your body so you can be as tight as possible, stabilizing the bar more.

With the head under the bar and grip set, start getting your bar to your shoulders by wedging into the bar on your shoulders and upper back (see figure 3.11*a*). Then step each foot, one at a time, directly underneath you and just inside shoulder width (see figure 3.11*b* and *c*). At this point, you should be positioned directly under the bar, your hands evenly spaced on it and squeezing tightly, your wrists stacked, and with both feet directly underneath you. Note that in this position, your elbows are the key to locking in your upper back and the rest of your torso. Think about taking your elbows and putting them in your back pockets—not driving them forward or back but driving them down and slightly back to create a shelf for the bar to rest on (see figure 3.12). This is what locks the bar in so tight it never moves. At this point, I want you to exhale, nice and slow. Then raise your head, look directly in front of you, and take a deep breath in. You are now ready to unrack the bar.

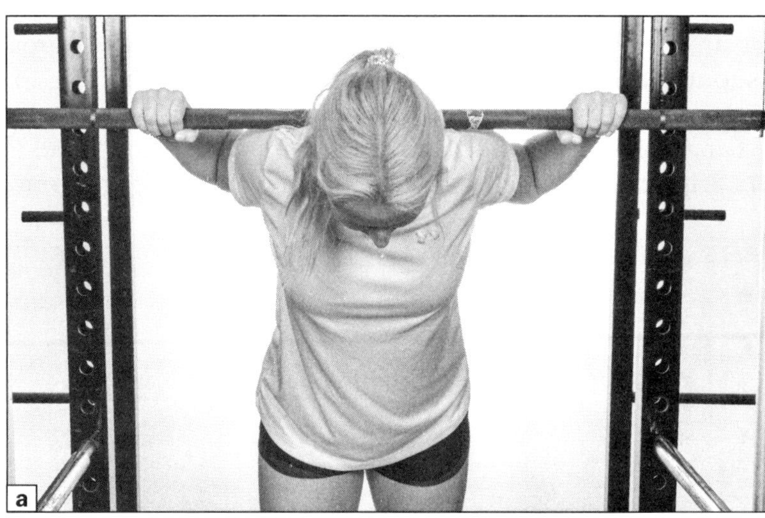

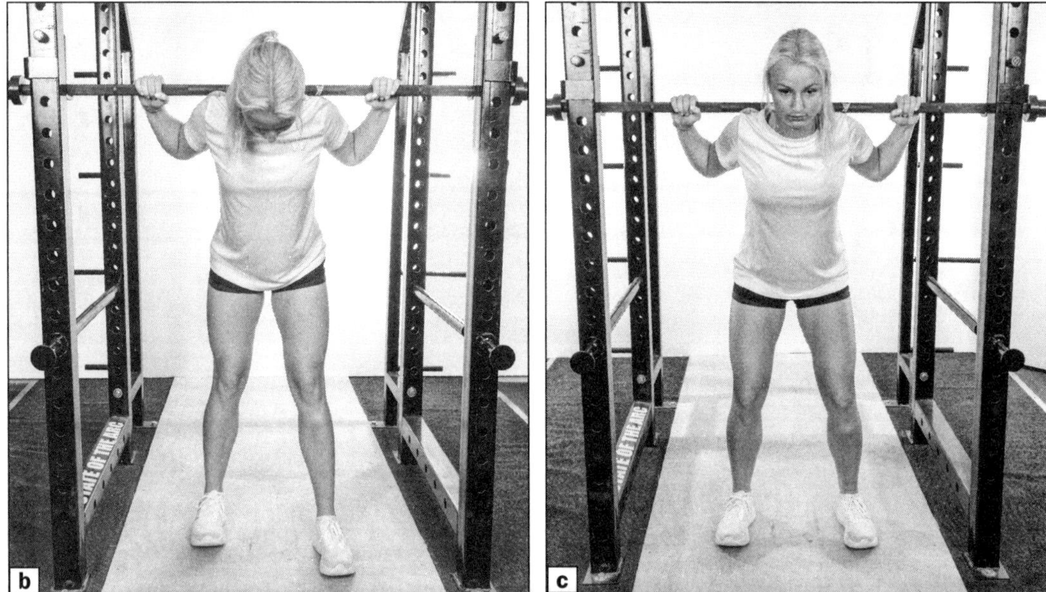

FIGURE 3.11 Process to get set up directly under the bar: *(a)* duck the head under and set the bar on the shoulders, *(b)* take first step under the bar, and *(c)* take a second step under the bar, bringing the feet even.

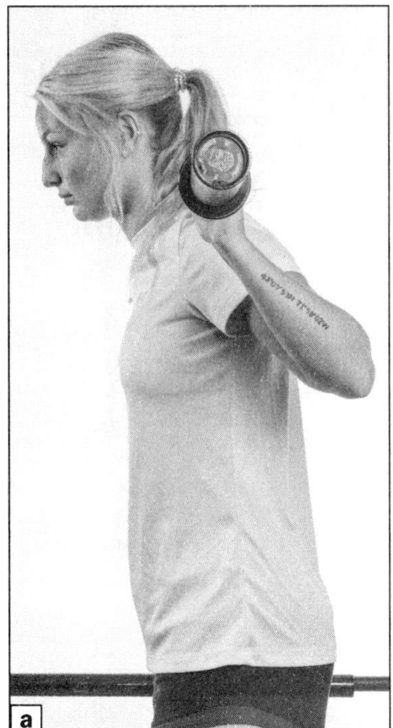
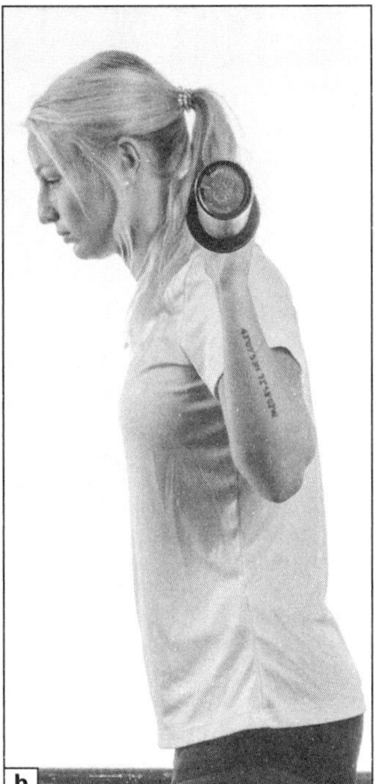
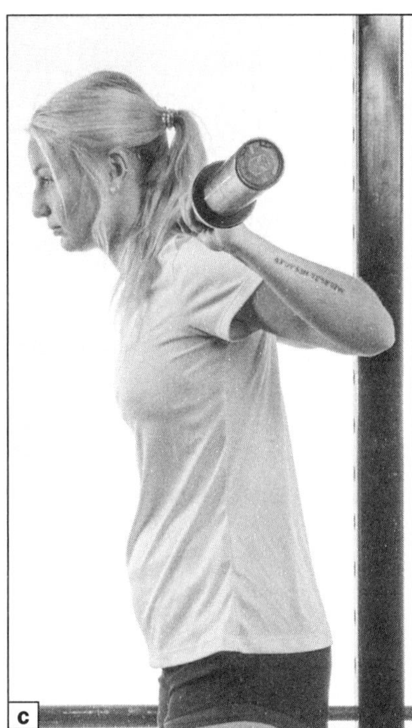

FIGURE 3.12 An example of *(a)* good elbow positioning at the start of the squat versus two examples of *(b and c)* poor elbow positioning at the start of the squat.

Unrack the Bar

The unrack should be sharp and just as diligently performed as the rest of the squat. However, this is where I see most people rush, so we're going to break it down into distinct steps (see figure 3.13). At this point, you already have a tight setup under the bar and have taken a deep breath in. Now drive through both legs, lifting the bar out of the hooks. Once you are standing up straight, don't move. Take a split second to let the bar settle while remaining tight underneath it. Do not breathe out yet. Walk the bar out by taking three steps. Just three and no more. All you need to do is get the bar away from the hooks holding it on the rack. There is no need to take the bar five feet from the rack to get started.

Once the bar settles and you can feel its weight sink into you a bit, choose the foot you are going to step with first and step straight back one foot length. Then step your other foot straight back, bringing it in line with the first foot. You should be well out of the hooks now, with enough room to squat safely. Your feet should be even with each other, just inside shoulder width, setting you up for the last step. Again, don't breathe out yet. Finally, step one foot out to widen your base to just outside shoulder width. This is the last step you need to take to be close to your final start position. At this point, your knees should be locked, your head and eyes facing forward, your hands and upper back still squeezing the bar and staying tight, and your belly full of air.

An important note regarding your head and neck in this start position: You don't want your head moving up and down during the squat movement, so it's best to find a spot 10 to15 feet in front of you to lock your gaze to. This should put your head and neck in a relatively neutral position and keep you from moving it during the lift.

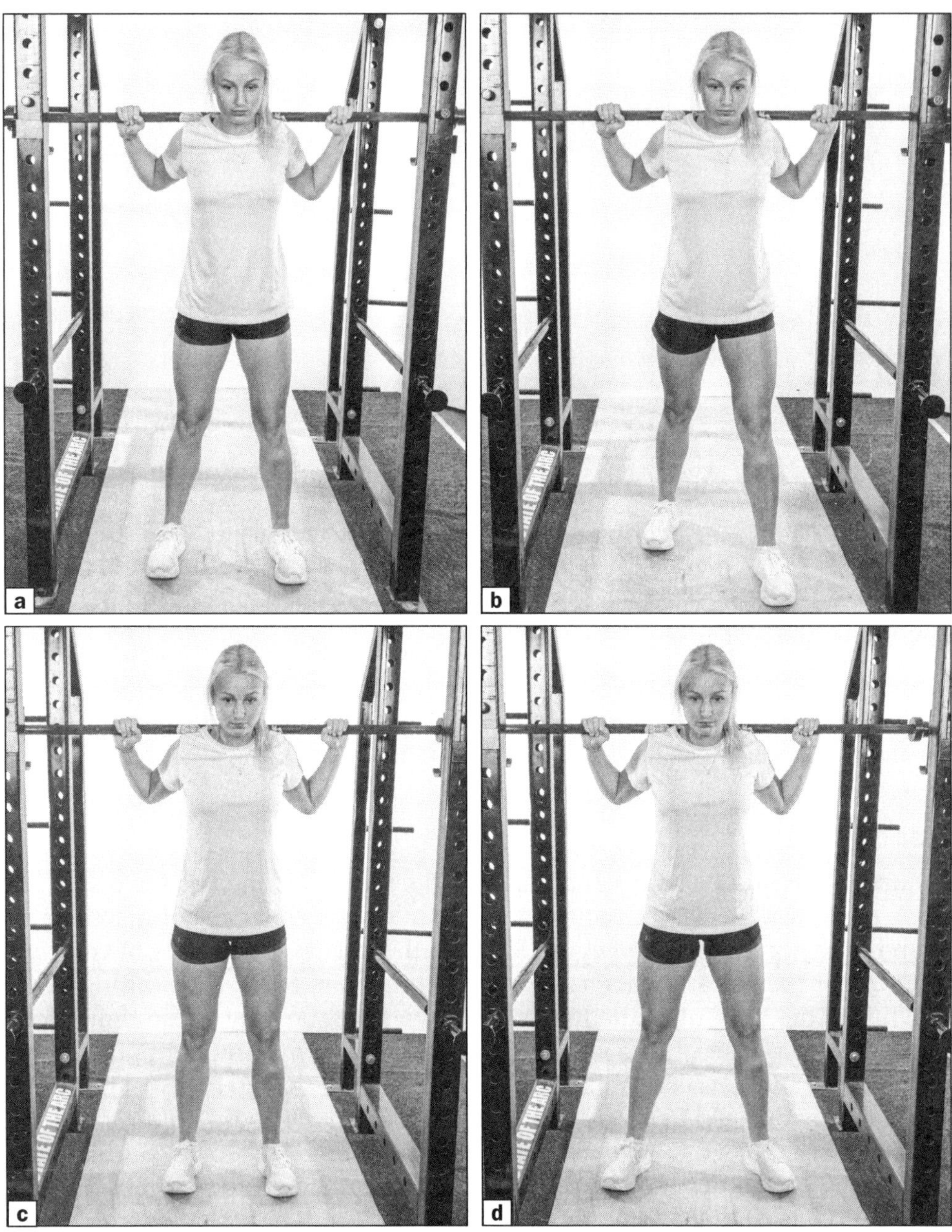

FIGURE 3.13 Unracking the bar should be precise and repeatable: *(a)* Stand straight up with the bar and let the bar settle; *(b)* take one step straight back with one foot; *(c)* take your second step straight back with the other foot, bringing your feet in line with each other; and *(d)* take one step sideways to get the correct width for your squat stance and set your gaze.

If you need to adjust your feet to turn them out, you can do that now as well. There is a high probability you have heard that you need to squat with your feet pointing straight forward, but in reality, a toe-out of 10 to 30 percent is normal for most lifters and is a good way to create a strong and stable base. It also tends to be a more comfortable foot position overall. All it takes is a slight outward rotation of the feet. As you get more familiar with this walk-out, you will start doing it naturally with each step you take.

Once the feet are in position, you should get them rooted into the ground. Think of your foot as having three points: your big toe, your pinky toe, and your heel. These three points create a tripod for the rest of your body to work from, and you need that as stable as possible. There are many ways to describe this, but think of it as trying to spread your foot out and to make it as big as possible while also trying to spread the floor underneath you with both feet (see figure 3.14). Envision yourself pulling your heels and feet away from each other so hard it rips the ground apart underneath you. To clarify, your feet should remain exactly where they are, but they will be firmly screwed into the floor at this point.

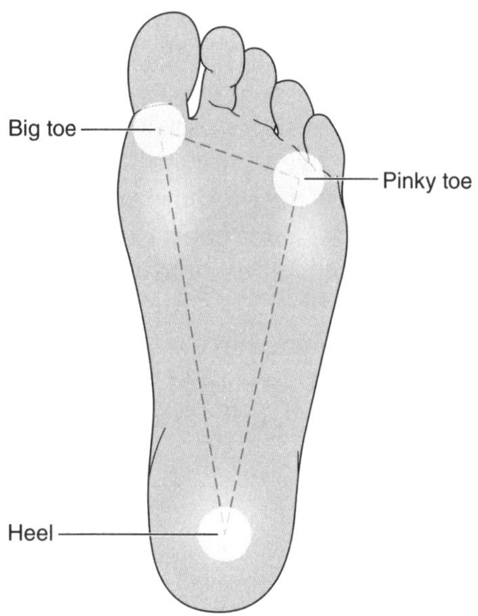

FIGURE 3.14 The foot as a tripod creates stability from the ground up.

So far you haven't exhaled, and there is a reason for this. That air is what creates the pressure to stabilize your torso. We call this *bracing*, and it's an important concept to learn early in the process. So what exactly does bracing do? *Intra-abdominal pressure* is the fancy term for what we are creating here. Bracing creates tension and stability through the trunk and stabilizes the spine and torso. This can be enhanced with the use of a lifting belt, and if you've ever used one, you've had that feeling of being more stable and stronger, even if you didn't know why. Check out the sidebar Learn How to Brace for more information on how to brace and create this intra-abdominal pressure.

Learn How to Brace

The common advice to fill your belly with air is only one part of the puzzle. To have a strong, effective brace, you need to create 360 degrees of pressure around your torso. A way I love to teach this is by using a belt, and it doesn't have to be a lifting belt to start. You can use the one holding up your pants right now.

To begin, place the belt around your waist at belly-button height. You don't want it super tight. On the contrary, you want it loose, with a little wiggle room. From here you are going to take a big breath in, slowly—like we talked about in the setup—to get ready to unrack. What you should feel is not just your stomach pushing out and into the belt but your whole abdomen and lower back beginning to push into the belt. Fill up the space between your torso and the belt, and have your torso pressing into the belt, locking it in place. If you need more feedback to feel this, grab a friend and have them put their hand in the belt at your lower back. That tends to be the hardest place to feel this. Now hold that breath and bear down. Feel the pressure build up and the belt get even tighter. The last step is to top yourself off with a short, sharp breath in through the nose, and then you'll feel what I'm talking about when it comes to tension and bracing. To learn this faster, do it a few times each day as part of your warm-up.

A word of caution: Some of you may get lightheaded when you first start doing this because you aren't used to the pressure you can create. There is no need to achieve that level of pressure early, so scale it back if you feel this way. Also, over time you will adapt and be able to handle more and more pressure as you get stronger (Blazek et al. 2019). The human body is amazing and can adapt to nearly anything you throw at it, so keep practicing your bracing.

We are almost ready to start squatting, but there is one more final step. As you are aware, at this point you haven't breathed out yet. Guess what? You aren't going to, yet. What you need to do first is top yourself off by taking a short, sharp breath in through your nose to get just a little more air and tension. This breath isn't going to go into your chest, as you can see in figure 3.15*a*. Rather, you want it to increase the pressure around your whole torso, as seen in figure 3.15*b*, where the shoulders and chest don't elevate.

Now you are ready to squat. This has been a lot of reading so I'm sure you're estimating that this setup and start position must take at least 5 minutes and that you are going to have to set a world-record breath hold! You'll be happy to learn that, in reality, it should take around 10 seconds, though it may take you slightly longer when you first start, as you feel out each step.

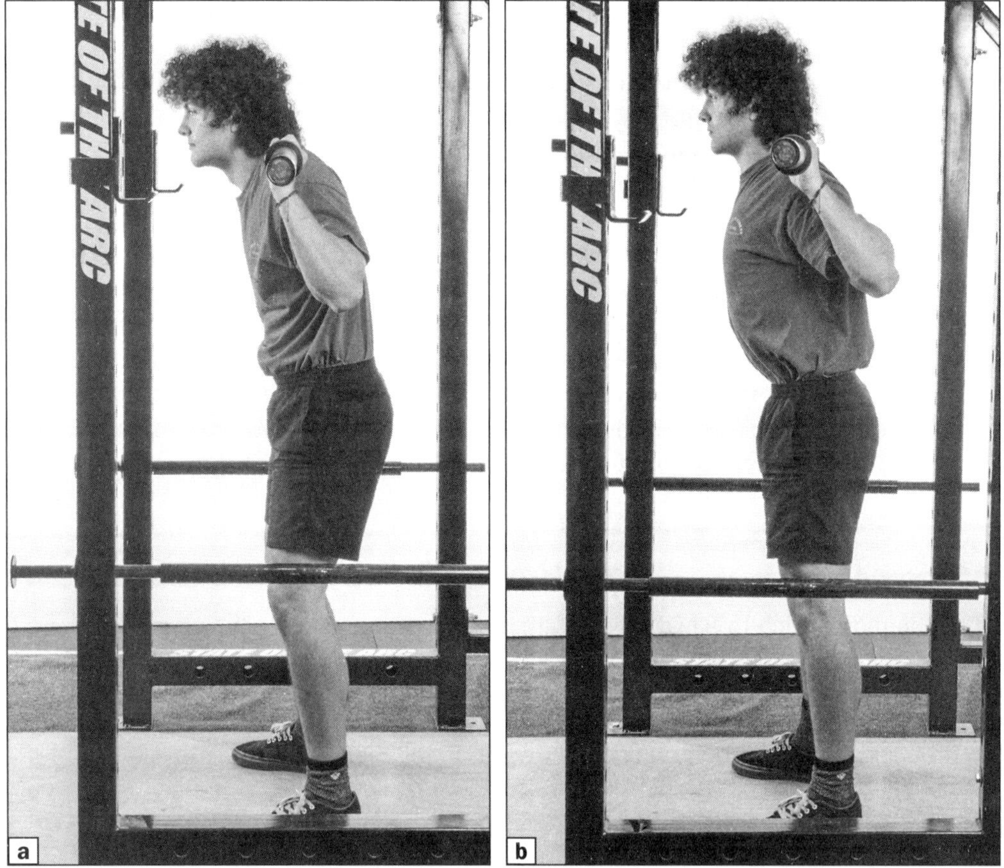

FIGURE 3.15 *(a)* A poor brace versus *(b)* a solid brace.

So let's take a minute to recap the start position, as shown in figure 3.16, that you will make repeatable for every session. At this point, this is how you should be positioned:

- The knees are locked.
- The eyes are forward with the head neutral.
- The hands are evenly spaced on the bar and squeezing it tightly.
- The upper back is tight, but you aren't shrugging into the bar ("elbows in back pockets").

- The core is tight and braced to stabilize you and the bar.
- The feet are rooted to the floor, slightly inside shoulder width, with the toes pointed out 10 to 30 degrees.

While this may seem overly complex, when it comes to walk-outs, this is as simple as it gets because it eliminates the guesswork and all the wasted movement and energy. Plus, it really pays off down the road, when the weight gets heavier or the reps get higher, if you can be deadly efficient with this part. Big lifts are made or missed at the setup. Don't rush it.

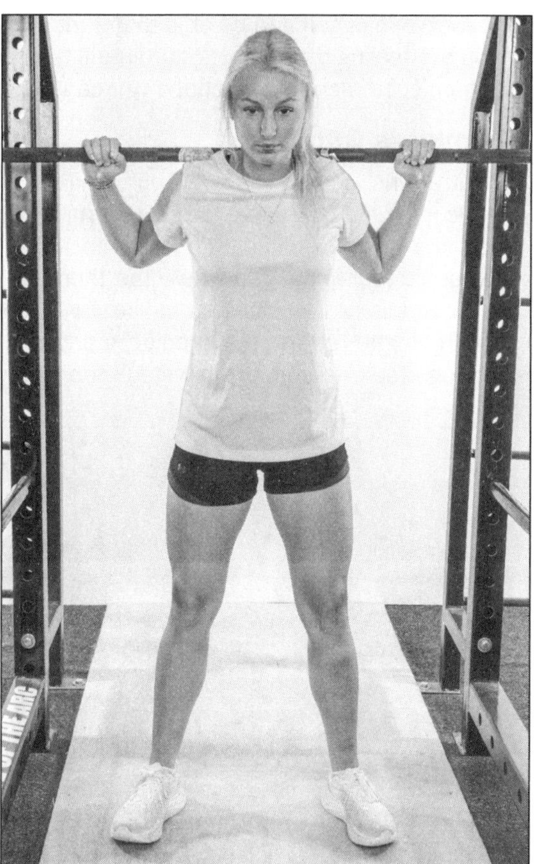

FIGURE 3.16 Walked-out start position for the squat.

The Descent

Here we go! It's finally time to get moving. I'd like you to think of the descent as loading a spring, and you are that spring. As you go down, the tension and pressure are going to build until you decide to stand up and take all that built-up energy and unleash it on the weight. Think about when you were in school and you would take the spring out of your pen, compress it, and shoot it across the room at your best friend. You will be that little spring. For a good visual of this, check out figure 3.17. To do this well, you must stay in position, know where your body is going go, and keep that bar going in a straight line. I am going to show you how to do that.

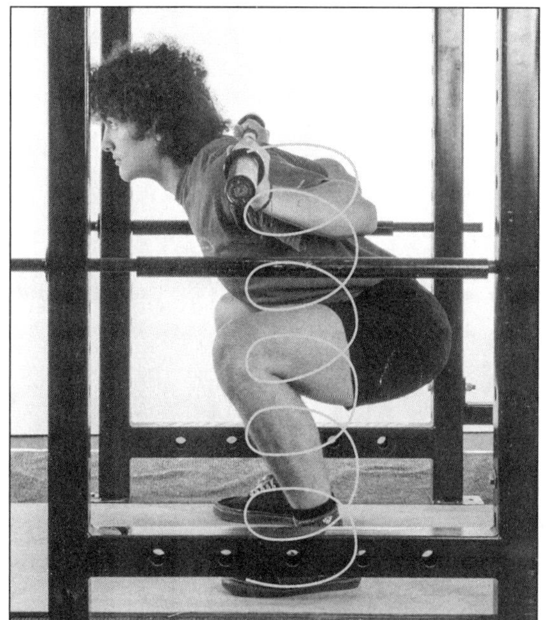

FIGURE 3.17 The lifter as a spring.

Start-Position Modifications

Not everyone is going to be able to get into this general start position, and that's okay. If you are feeling discomfort or an inability to get into the position outlined here, these are some common modifications you can make to help get into a better start position.

Thumbless Grip

A neutral wrist position can be a challenge for those who lack the required mobility. The most common problem is a lack of external rotation in the shoulder, which makes getting under the bar more difficult or uncomfortable. A good way to get into a better position is to use a four-finger grip where the thumb is not wrapped around the bar (see figure 3.18). This is not a suicide grip, like it would be in the bench press, because the bar is still going to rest on the shoulders and upper back. But it will give those who need it enough room to comfortably stack the wrists and keep a tight squeeze on the bar.

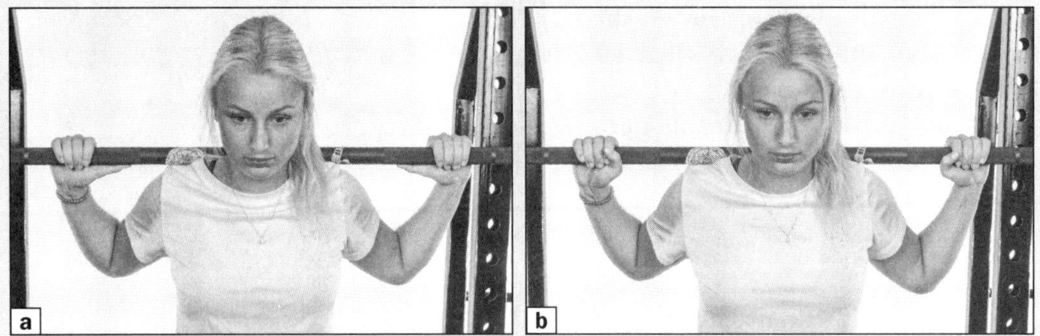

FIGURE 3.18 *(a)* Four-finger grip with the thumb still in contact with the bar but not wrapped around it compared to *(b)* a full grip around the bar.

Wider Grip

Some lifters may have to widen their grip on the bar for similar reasons. For example, shoulder mobility may limit how closely together their hands can grip the bar while still being able to comfortably get themselves under it. If this is the case, widening the grip one hand width at a time is a good strategy to find proper grip width (see figure 3.19). The trade-off with this is that it will be slightly more difficult to get the elbows locked down as tight, and you can expect to see them pointing back more the wider the grip goes.

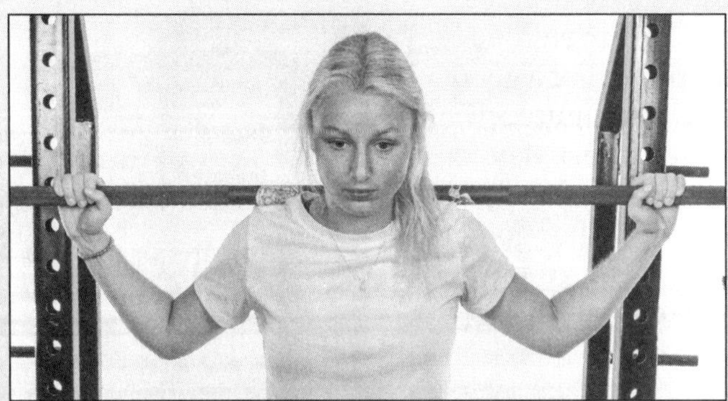

FIGURE 3.19 A wider grip position on the squat to accommodate shoulder range of motion.

Stance Width

At times, having the feet set just inside shoulder width will feel uncomfortable. Not to worry. If you walk the bar out and get the feeling that your feet aren't in the right position, move them to where they feel better, remember to root them into the ground like a tripod, and you will be fine.

The descent starts in two places: the hips and knees. To get the descent going, bend the knees and break at the hips at the exact same time (see figure 3.20). The hips go back and down, like you are sitting in a low chair, while the knees bend and move forward. That's right—the knees are going to go forward. If you are a tall lifter or have long legs compared to your torso, you can expect your knees to travel forward more than other lifters. This is nothing to worry about as long as the feet stay firmly planted on the ground. You are going to achieve this by continuing to spread the floor with your feet the entire way down, just like you did in the start position.

About halfway down is when many people start allowing the bar to bend them forward and get out in front of them. This throws off the bar-lifter unit and moves the center of gravity to in front of the foot. The leverage here is poor, so you don't want to allow that change in torso position to happen. Even though you are on the way down with the bar, you aren't just going for

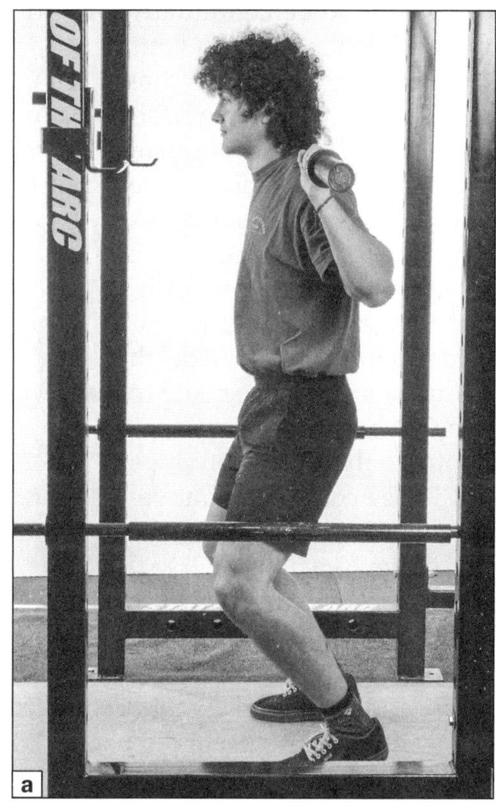

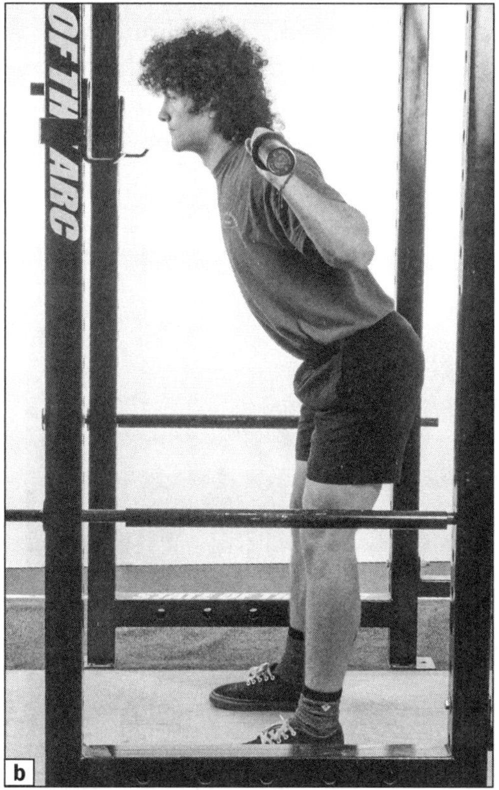

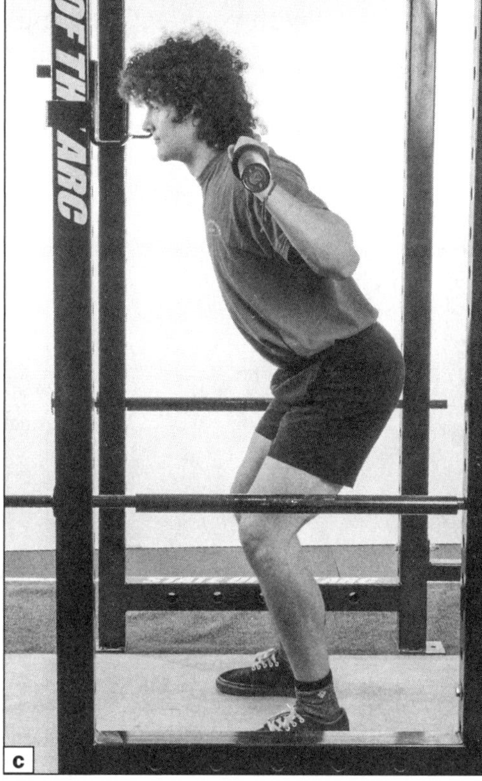

FIGURE 3.20 Comparison of *(a)* the knees improperly breaking first and *(b)* the hips improperly breaking first versus *(c)* the hips and knees breaking at the same time. Notice the change in the position of the lifter and the bar.

a ride with the bar being the driver. You are in control here. The goal is to be continually driving into the bar with your torso and upper back so that you can keep your torso position stable. This is more than just a chest-up position. Once you start the movement, your head, neck, and shoulders should act as one big unit, fused together like a block, never to be separated, till death do them part. You are going to take that block and keep driving it into the bar as your hips and knees control the movement of you and the bar on the way down (see figure 3.21).

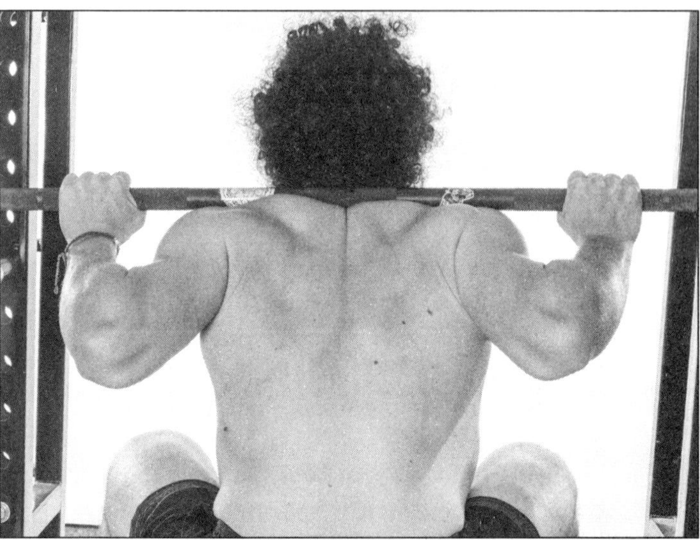

FIGURE 3.21 The head, neck, and shoulders should act as a unit, pushing back into the bar.

We are almost there, to the bottom of the squat, but we aren't done. A common error I see with the final few inches of the descent is letting all the energy and tension the lifter just built up go out the window. It would be like taking that spring and watching it wobble at full compression, only to throw all that energy in one thousand different directions. You must stay tight all the way through the lift (see figure 3.22). That means no breathing out and no letting go of your brace. As you approach the bottom of the descent, it's also paramount to keep spreading the floor apart with your feet, keeping that tripod planted. There shouldn't be a distinct change of speed here. It should look the same all the way to the bottom of the movement. Yes, tension and pressure will be high, but if you keep that tension, the rest of the lift becomes much easier. You are now at the bottom of the squat. It's almost time to stand up.

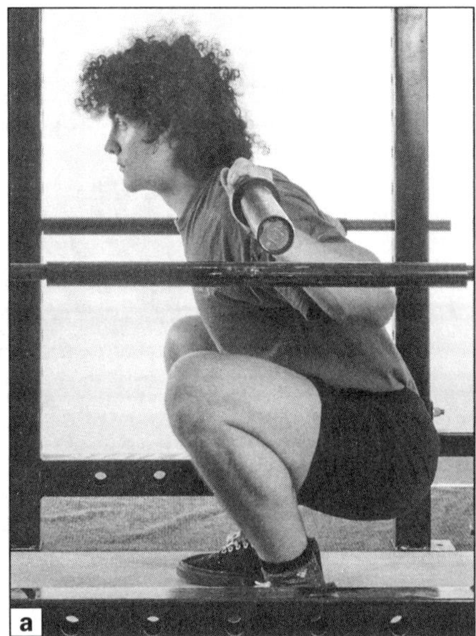

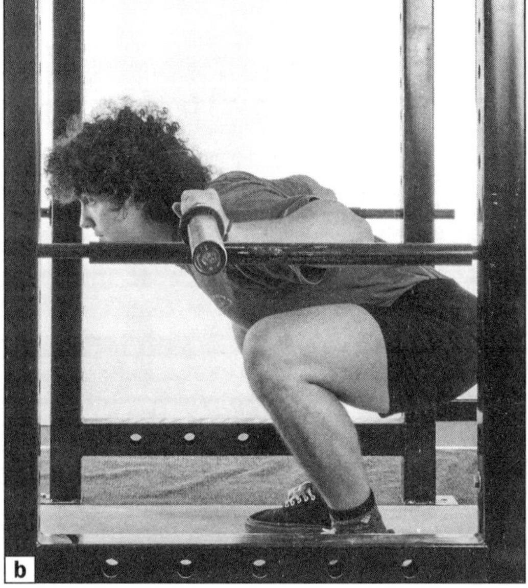

FIGURE 3.22 *(a)* Good tension allows you to maintain position. *(b)* Losing tension means losing position—sometimes completely, like in this example where the athlete loses the bar going forward.

Descent Modifications

There are some key modifications that can be made in the descent to make the movement more efficient for certain people. The most useful are changing the stance width and using an external support like a box or chair. Let's look at both.

Stance Width

Stance width affects the travel of the hips and knees during the lift. It can be used both as a way to get lower in the squat and as a way to work around discomfort. A general rule of thumb here is that the wider the stance, the less the knees will move forward, the more the shins will stay vertical, and the more the hips will have to sit back (see figure 3.23*a*). The opposite is true for a narrower stance, where the knees will drive forward more (see figure 3.23*b*). The mobility demand on the ankles to let the shins travel farther forward is greater, and the hips will sit more straight down rather than back. So a wider stance is more hip dominant, and a narrower stance is more quad dominant.

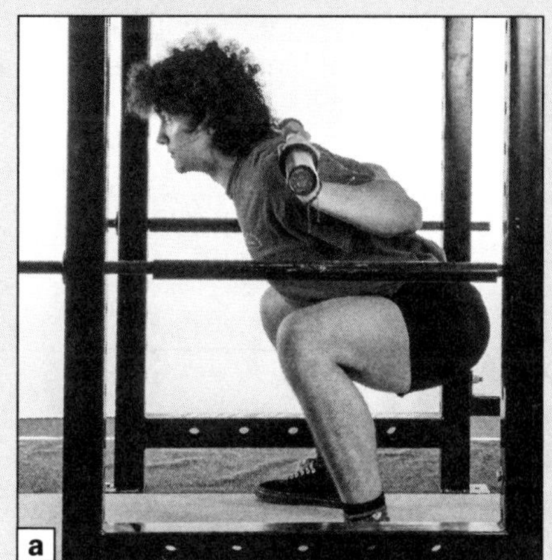

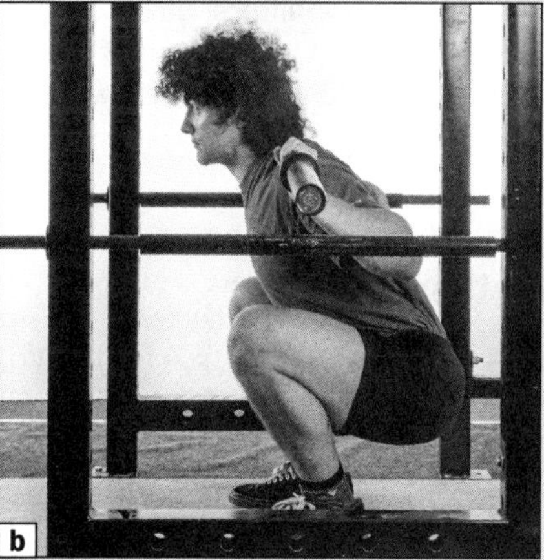

FIGURE 3.23 Positional differences in the squat between *(a)* a wide or *(b)* narrow stance.

This is pertinent if you experience discomfort in either the hips or the knees, because you can modify the stance width to load the weight more on one or the other. As always, if the discomfort persists or doesn't resolve in a few days, it's best to get it checked out by a professional.

External Support

External support, or an external frame of reference, is a great way to build confidence in the squat and to learn the positions. Especially for beginners, starting with a high box (see figure 3.24), and then gradually lowering the box over time, can provide a mental safety net and allow them to gradually build the skills and range necessary to squat to deeper levels. The target depth will vary based on individual goals. Powerlifting depth for competition means getting the crease of the hip just below the top of the knee. But not everyone needs to squat to powerlifting depth on their first day, so use tools to meet yourself where you are.

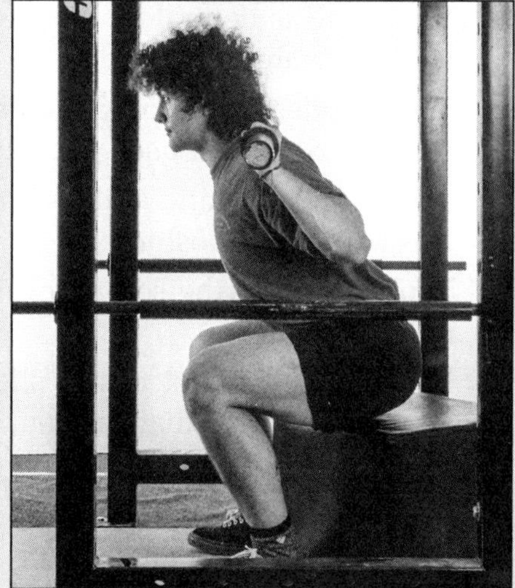

FIGURE 3.24 A great way to find depth in the squat is using a box.

Should I Bounce Into and Out of the Bottom of the Squat?

This actually was the way that I used to squat, and I found out very quickly that it has very unique purpose: namely to practice the timing of the bottom position of a snatch or a clean in Olympic weightlifting. This kind of bounce technique has massive utility there, but I've found it to be limiting when the goal is hypertrophy or lifting as much weight as possible. Here's why: The bounce at the bottom is done one of two ways. The first is a passive drop, where the lifter momentarily relaxes, specifically the legs, to create speed and a rebound effect out of the bottom of the squat. The other, my preferred method, is a more active pull into the bottom, where the lifter maintains tension but uses the hamstrings to pull down with more speed, creating a similar rebound effect.

Can people move extremely heavy weights like that? They sure can, but they will always be limited by how fast they can relax their legs, in particular their quads, and then regain the tension and force required to move the weight. Hypertrophy is best driven by a full eccentric range of motion creating complete stimulus to the muscle. Those who squat the most weight, like powerlifters, utilize a similar full eccentric range of motion to capitalize on the stretch reflex. A bounce out of the bottom of the squat isn't recommended unless you are using the squat for Olympic weightlifting purposes.

The Bottom, or Hole

All that's left is to stand up, right? Wrong. At this point you are in the bottom of the squat, or the hole, and it's important to know what this should look like in order to evaluate your performance in the descent and to be successful on the way up. Let's take a look (see figure 3.25 for an example of proper positioning in the hole):

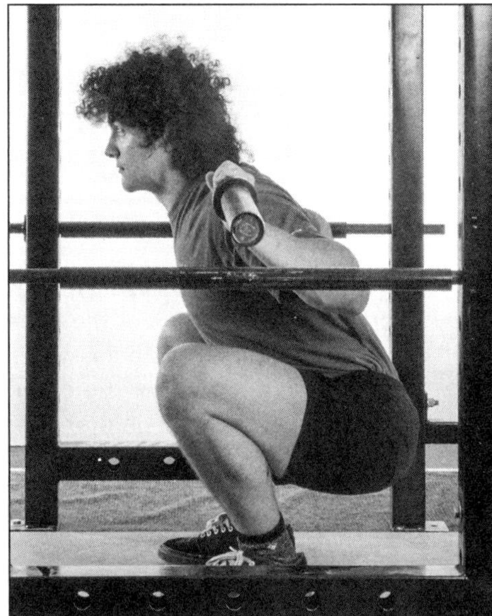

FIGURE 3.25 Ideal position at the bottom of the squat. Remember that depth will be goal dependent.

- Your head is neutral, and your eyes are looking straight forward.
- Your hands are gripping the bar tightly, with elbows in the back pocket.
- Your back is flat and at the same angle it was at the start position.
- You inhaled at the setup and still have not exhaled.
- Your knees are flexed and slightly forward (remember that this can vary forward or backward depending on stance width and leg length).
- Your hips are back and down.
- Your feet are flat on the floor and remain active. Keep spreading the floor.

The bottom of the squat is a static position that you must maintain as you start to reverse the weight. It's also the scariest part of the lift for beginners because it is foreign, and they suddenly realize that they now have to actually lift the weight. Don't panic. Stay tight here. Don't throw away these positions, and you will be set up for a great finish to the squat.

What About "Butt Wink"?

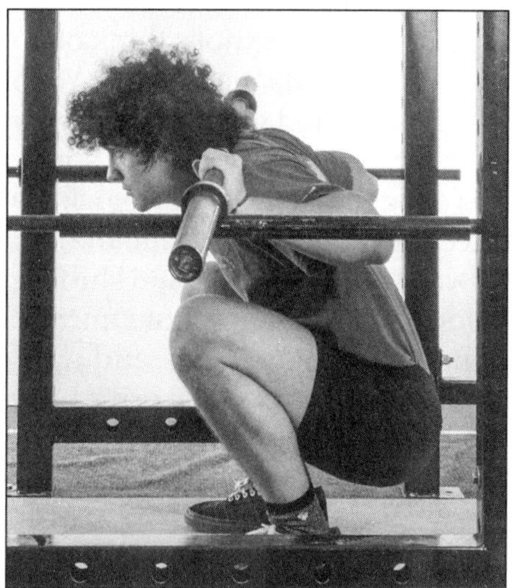

FIGURE 3.26 Butt wink.

At the very bottom of the squat, some lifters experience a change in position called the "butt wink," where their hips tuck under and cause the lower back to look rounded, giving the appearance of lost position (see figure 3.26). Many lifters have spent a lot of time trying to conquer butt wink without success. I want to save you that time.

Whether butt wink is injurious or even important is a back-and-forth debate in the strength-training world, and it's one not likely to be settled anytime soon. But with the right information and tools, you can learn to navigate and manage it, along with other issues like it.

Butt wink is just not that big of a deal. That may sound like a radical take, but hear me out. It's mostly caused by one of two things: a lack of mobility in the hips and posterior chain or a tissue accommodation when the head of the femur runs out of room in the hip socket as it flexes during the descent, pushing the pelvis back and around to make room.

No amount of mobility work is going to change the structure of your femur and its relationship to your hip, but a tissue-accommodation issue can be addressed with a change in stance position. If you experience butt wink due to mobility or range of motion issues, your first step should be to do more squats, because the most effective way to address the problem is to spend time on it.

I had a lifter with such a substantial butt wink that it changed the position of the bar and caused it to start coming forward. We modified her squat so that the point in the descent where she started to lose position became her new bottom position. On one squat day she would go to this depth at a normal tempo, and on the second squat day she would pause for three seconds there. In two weeks, we reset her bottom position about two inches deeper, and two weeks after that, we were back to full depth, with no more bar-path issues and negligible butt wink. It really can be that simple. Not only with butt wink, but with many issues related to the bottom of the squat. When in doubt, spend some more time there.

One thing you can control is your anterior and posterior pelvic tilt, or the extent that your pelvis rotates forward or backward as you squat. The primary issue is with anterior pelvic tilt. To be clear here, anterior pelvic tilt is not a bad position and it's not inherently injurious. But it can affect the depth of your squat and your hip flexion.

When the pelvis is in anterior pelvic tilt, it puts the femur in relative flexion since these are the two bones that make the hip joint. While squatting with anterior pelvic tilt, some people will feel a lot of hip tightness because the APT causes the pelvis and femur to reach that point of tissue accommodation faster, creating a false positive and resulting in a butt wink. The hip joint or musculature around it feels tight, but in reality it is not. The issue is the position of the pelvis, which can be easily corrected with better bracing, remembering to squeeze the glutes in the start position of the squat, and making sure the hips and knees move at the same rate.

The Ascent

Now it's time for the fun part: lifting the weight from the bottom to the top and standing tall, having conquered another rep.

To get out of the hole, think of yourself as that spring again, but this time with a rocket pack attached to you. You must now overcome the movement of the bar going down and get it going up by driving through the floor aggressively with your legs and continuing to spread the floor with your feet. At the same time, you are going to drive the block you made with your head, neck, and shoulders, directing it up and back into the bar. This is going to keep the bar from pulling you forward out of the hole and shifting your center of gravity to in front of your foot.

Ideally, the ascent should mirror the descent when it comes to positions. As you stand, the wrists, elbows, and where you are looking all stay locked in and don't move around. When you drive up and back into the bar with that block, your torso will stay in position as the bar moves upward (see figure 3.27). The only things that should be moving are your knees and hips extending and the bar going up.

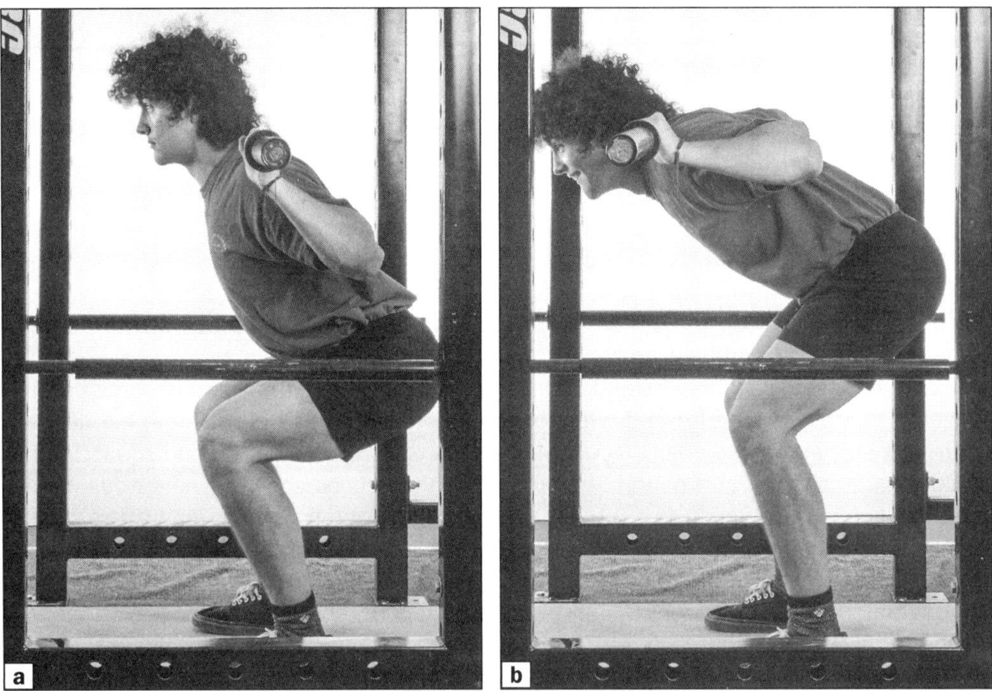

FIGURE 3.27 *(a)* When the ascent is executed correctly, the bar will stay in position. *(b)* When done incorrectly, or when a loss of tension happens, the bar will move forward and leave you in a more difficult position.

It's time to circle back to bar speed for a moment. During the ascent, it is normal to experience two speeds. The first pop of speed is coming out of the hole, then the bar tends to slow down about halfway up. That second pop of speed comes from driving your hips forward aggressively to get back to the start position. A good way to think about it is to lead with the chest and hips on the way up. Get the chest up and get the hips forward. As you approach the start position again, the bar will slow down one last time as you hit the brakes coming to a full stop. There is no reason to force past this natural slowing and risk having the bar thrown off you.

At this point, you are now back to the start position and will either repeat the process over and over for the number of reps you need to hit, or rerack the bar.

To rerack the bar, do not start by looking side to side to try to find the hooks (see figure 3.28*a*). Rather, you should walk straight forward, keeping the eyes forward, and bring the bar in contact with the rack (see figure 3.28*b*). Once you feel like you are in contact there, keep pressure on the rack, and then you can look to make sure you are in. Far too often I see lifters look to one side and the opposite side of the bar drifts backward and out of the hook. Then they go to place the bar down and they only have one side of the bar in the rack. Be safe; make contact and maintain pressure on the rack, then set it down in the hooks.

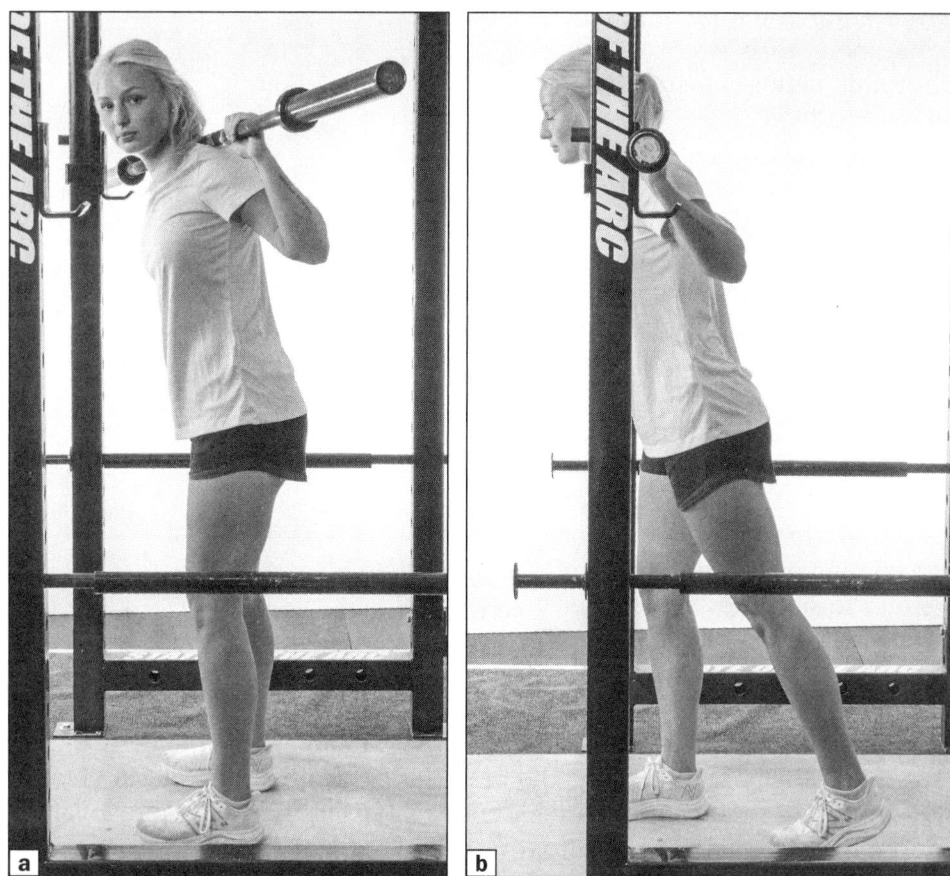

FIGURE 3.28 *(a)* When you look side to side, the bar can drift away from the rack and miss the hooks. *(b)* Keep the eyes forward, contact the rack, then check to make sure you are in.

It is worth taking time here to note that when first starting out, the most common errors I see on the ascent are knee cave, or knee valgus, and the hips rising faster than the bar, which is known as a "good morning squat." Let's break down how to address each.

Knee Valgus

Knee valgus is when the knees cave inward during the squat (see figure 3.29). It can look pretty cringe, and knee valgus has been demonized as a cause of injury, but we don't have a ton of evidence to support that. However, I will argue that when the knees cave inside the hips, the potential to lose a ton of power and leverage presents itself. No amount of banded clamshells is going to help this so, as you've guessed it if you made it this far, we're going to address it with more squatting.

There are three primary factors that lead to knee valgus: a lack of tension, a lack of skill, and a lack of strength. There are times when the simple reminder to spread the floor and keep constant tension in the feet solves the problem. A really effective method to practice this is to add a slow tempo on the way down and up. A tempo of around three seconds each way can help groove this better. Tension helps maintain position.

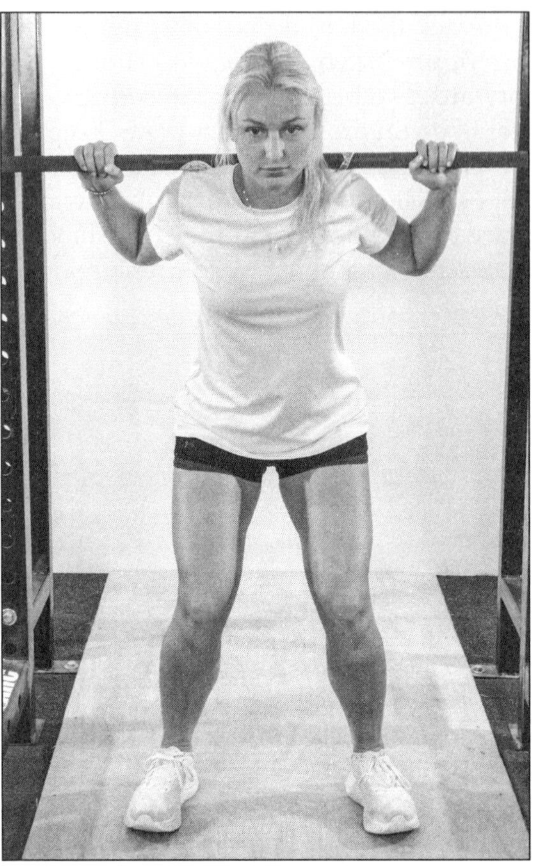

FIGURE 3.29 Knee valgus is when the knees cave inward in the ascent of the squat.

The other factors are skill and strength, and we aren't talking gluteus medius strength, as many will claim. Sometimes the weight is just too heavy, and the brain uses knee valgus to get out of a sketchy situation by recruiting the hip adductors to join the party to try and get more hip extension. The hip adductors are honestly the unsung heroes of the squat. In the most common cases, they help with hip extension when coming out of the bottom of the squat to start the ascent when the hips are beyond 90 degrees of flexion. This is how the adductors are supposed to work. Knee valgus, however, happens higher up in the range of motion where the hips are at smaller degrees of knee flexion and the adductors are kicking in in an attempt to keep the hips closer under the bar. Essentially, the brain pulls in the adductors to get more hip extension so that the hips can get under the bar and into a more leveraged position. In these cases, it's best to lower the load, get good consistent reps in with limited valgus, and build that skill set while also building the strength base needed in hip extension to succeed.

Good Morning Squat

The good morning squat is the most common error I see. It's when the lifter starts the ascent of the squat and their hips rise quickly, folding them forward and pushing the bar forward as well (see figure 3.30). If you see yourself doing this, don't beat yourself up about it, because we all have done it. There are two causes I want to cover here: poor bracing and upper-body tension, and speed.

The head, neck, and shoulders block that we mentioned earlier is crucial here as well as an effective brace. Without both, the bar will drift forward during the ascent of the lift, resulting in a good morning squat as the center of gravity of the bar-lifter unit moves out to in front of the foot. Once it's there, it's not easy to bring it back to where it needs to be. This means that preventing a good morning squat starts with the start position.

Tension has to be built there in addition to starting with the correct torso angle. If you are squatting low-bar and trying to stay upright like a weightlifter, this is going to manifest on the ascent as the hips shooting up at a faster rate than the bar. Revisit the setup as the first step to correct for this.

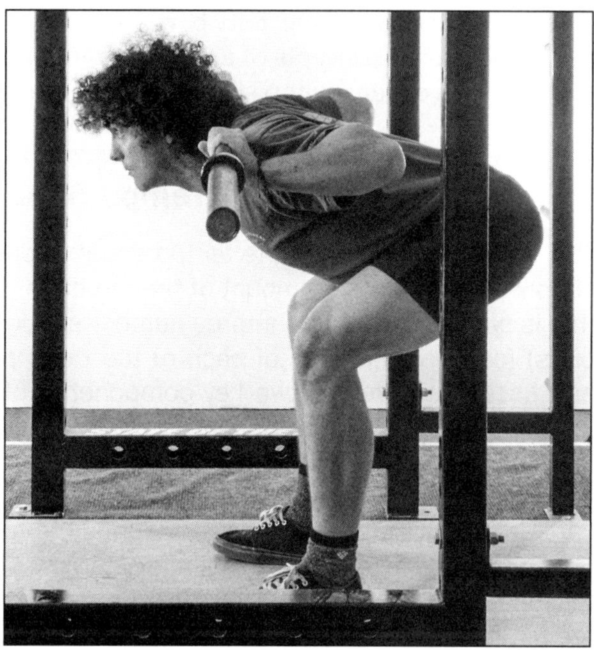

FIGURE 3.30 A good morning squat is when the hips rise too fast and the bar and lifter get pushed and folded forward.

Lastly, one thing I see people do far too early in their training life is adding speed to a movement. Remember when I mentioned how slowly Stan Efferding descends in his squat? When you are starting out, moving slowly is going to help you learn what you are doing. Many times, I see a new lifter do a good morning squat simply because they are trying to move too fast. Slow down, focus on what you are doing, and know you are building a house brick by brick, session by session. Slow is smooth, and smooth is fast.

Squat Variations

Some of you might be thinking, "What do I do if I can't squat in the positions as you have described them here?" No problem. It's time to find out how you can squat and start there. That's your entry point. To do that, we use slight variations of the movement. This is how we progress and regress the barbell back squat to other movements that can be easier or harder than the original, and also help you find *your* way to squat.

Here's the catch though. While progression and regression are what is technically happening when you use these variations, I don't like to think of it that way during training, especially with new lifters or people working through injury. There is already a barrier of "I can't" bouncing around in their head, and the thought of regression can fuel that. Avoiding these terms and placing the emphasis on finding an entry point and variations that align with where they are in their training, keeps the focus on what *can* be done and on making good training decisions. With that said, let's look more at specific variations for the squat.

Variations of the squat can be very useful in many cases. They can help build your positions, accelerate learning, spice up your training, and break through plateaus. But first, let's define a variation. Using the squat as the example, a variation is something that has many of the same components and guidelines of a high- or low-bar squat but with select differences that elicit specific responses. These could be a specific tempo, stance width, bar position, the use of additional equipment, the use of specialty bars, or a combination of any of these. However, the foundational concepts of execution remain the same. Now that that's out of the way, let's cover my top six variations for the squat.

Tempo Squat

As I've alluded to earlier, the tempo squat is one of the best teaching tools. It's simply assigning a set amount of time to each phase of the lift. In programming, this is typically written as a three-number sequence, indicating the count (in seconds) for the completion of each of the three phases of the lift (descent, hole, and ascent). There are two key components of tempo squats that make them effective. The first is time spent in positions. This is a huge teaching tool that can help an athlete feel each part of the movement and learn the positions in a controlled manner. The other component is that they are hard. Adding a tempo can make light weight feel heavy, ensuring the training session still has considerable challenge even if it is mostly for learning. This can be especially important for those dealing with injury. Nothing is more frustrating than being injured and feeling like training is too boring or too easy to be effective. Being able to train hard with significant challenge can be motivating.

When it comes to tempo, I like to start with a 3-1-1 tempo, focusing on maintaining tension during the longer eccentric of the descent. If you find you lose position on the ascent, a 3-0-3 tempo is great to focus on the descent and ascent looking the same. The most common counts I use are 3 and 5 seconds. In my experience, any longer than that feels harder but doesn't provide any added benefit. I suggest staying disciplined either by counting with "Mississippi" or using a metronome.

Box Squat and Pin Squat

The box squat and the pin squat are also amazing learning tools and can be used to turn an already good squat into a great squat. These are a couple of my most used variations with athletes and why I like them:

The first thing box squats and pin squats do is allow you to control the range of motion. If you lose position or have discomfort at a certain point, you can easily set up a box or pins at that point. For example, some people feel discomfort with deep squats. Using a box or pins can limit that range of motion before they get to that depth, helping them to continue squatting without discomfort (see figure 3.31). This gives us a ton of flexibility to program around injuries and to learn very quickly how to improve positions.

So how do box and pin squats help us learn faster? We talked about spending time in positions, and this builds on that. If you have a breakdown in a certain position, more reps at that position is going to help. Having a physical constraint, such as a box or pins, right at that position can give you those reps. Additionally, the box and the pins give direct feedback that can give your brain more information during the movement, like where your body is in space. They are also great for learning to stay tight; nothing teaches that better than a barbell smacking into the safety pins and nearly jumping off your back. A nice gentle touch of the bar on the pins means a much tighter athlete at the bottom of the squat.

There are some distinct differences in execution for each of these—the box squat and the pin squat—so let's break them down.

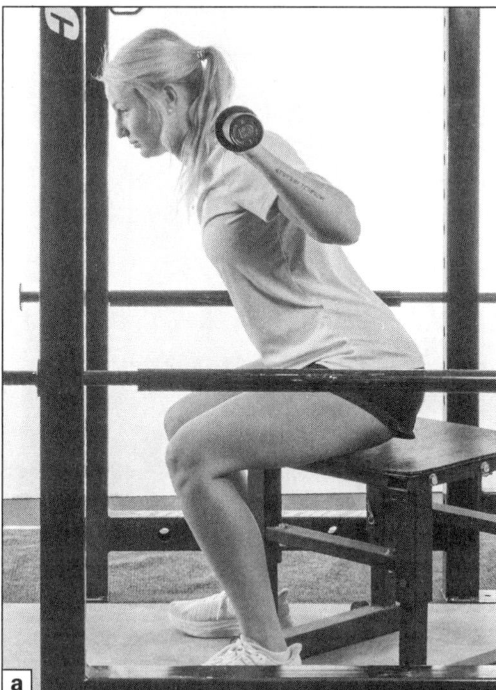

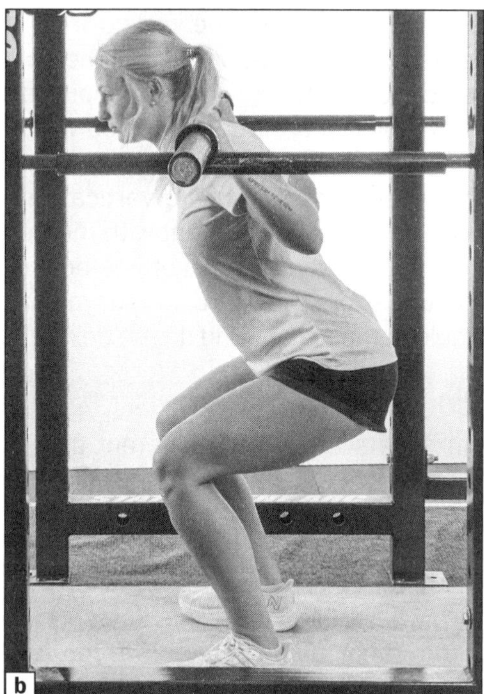

FIGURE 3.31 Use *(a)* a box or *(b)* pins to limit range of motions that may cause discomfort.

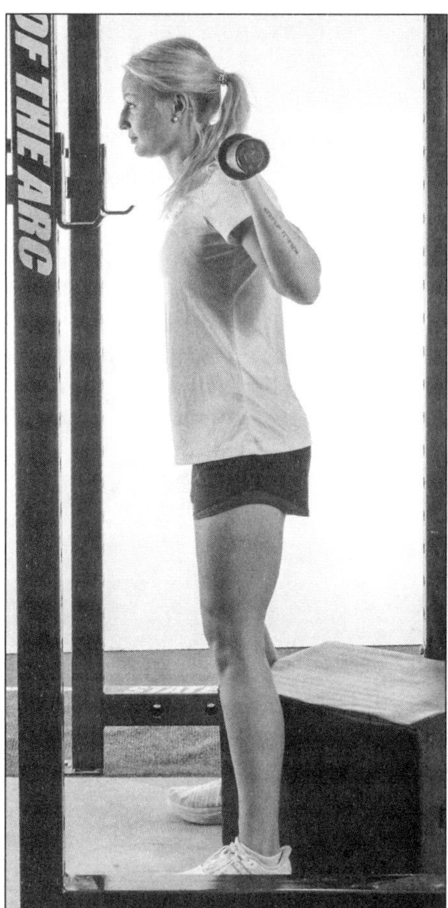

FIGURE 3.32 Setup for box squat.

Box Squat Execution

For the box squat, select a box that is either the height of where you break parallel *or* the height where you lose position or have discomfort. Make sure the box is angled so that you can straddle it (see figure 3.32 for an example of an angled box). This will allow you to be closer to the box and increase safety.

Everything from the walk-out to the start of the lift is the same as with a regular back squat. With a box squat, however, you need to sit back more on the box when you're in the hole. Think about aiming the middle of your hamstrings at the front edge of the box. When you feel yourself touch the box, stay tight and sit all the way down to it (see figure 3.33). Don't just tap the box; you should sit to it fully while keeping all the tension you have built. If you watch video of yourself doing it, you will notice that your shins stay more vertical this way, which is what we want with the box squat. Once you've been on the box for a count, explode upward as you typically would in the ascent and do the next rep.

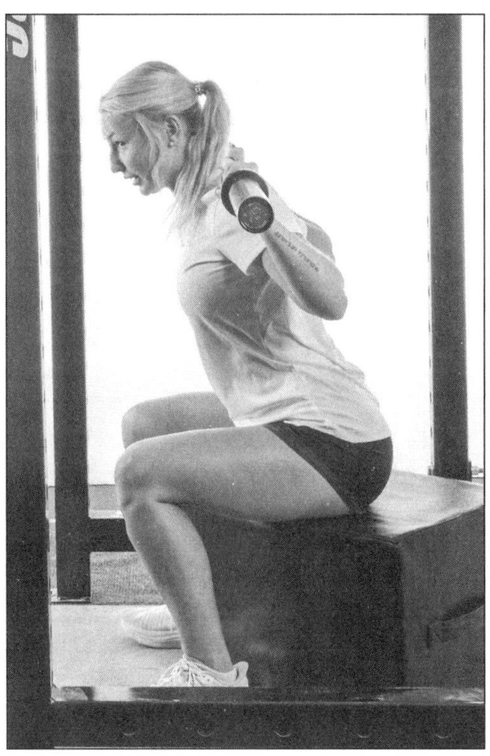

FIGURE 3.33 When you feel yourself touch the box, don't relax on it. Stay tight and sit back.

Pin Squat Execution

Pin squats are slightly different than a typical back squat in that they have the ability to separate the bar from the lifter. This is a distinction from the box squat, where the box supports the bar-lifter unit as a whole. Pins only come into contact with the bar, so if you go down too fast or aren't under control, the bar can be completely removed from you and end up staying on those pins. This is precisely what we want though, because that is going to teach you better control and how to maintain tension in the hole, if that is the position where you are lacking. We can also control range of motion with the pins in the same manner as with the box.

For the pin squat, set the safety pins/bars/straps in the rack at the height that is just below where you break parallel *or* where you lose position or have discomfort. At the start of the lift, squat as you normally would and bring the bar down to the pins with control (see figure 3.34). Just like with the box squat, don't try and tap the bar down; it will just bounce and throw off your balance. Let it get to the pins and settle for a second before you explode back up. Then do the next rep.

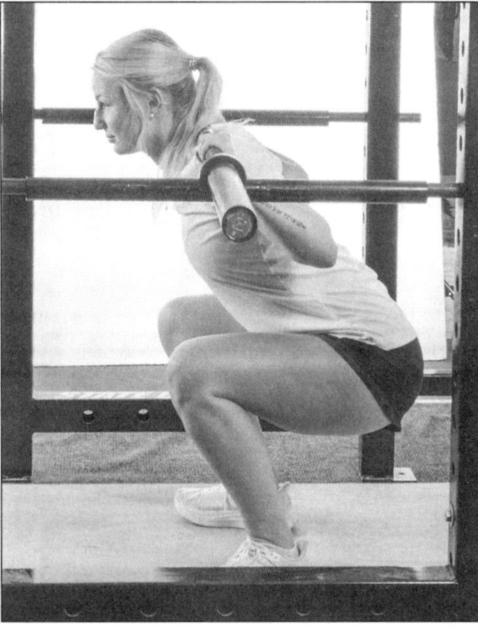

FIGURE 3.34 Example of well-set pins where the bar makes contact at full depth in the squat.

A quick note to head off confusion. You may look up a pin squat online and find a video of it starting from the bottom of the lift and think, "Hey, that's not what my book said! This must be *wrong*!" Before you go flame the comments section, this is called an *Anderson squat*, and it is a variation of a pin squat. It's an incredible lift but can also be difficult to set up and execute for many lifters. For that reason, I opted to not highlight it here directly.

Wide-Stance High-Bar Squat

The wide-stance high-bar squat is an exceptionally difficult variation because it accentuates one of the most common faults in the squat, which is the hips rising early out of the hole resulting in a good morning squat. This is due to the position of the bar and the wide stance creating a smaller area of base anterior to posterior, or front to back. Yes, it's wider and more stable side to side. However, the wider stance requires the feet to turn out more, decreasing the front-to-back stability under the lifter and creating a very low margin of error for forward or backward movement of the bar during the lift (see figure 3.35).

So if it accentuates an error, why use it? Shouldn't we look to build perfect technique by practicing it? Let's circle back to some motor-learning principles we discussed earlier.

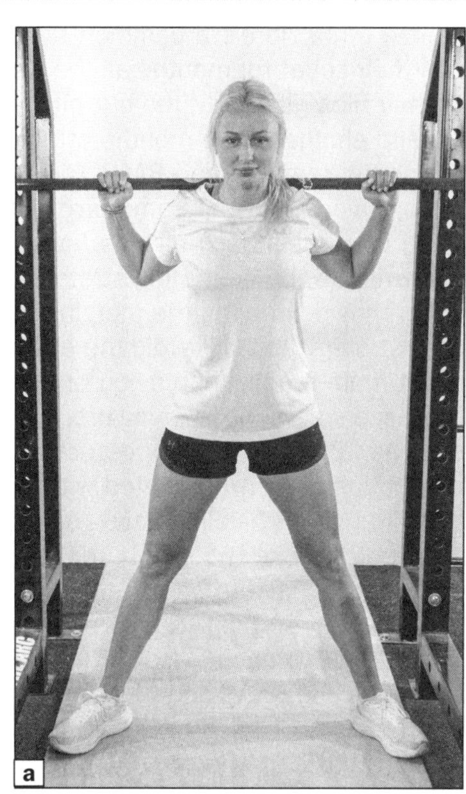

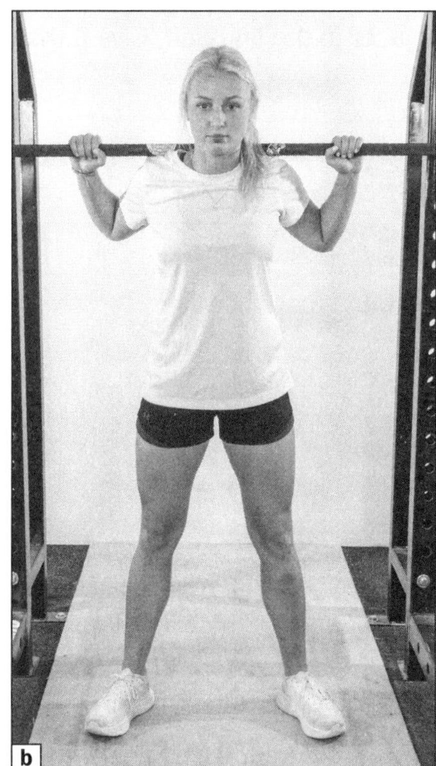

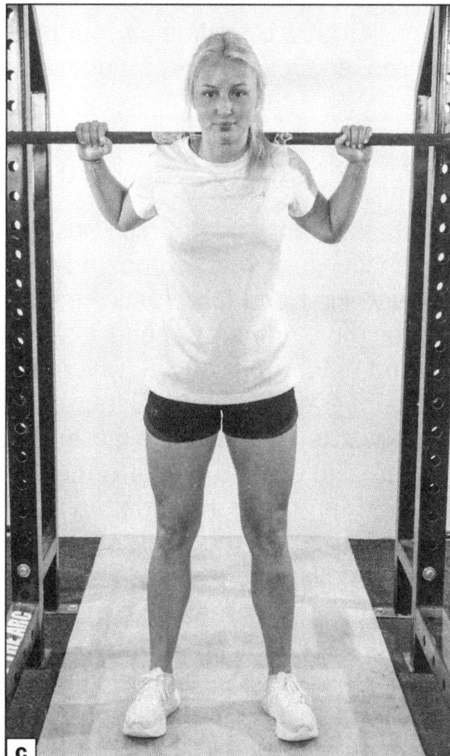

FIGURE 3.35 Typical area of base created by the feet for *(a)* the wide-stance squat compared to that of a *(b)* a typical squat stance or a *(c)* narrow-squat stance.

The brain learns through error. Practicing good technique is one aspect of the motor-learning puzzle. For the brain to learn completely, however, it needs to experience error. Here's a common scenario that many lifters experience: They work on their squat for months all the way up to a test day. Once the weight gets heavy, their hips rise early, the bar pitches them forward, and they miss the rep. They spend another three months attacking this with their usual squat until they get to another test day and BAM! They may have added a few pounds from the sheer work alone, but the same error shows up and leads to failed lifts. A variation like the wide-stance high-bar squat solves this by allowing the learning of the movement while promoting strategies to be successful. By using a variation that inherently decreases the margin for error, your movement pattern is guided toward a strategy that will avoid the error. Additionally, if the error does occur, you will feel it more readily than if you only practiced technique by using the primary lift. This accelerates the learning process by constantly allowing you to go through a heightened process of error detection and correction. It also strengthens the muscle groups directly correlated with those strategies. It teaches you to squat better while flat out helping make you physically stronger.

There are a few key notes when it comes to execution of this movement. The stance does not have to be extreme. You can start one or two foot widths wider than your current stance. The bar position will be the high-bar position described earlier in the chapter. The rest of the guidelines to execute a back squat apply here with one additional note. When you are first starting with this variation, give yourself time to get used to it and don't force depth. The wider stance can put the hips in a position where you may have less range of motion to play with before feeling a restriction or discomfort. There is no need to push past this; this range of motion will grow over time as your body adjusts to the lift itself. Give it the time it deserves, and it will blow up your squat.

Front Squat

Next up is the front squat, which has some unique challenges when compared to the back squat. First and foremost, the load is going to be more difficult to handle because it is placed out in front of you, which alters the center of gravity of the bar-lifter unit and also requires you to maintain a more upright torso (see figure 3.36). This difficulty is also the reason the front squat can be an important builder of the back squat. With the weight pulling you more forward, the upper back has to work harder from a slightly more disadvantaged position, which will build strength there. This can help decrease upper-back rounding in the back squat, which is a common fail point.

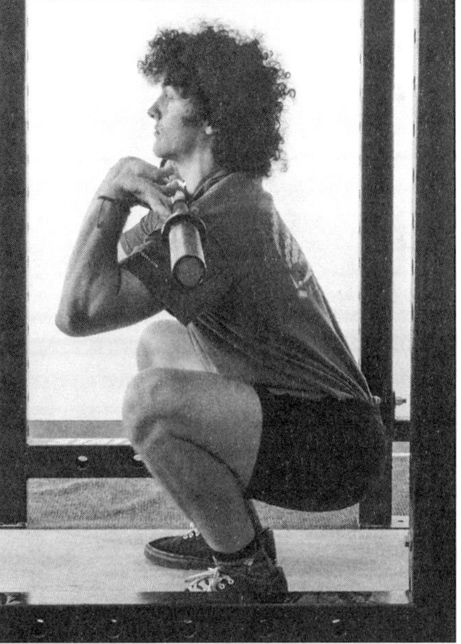

FIGURE 3.36 Body position in the hole of a front squat (note the more vertical torso).

Additionally, the more upright torso angle helps to overload the quads more during the movement as a result of the increased forward knee travel and relative knee flexion. At times, the quads become the weakness in the squat, and having something like a front squat to work them more directly can address that weakness faster. I've also had athletes with back pain who experience less of it with the front-squat variation due to the bar being loaded in the front, the overall weight being lower than with the back squat, and the more upright torso position. That position and the lower weight tends to allow them to control the flexion or extension in the back that may trigger their discomfort. I'm a big fan of being able to find ways to train around discomfort and train hard. If front squats are asymptomatic, then I'm using them.

For the front squat, the start position is what's most different from the back squat. For newer lifters, I prefer the arms-crossed rack position over the typical Olympic weightlifting position because the required wrist and shoulder mobility for the Olympic position can be hard for many (see figure 3.37). Unless you are going to be doing an Olympic clean, I don't find a ton of utility in the traditional Olympic front-rack position.

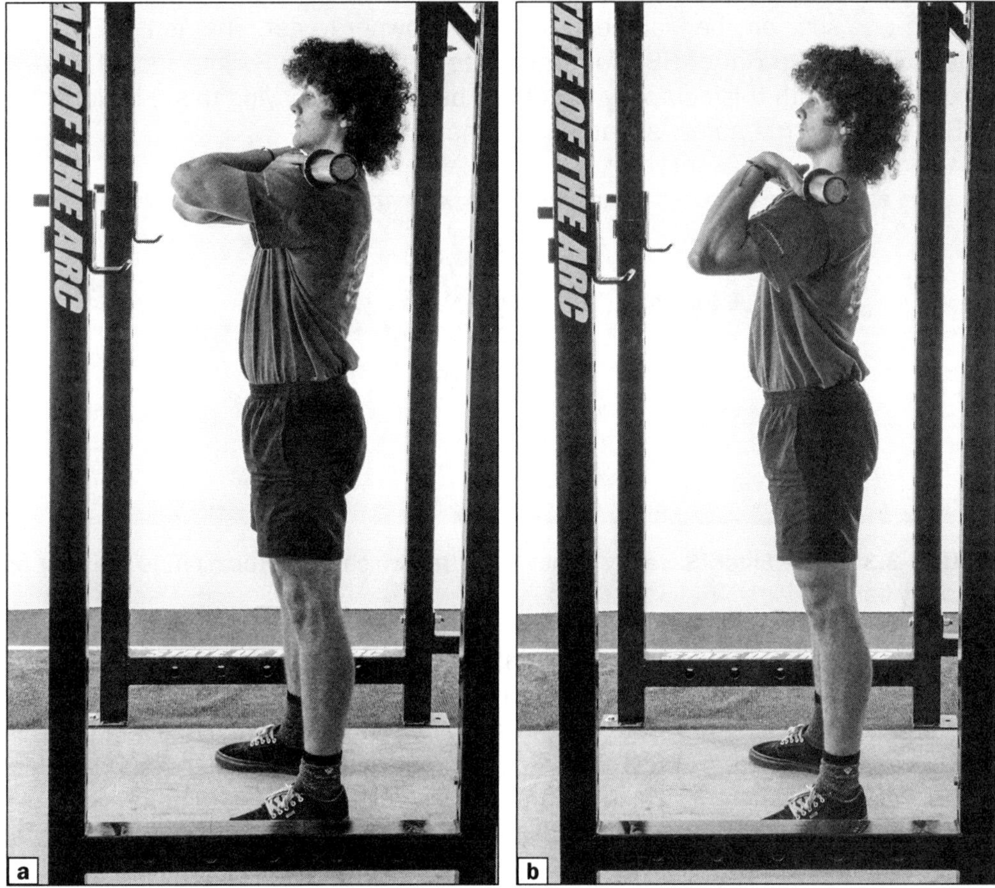

FIGURE 3.37 Front-squat rack positions: *(a)* arms crossed and *(b)* Olympic.

To get under the bar, step toward it until the bar comes into contact with your throat. From here, duck your shoulders under the bar and then cross your arms over the bar, securing it to your shoulders. The bar should be touching your throat and your deltoids. It will depend on your size, but for most it will be right behind the front deltoid. From here, the unrack is the same as with the back squat. Take a deep breath, lock down the lats to drive the shoulder blades into your back pockets, drive the bar up and out of the hooks, and take your steps. Everything else stays the same as the back squat. Hips and knees move at the same rate, but it will feel different with the more upright torso angle. This is normal, and the first few times you may feel yourself fighting the balance of the bar pulling you forward. The same may happen when you're getting out of the hole; you may feel the upper back start to round more with the bar in this front-rack position. Resist that by thinking about the same cues as with the back squat: drive the head, neck, and shoulders as a unit up and back.

The front squat is a massively underutilized variation for the building of the back squat. It's great as a secondary lift during the week or as a main movement during the off-season. Many lifters overlook it, but if you do, you could seriously be missing out on some amazing progress.

SSB Squat

If you have a home gym, there is one specialty bar you need. If you go to a gym, there is one specialty bar you need to beg the owner to get. That is the EliteFTS Safety Squat Yoke Bar or SSB for short (see figure 3.38). For the record, I have no affiliations with this company or get any benefit from saying this. I believe the SSB is the only true safety squat bar out there.

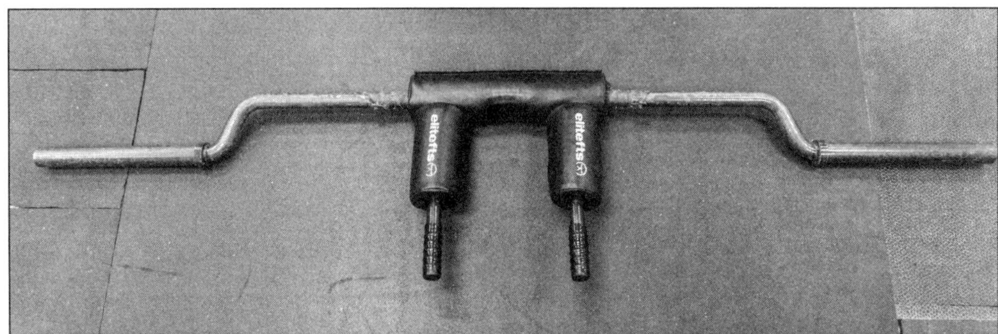

FIGURE 3.38 The EliteFTS Safety Squat Yoke Bar, which, in my opinion, is the king of specialty bars.

The SSB doesn't require your hands and shoulders to be in the same position as in a straight-bar back squat. It has handles and it sits more like a yoke on your shoulders, taking pressure off the shoulder joints while still having the bar on your back (see figure 3.39). This doesn't mean that it's easier. This bar also has a small camber to it, which means the weight will be slightly more forward during the movement than with a straight bar. This creates the perfect storm of a bar-lifter unit that is more forward like a front squat, the overload of a back squat, and the comfort of a custom bar that can accommodate for shoulder range-of-motion limitations.

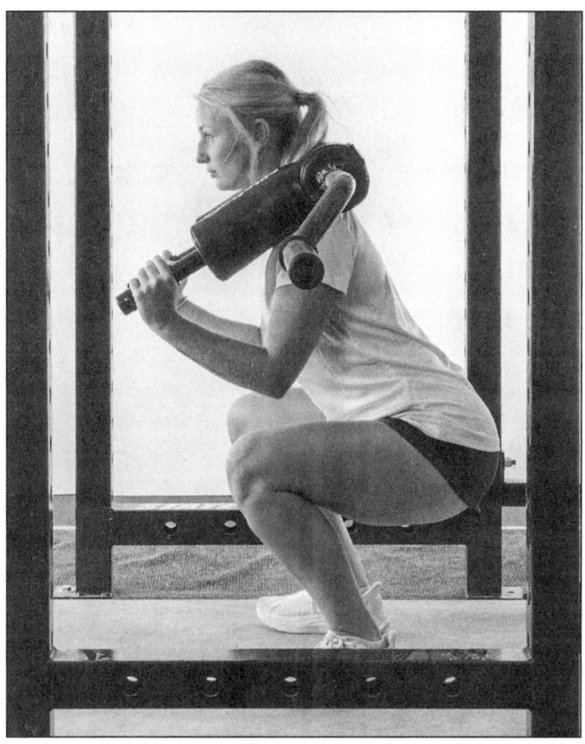

FIGURE 3.39 The SSB changes the dynamic of the bar-lifter unit by bringing the weight slightly forward, bringing the center of gravity slightly forward with it.

Similar to the front squat, the SSB squat will strengthen the upper back as it tries to push you forward with the camber of the weight. For lack of a better way to describe it, the bar itself smushes your upper body more than any other bar can. It does this with the way the weight is cambered. This creates a lever that can force more forward flexion of the upper back. Essentially, it's able to take your head, neck, and shoulders and fold them forward more.

Since the SSB has handles, you start by grasping them and then getting under the bar. The thickness of the padding should go across the shoulders. A common error I see when people first use this bar is riding it too high up their neck or using the bar backward. Because of all the different brands, check out figure 3.40 to see what it should look like when in the proper position and facing the correct direction.

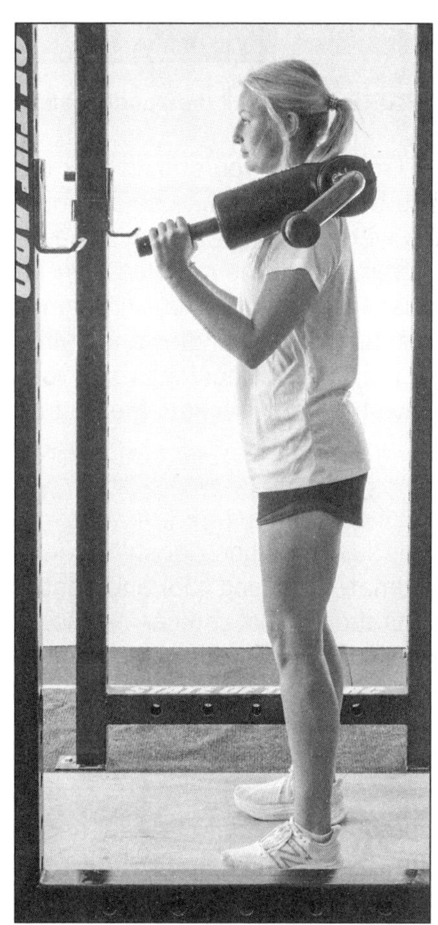

FIGURE 3.40 Proper SSB position on the shoulders and what it will look like when using it correctly.

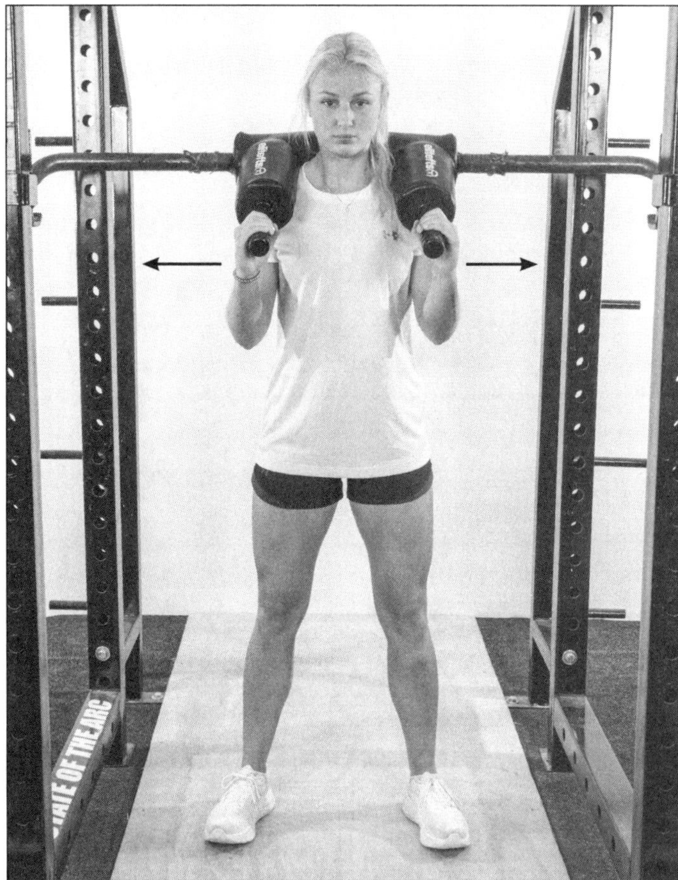

FIGURE 3.41 Pull the handles apart like Superman to get the most out of the SSB.

From there, you should lock down tension by driving the shoulder blades into the back pockets like before, but because the arms aren't in the same position as with a straight bar, this may not feel as tight. That's when we want to take advantage of the handles. I've heard lots of ways people like to use these like pushing them up or pulling them down, but when you first start out, think about grabbing those handles and trying to pull them apart like you are Clark Kent trying to tear off your business suit to become Superman (see figure 3.41). Once you have the bar unracked, the rest of the movement is the same as the back squat.

Goblet Squat

This last variation doesn't even use a barbell! I find the goblet squat to be the ultimate teaching tool and vastly superior to the bodyweight squat. Its biggest limitation is that you can only load it with as heavy a dumbbell or kettlebell as you can hold. It has one big benefit though; the dumbbell in front of the lifter helps create a counterbalance, keeping the lifter in a better position. Let me explain.

A common error in bodyweight squats is folding forward. Many times it's because people haven't squatted very much, and they don't know how it's supposed to feel. With the goblet squat, if you fold forward it becomes difficult to hold on to the dumbbell and it just feels wrong. The weight being in front helps people naturally stay more upright and learn what the positions of the squat should feel like (see figure 3.42).

When first learning how to squat, many people turn to the bodyweight squat as their first variation. This makes sense since it's unloaded, but for most, balancing is difficult and they may get discouraged. I mean, if you can't keep from falling down with no weight, how can you stay standing if you add some? This isn't actually the case though; you can see immediate improvement in the squat pattern by adding even a 5- or 10-pound dumbbell. With this, reps and confidence can be built up, leading to the use of the barbell once the athlete is confident and strong enough.

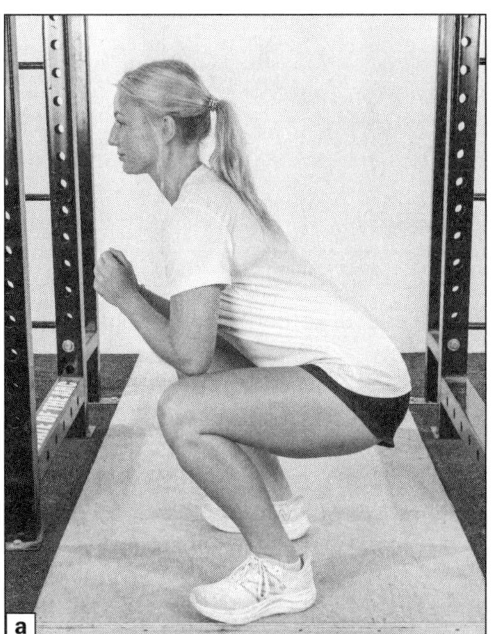

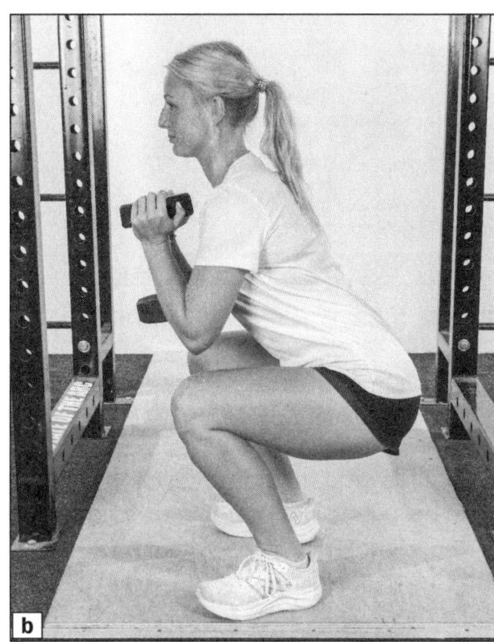

FIGURE 3.42 Compared to *(a)* an unloaded squat, the counterbalance effect of *(b)* the goblet squat is what makes it an excellent teaching tool.

For the goblet squat, simply grab the dumbbell or kettlebell that you are going to use and bring it up to your chest. If it's a dumbbell, hold it vertically from right underneath one of the ends so it's parallel to your torso (see figure 3.43*a*). Bend your elbows enough so that it's resting in your hands more than being held up by your arms. If you are using a kettlebell, the same applies but you will hold it by the horns (see figure 3.43*b*). From here, the rest of the movement is the same as the back squat. If you are stepping into the gym for the very first time, or teaching someone who is, you can't go wrong with a goblet squat.

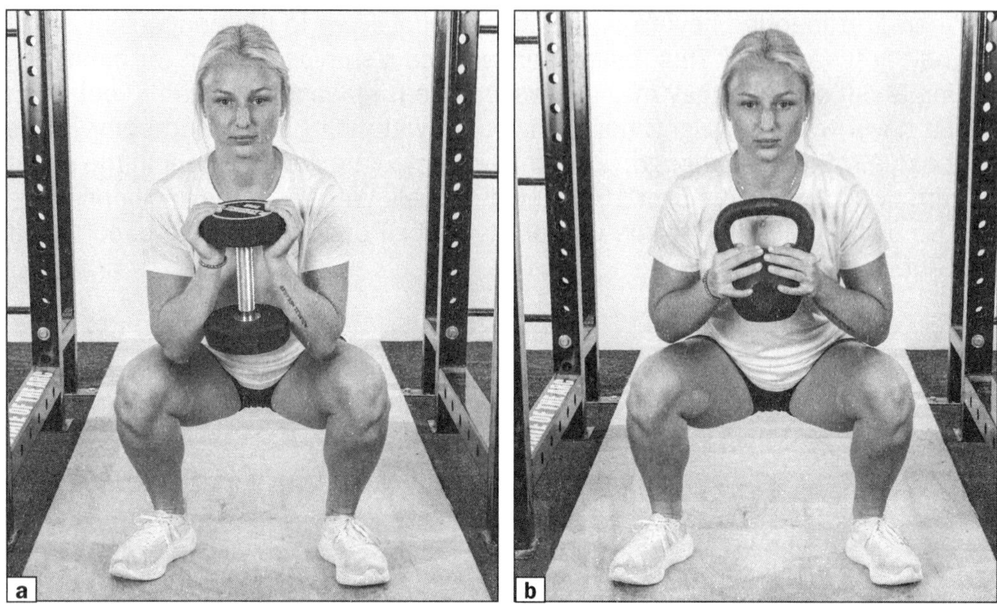

FIGURE 3.43 The proper way to hold *(a)* a dumbbell and *(b)* kettlebell in the goblet squat.

Warming up for the Squat

As we covered in chapter 2, there is no need to get fancy or crazy with warm-ups. However, I do want to provide you with some of my favorite warm-up exercises that are specific to the squat and to the limitations I commonly see. Let's cover the five that I use most often.

Half-Kneeling Arm Circles

Two common complaints I hear when people start squatting are tightness in the shoulders when getting under the bar and tightness in the hips during the movement. Half-kneeling arm circles can help with both. This is a strength book, not a mobility book, so we aren't going to dive into that rabbit hole. What I will say is that many of those sensations you feel around tightness are less related to tension in the actual tissue and have more to do with how well you tolerate those ranges of motion.

For half-kneeling arm circles, find a wall that is clear of equipment. I also suggest a smooth wall, because you will be dragging your arm on the surface. Lower yourself onto the knee closest to the wall. Both your bottom and top knees should be bent at 90 degrees (see figure 3.44*a*). There is no need to lean forward. Remain tall and you should be close enough to the wall that your shoulder is just touching it. Extend the arm closest to the wall straight out in front of you with your palm facing away from the wall (see figure 3.44*b*). Squeeze your glutes tight and you should feel a decent stretch in the front of your hip. From here, bring the arm overhead as you work it around in a circle on the wall (see figure 3.44*c*). As your arm gets around behind you, allow your hand to naturally turn toward the wall so your palm is facing the wall (see figure 3.44*d*). Keep working your arm around and as it approaches your hips, you can turn your hand back over (see figure 3.44*e*). Do this for five to eight reps on each side and then move on to the next part of your sequence. If being this close to the wall is too hard or you aren't able to get your arm all the way around in the circle, slide away from the wall until you can.

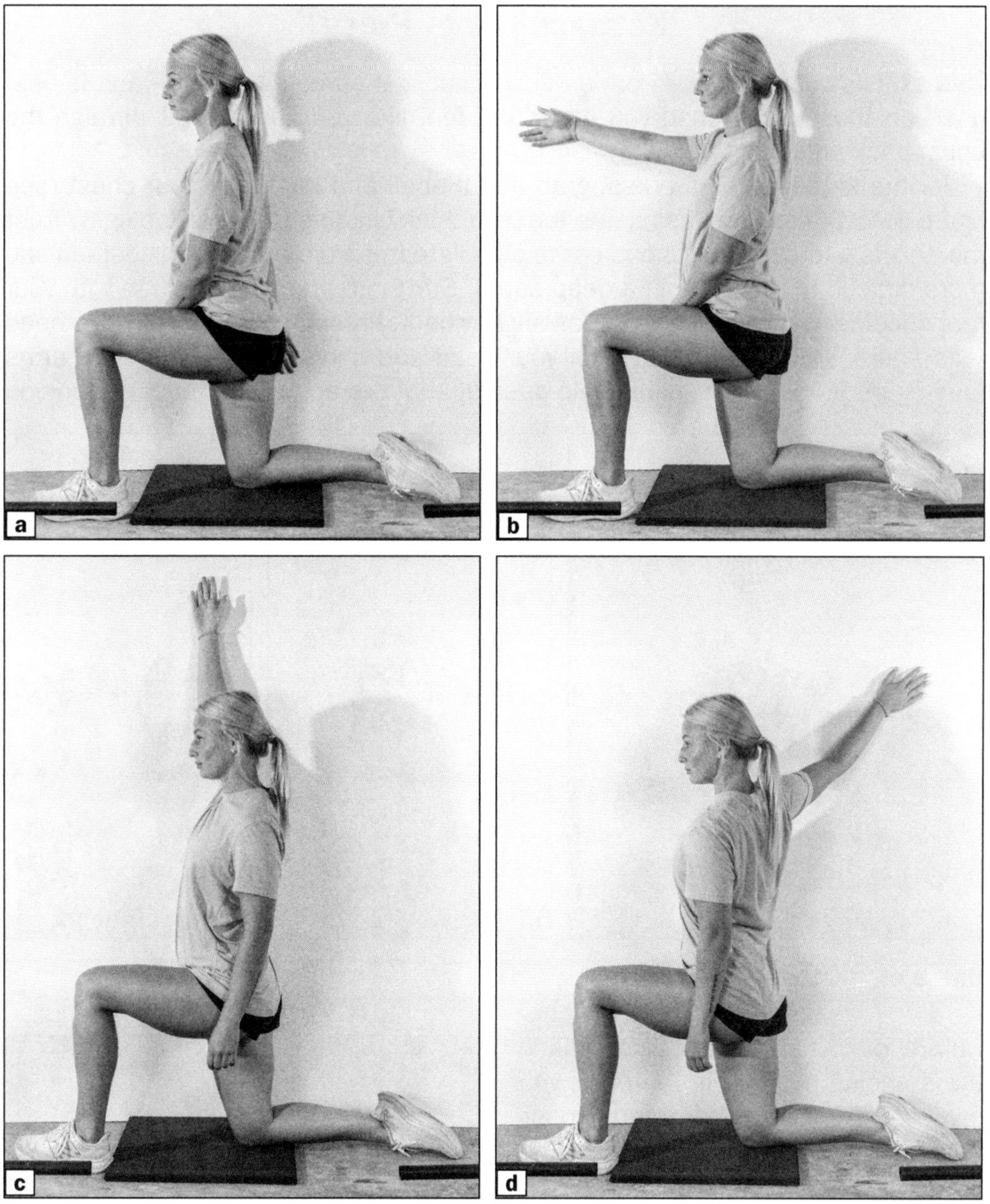

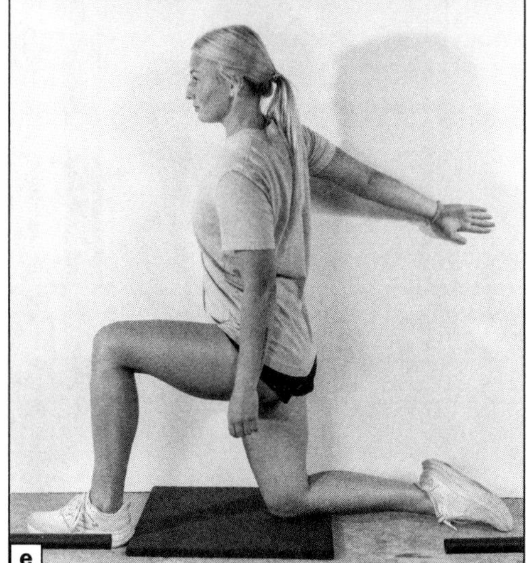

FIGURE 3.44 Half-kneeling arm circle.

Kettlebell Sots Press

This exercise can be done from a deep squat or a standing position and is best used on those days when you just don't feel like you can extend through the upper-back area.

For the kettlebell sots press, grab a kettlebell and hold it at your chest (see figure 3.45*a*). I suggest using one that you think is going to be far too light. Trust me, this is a tough one. It's easiest to complete this from a standing position and more difficult to complete in a deep squat. Start in a standing position with your feet shoulder-width apart and knees slightly bent. Press the bell directly overhead (see figure 3.45*b*) and then push your head and shoulders through your arms (see figure 3.45*c*). This should help open up that thoracic (upper back) extension

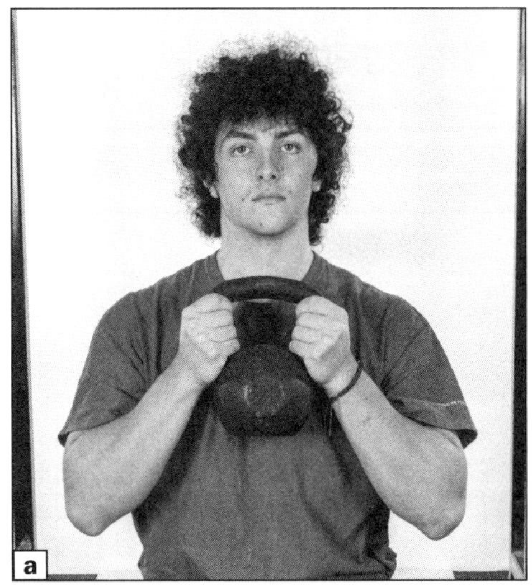

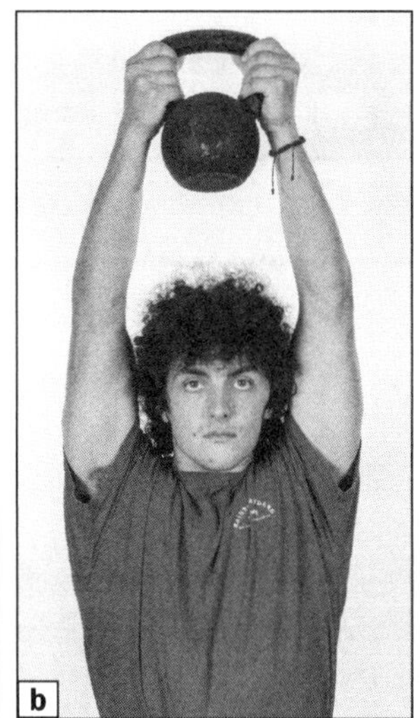

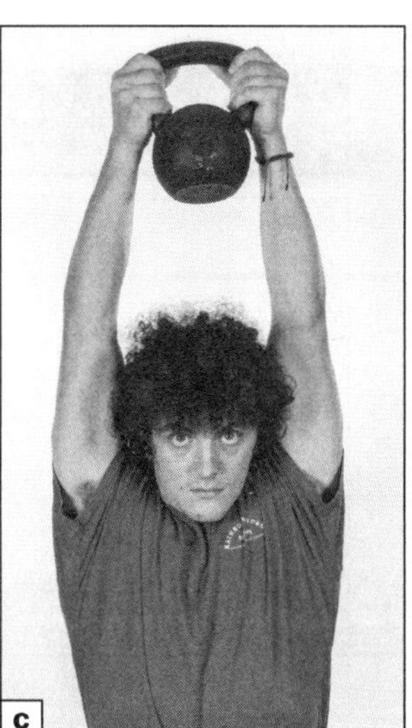

FIGURE 3.45 Kettlebell sots press.

we are looking for. If performing this in the standing position is too easy, you can move right to a deep-squat position the same way you would with the goblet squat, or even use a chair or low box to go into a seated position (see figure 3.46). This will be much harder for most, so master the standing position before attempting the deep-squat position. Five to eight reps tend to be enough, then you can move on to the next exercise in your warm-up cluster.

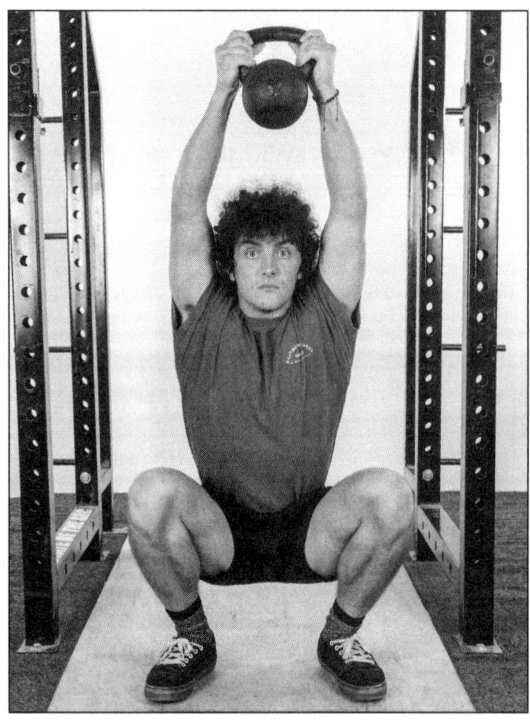

FIGURE 3.46 Kettlebell sots press in the deep-squat position.

Cossack Squat

The Cossack squat is one of my favorite lunge variations of all time. This is a great way to work your hips and knees through a full range of motions that are close to the positions you will use in a back squat, and it's something you can scale easily. I like to start with just body weight, progressing to a dumbbell or kettlebell like with a goblet squat, and finally to an empty barbell.

For the Cossack squat, stand tall with the feet about one-and-a-half shoulder widths apart (see figure 3.47*a*). From here, lunge down to one side, keeping the heel flat and squatting down as far as you can (see figure 3.47*b*). The opposite foot's heel is down, but the rest of the foot is allowed to rotate up toward the ceiling. Hold on to something like a pole or a rack for balance if needed. Hold this position for one to two seconds and then switch directly over to the other side. I don't have athletes do this weighted as a warm-up when they first start with them; I prefer them to go through as large a range of motion as possible instead. The Cossack squat is great to help with squat depth and groin and hip tightness in the squat, and it gets the heart rate higher than the other options we have covered so far.

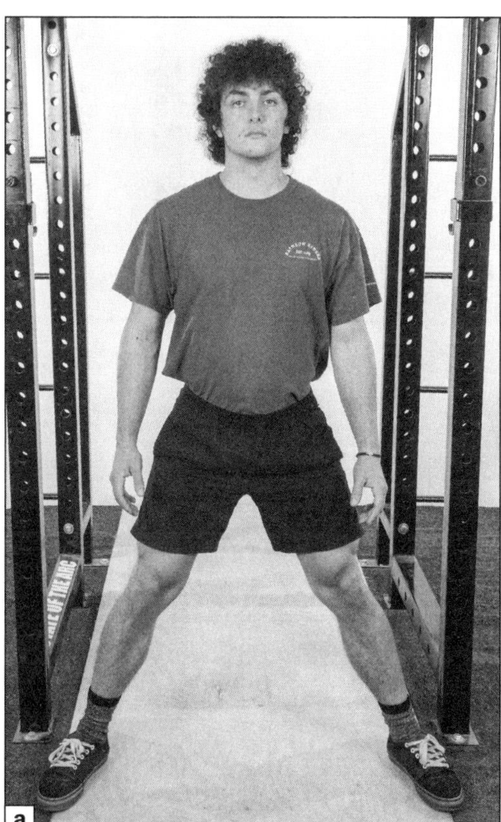

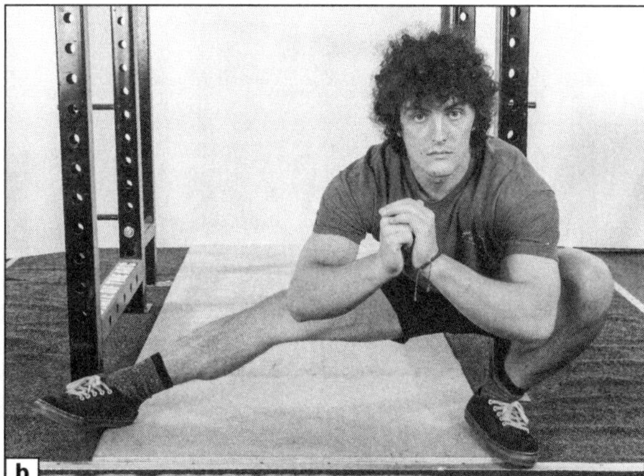

FIGURE 3.47 Cossack squat.

Barbell Good Morning

The barbell good morning tends to be a staple in some people's training as an accessory lift, but I love it as part of the warm-up as well, especially for those with a history of back injury, who can use this to gauge how they are feeling and adjust their training accordingly. I don't load these past the barbell for warm-up purposes when people first start out. The goal here is to get the posterior chain warmed up by loading the hips and back directly.

For the barbell good morning, start with an empty bar in the same preferred position that you would for the back squat (see figure 3.48*a*). The difference is that to start the good morning you will push your hips straight back, just like when you are trying to shut your car door with your butt (see figure 3.48*b*). Keep tension in the upper back just as you would with the squat and keep pushing the hips back. Stop when you feel a big stretch in the hamstrings, your torso is parallel to the floor, or you reach your maximum tolerable range of motion, whichever comes first. No need to push past these ranges or add a ton of weight when using this as a warm-up. Remember, this is to set up the big lifts for success.

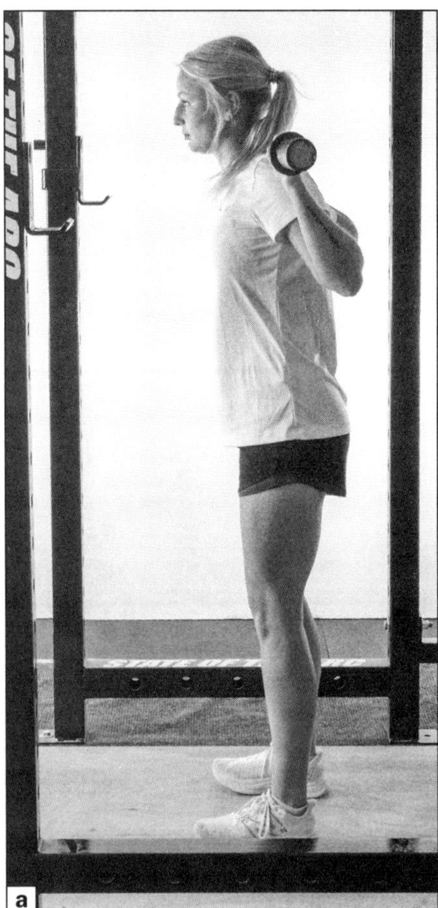

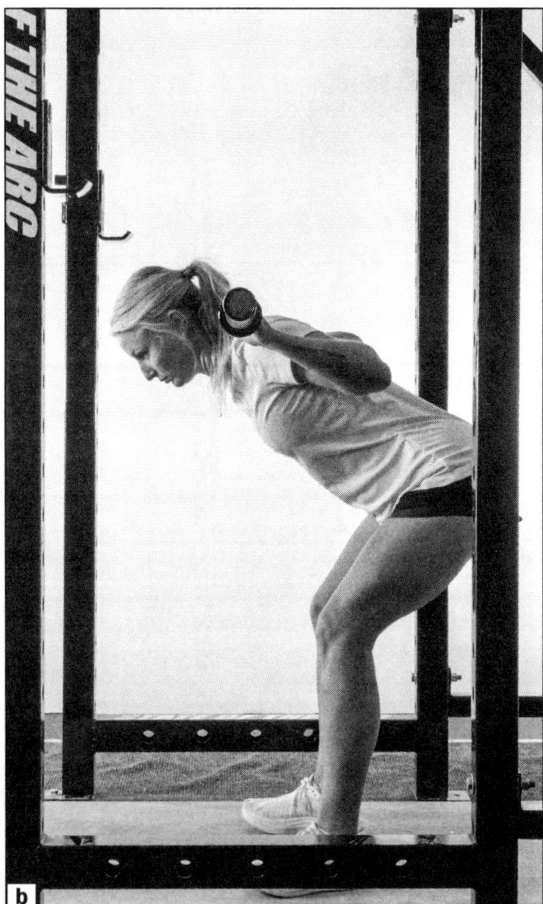

FIGURE 3.48 Barbell good morning.

Lateral Step Down

Last but not least, the lateral step down is my go-to for people who have knee discomfort, want to work on ankle range of motion, or want a little extra quad work. It's great because it's also massively scalable, from a 2-inch block all the way up to a 24-inch box. The key is control.

For the lateral step down, start by standing tall on a box, block, or step (see figure 3.49*a*). I like to use body weight only for this as a warm-up. It's important that whatever you are standing on is stable, and hold on to something like a pole or rack for balance if needed. This isn't a balance exercise but a way for us to strategically load certain tissues. Bring one leg off to the side, hanging it off the box, and keep the other foot nice and flat throughout the entire movement (see figure 3.49*b*). Slowly lower yourself down by bending the knee of your standing leg until you can touch the heel of the other foot on the ground (see figure 3.49*c*). Keep as much control as possible, sitting the hips back and bending the knee the same way you would in a squat. I want the tempo to be a solid three Mississippi-count seconds on the way down. Tap the heel on the ground and then come back up to the starting position. Eight to ten reps here tend to be enough to get moving.

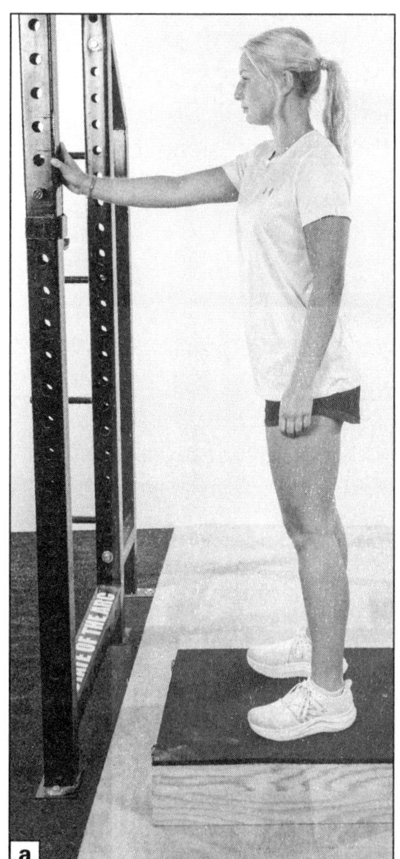

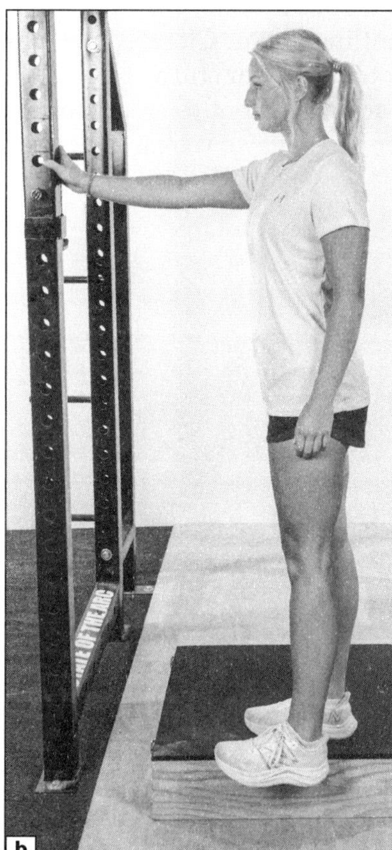

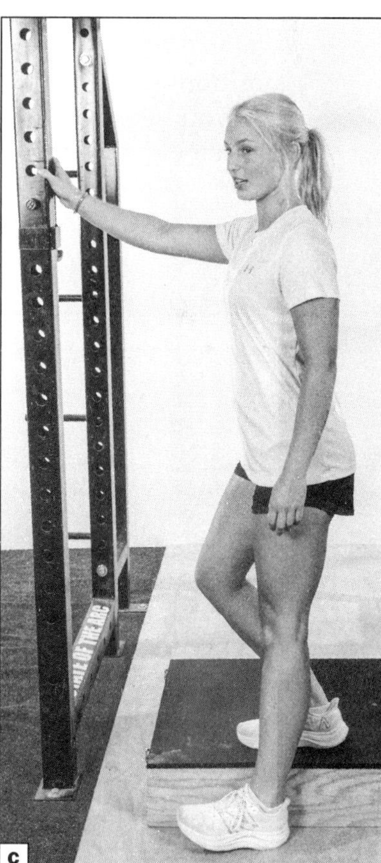

FIGURE 3.49 Lateral step down.

Remember the concepts from the warm-up chapter. Each exercise that we select should address either a physical restriction like range of motion or some form of discomfort. There are more exercises than the five I have introduced here, and you are more than welcome to try any of them. In reference to these five though, here's what each of them can help address.

- *Half-kneeling wall circle:* shoulder or anterior hip tightness
- *Kettlebell sots press:* shoulder or thoracic extension range of motion
- *Cossack squat:* hip range of motion and anterior knee pain
- *Barbell good morning:* lower-back pain and hamstring tightness
- *Lateral step down:* anterior knee pain

Mission complete. You now know everything you need to know to get started squatting effectively and safely. Here is my challenge to you though: Plenty of people can read a book and think they've got it figured out. The difference between thinking you know something and actually knowing it is implementation. Take this knowledge and go apply it. Go to the gym and get under a bar and pay attention to how you are doing that. Design your repeatable setup. Get a few reps in, thinking about each phase of the squat. Film yourself and watch it back. Are you in the positions we outlined here? Close? What's the bar path look like? Are positions slightly different but the bar still a straight line? Yes? Good. No? What can you take from this and implement to create the change you need? Go and implement now, then turn the page so we can talk about the bench press next.

Chapter 4

The Bench Press

For most, the bench press is their first introduction to strength training, and it is by far the most accessible piece of equipment you can find. You may go on vacation and really struggle to find a good squat rack, but every gym in the country has at least one bench press. Because of this, most people think that the bench press is an easy upper-body movement to master. This isn't completely accurate. It could be argued that of all the lifts, the bench press has the smallest margin for error at higher loads. It's the lift with the most abrupt ceiling: You feel like you are on fire in the middle of the set, then you add five pounds (2 kg) and suddenly everything just stops. You try to press the bar up from your chest, and nothing happens.

Another misconception about the bench is that it is only about the upper body. It's true that the primary movers of the lift are the arms and the chest, but this is not an upper-body-only movement. With the squat, you need to create tension in the upper body to keep the bar stable and to be successful. With the bench, the lower body needs to be tight and stable to allow those big prime movers of the arms and the chest to do the most work. If you want a big bench, you have to be able to use your legs.

I don't want to scare you away from this lift; I just want to make it clear that this is the lift that most people overlook, and this is the chapter that many might skip over because they think already know what they're doing. As a coach, I have to do the most correction of bad habits with lifters on the bench press. Take this lift seriously right from the start, and if you've already been benching for a while, jump into this chapter ready to learn and refine. It will pay off with immediate improvement and greater long-term progress.

Reasons Why You Should Bench Press

An old strength coach once told me that the bench press is like the squat but for your upper body. That might sound far-fetched, but it's not completely off base. The bench press is the cornerstone of most upper-body development programs and sports-performance programs, and it is a competition lift in powerlifting. It's also the main lift in the Paralympic Games for weightlifting, and if you have never watched that, it is a truly amazing sight to behold. The fact is, there isn't a pressing movement for the upper body that can progress to the extreme levels of weight that the bench can. It stimulates a massive amount of muscle, it can be built to high loads, and with the right precautions, it can be very safe. There is a reason it is held in such high regard.

What's more, nearly all sports have some level of contact. Football, soccer, MMA, baseball and softball, and volleyball are all sports in which athletes can benefit from improved pressing power. The first three are obvious: blocking in football, contesting and pushing around for the ball in soccer, and throwing a punch in MMA. But the benefits of bench pressing can be seen in the intangibles as well. For my volleyball fans out there, this scenario is for you: Imagine a fast-paced, back-and-forth game of volleyball. Many high-level teams have a defensive specialist called a *libero*, and their job is to dig the ball out when it gets deep in their zone. They're the one who is diving all over the place, getting under the ball just before it hits the ground, and then popping back up just to dive again and dig that ball out. Do you think that athlete can benefit from more pressing power to help them to get off the ground faster? How about more upper-body strength and endurance to be able do it repeatedly over multiple games and then be ready to play again the following week? Or maybe you aren't in this for sports. Well, is being able to get up off the ground important? Is being able to push furniture around the house helpful? There are countless other examples of how building general upper-body strength through the bench press can benefit you in your everyday life.

The bench also offers a unique opportunity for improving body composition by building muscle. You won't become a bodybuilder overnight; it takes decades of hard training to get that big and that jacked, and you have to train specifically for it. What I'm talking about here is gaining enough muscle to change your physique. Every single elite bench presser in the world has jacked shoulders, triceps, and forearms. Muscle takes up space and spreads out all the other tissues around it. The skin and fat tissue gets spread tighter, and your arms end up looking better.

And a final reason why you should bench press is that there is something about being able to bench well that creates a swell of confidence. The bench press is the common measuring stick in every gym in the United States. Whether you are new to it or not, you've probably heard the question "How much you bench?" The bench is the most common piece of equipment, and this is the question that's most commonly asked. I don't think everyone needs external validation to feel good, but when you progress in the bench, everyone sees it. Whereas the squat and the deadlift may not be performed by every gym-goer, most have a frame of reference for the bench, and they understand the work you are putting in to make it better. On top of that, there is something about having that bar in your hands and just punching it off your chest that makes you feel like a rocket ship.

Elements of the Bench Press

In this section we are going to cover the key elements of the bench press, including the phases of the bench press, what the positions are and how to get into them, and how to perform the barbell bench press. These concepts build on one another, just like with squat, and you can build an exceptional bench press once you understand and master them.

As with the squat, there is no perfect bench press. But there are some universal guidelines, which we will cover here. It bears repeating, though, that just like with the squat, your bench is going to look like *your* bench. We need to nail the basics, but there will always be things unique to you in there. On top of that, benches come in a wide array of quality. Some are rock solid, and some are as slick as a Slip 'N Slide. The fundamentals will still apply, but there may be limitations to some of them based on what you are training on. That's okay. There are ways around some issues, and there are others you'll have to live with. But none of them are deal-breakers for performance.

Bar-Lifter Unit

The first concept we need to cover is the bar-lifter unit. For the bench, this will be created once the bar is in your hands and out of the rack, and you are in the start position. Unlike the squat, the bar will be doing most of the movement during the bench press, and because you're lying down on the bench, the center of gravity doesn't involve your whole body. The bar-lifter unit becomes the combined mass of the bar and the weights as well as your hands, wrists, and arms down to your shoulders. This puts the center of gravity directly under the bar and over your shoulders in the start position. This will change based on the individual anatomy of the elbow and the technique of the press, which is where bar path comes into play.

Bar Path

Bar path is a hotly debated topic in the powerlifting world. What is the ideal bar path in the bench press? Is it a straight line up and down? Or does it present more like an angle as the bar comes down to the chest and then back up toward the face? At this point, I have seen enough evidence from both sides of the argument to say that it depends and that neither side is wrong. Whether the bar has some horizontal movement or not, the goal is to move it in a straight line from point A to point B. But it should never be pushed down toward the feet. As soon as that happens you lose leverage and are in a position that is difficult to press from. From my perspective, there are two acceptable bar paths: completely vertical (see figure 4.1) or vertical and slightly back (see figure 4.2).

Bar Positioning

The bar will be doing most of the movement during the bench press, and the center of gravity doesn't involve the whole body, but that doesn't mean that the bar position through the lift doesn't matter. To create the vertical or vertical-but-slightly-back bar path, the bar, the wrists, and the elbows all have to stay in alignment. What we are looking for here is for the barbell to stay directly over the wrists and elbows through the entire bench-press movement (see figure 4.3).

When looking at this for yourself, you'll see there are three possible positions: the bar stacked over the elbows, the bar in front of the elbows, and the bar behind the elbows. Imagine dropping a line straight down from the barbell. If that line drops down directly to over the elbows, you are in a great spot. If that line drops down to between the elbows and the shoulders, then the elbows are *in front* of the barbell (see figure 4.4*a*). If the line drops down to where the elbows are between it and your shoulders, then the elbows are *behind* the barbell (see figure 4.4*b*). To

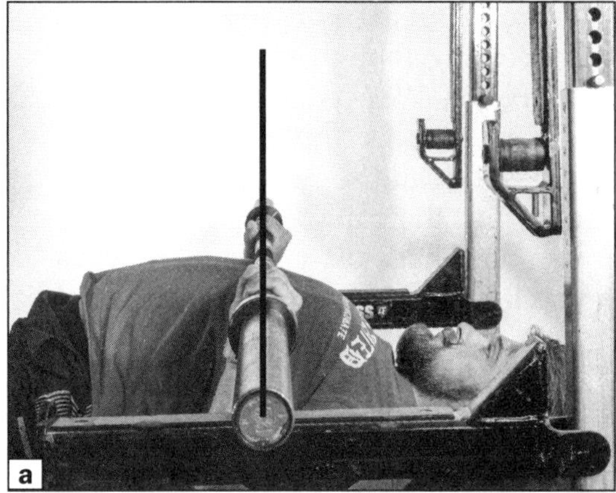

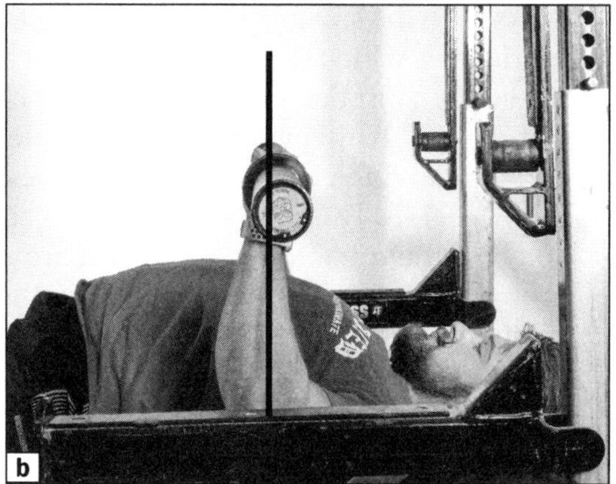

FIGURE 4.1 Vertical bar path in the bench press.

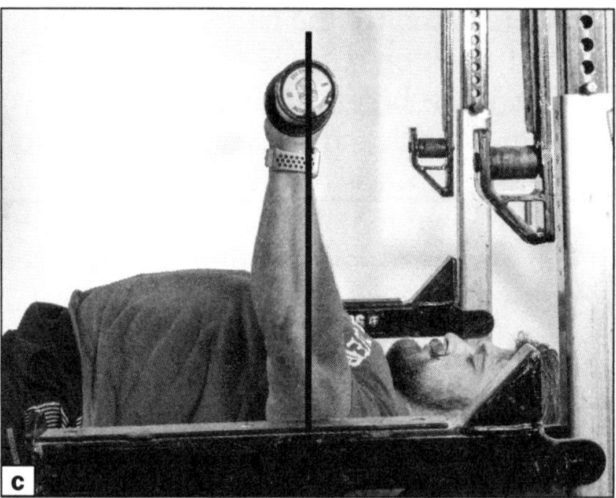

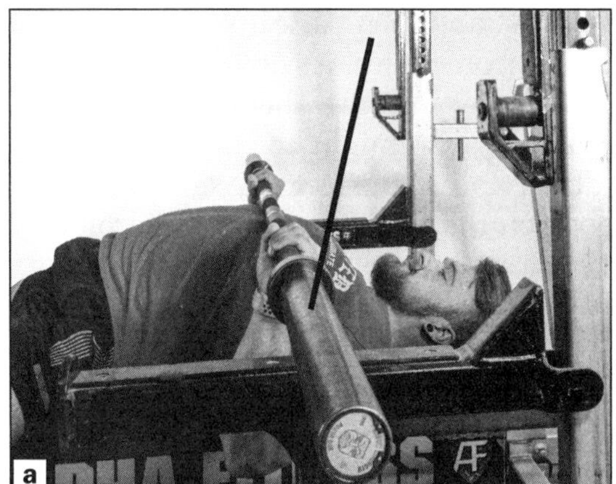

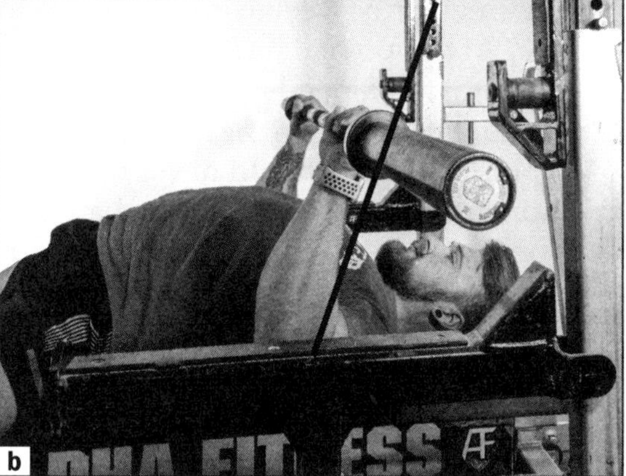

FIGURE 4.2 Vertical and back bar path in the bench press.

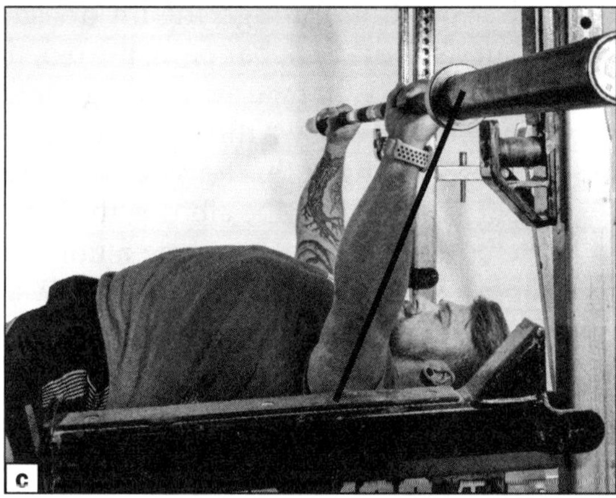

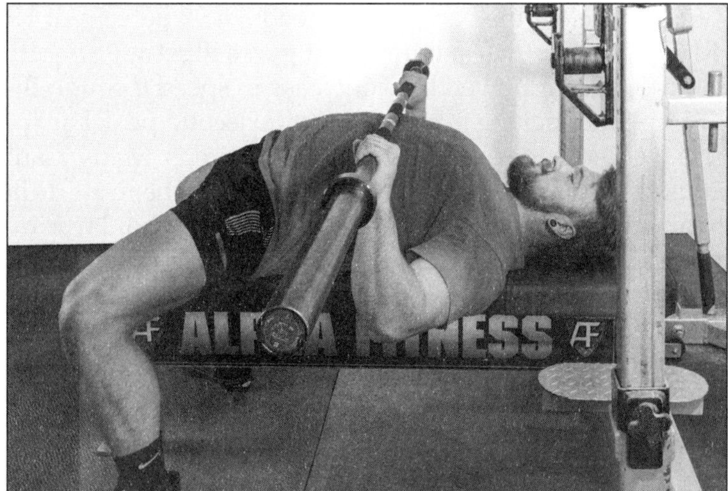

FIGURE 4.3 Barbell, wrist, and elbow alignment at the bottom of the bench press.

be clear, it is possible to press in both of these positions, but it is not the optimal position, and it will eventually limit progress toward achieving your bench-press goals. Keep that in mind as you start learning this movement, and try to keep the development of bad habits to a minimum.

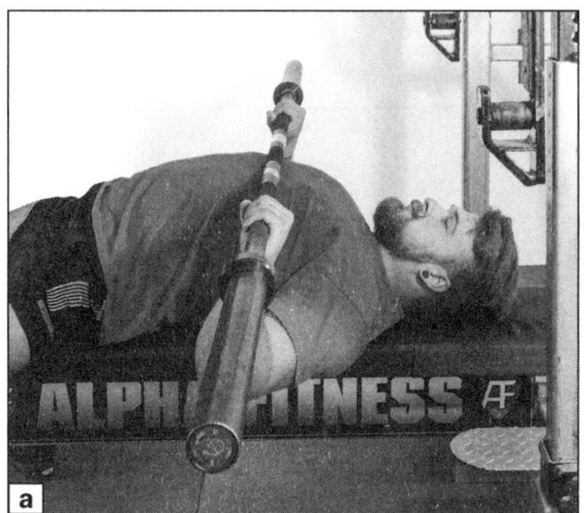

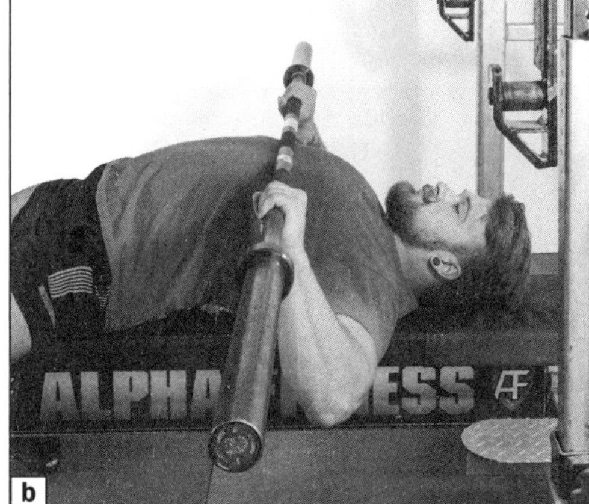

FIGURE 4.4 The elbows positioned *(a)* in front and *(b)* behind the barbell.

Bar Speed

Every lift has a sticking point, and the bench press is no different. Understanding the sticking points for each lift is a valuable tool for understanding how your training is going. If you are running into typical sticking points and the bar speed is dropping off in an expected way, there is no need to panic and change everything. If you are getting stuck in other positions, then that is a sign to take a deeper look into your training and technique.

For the bench press, the common sticking point is halfway up. This is where you will see a pronounced decrease in bar speed, especially at loads over 90 percent of your 1RM. You can see this in figure 4.5. Figure 4.5*a* and 4.5*b* show the bar speed at loads of 70 percent of 1RM and 80 percent of 1RM, respectively.

Figures 4.5*c* and 4.5*d* show the bar speed at loads of 90 percent of 1RM and 100 percent of 1RM, respectively. The latter two figures illustrate an initial peak bar speed right off the chest, followed by a decrease in speed through the middle of the lift and through the sticking point, and then a second peak bar speed toward lock-out where we find better leverages with the triceps. Many assume that the sticking point is right off the chest since this feels like the most difficult part of the press when you are first starting out. But this doesn't hold true over the long term. The pecs and anterior deltoids increase in strength rather quickly to create more speed off the chest, and that will help to drive the bar through the sticking point that occurs halfway up.

A great rule of thumb when evaluating your own bench press and looking at bar speed during the lift is that if you miss the lift right off the chest, the weight is too heavy by a large margin. If the bar slows down and gets stuck right at the midway point, the bar is still too heavy, but you're much closer to a complete rep, and it will be a good rep with more training.

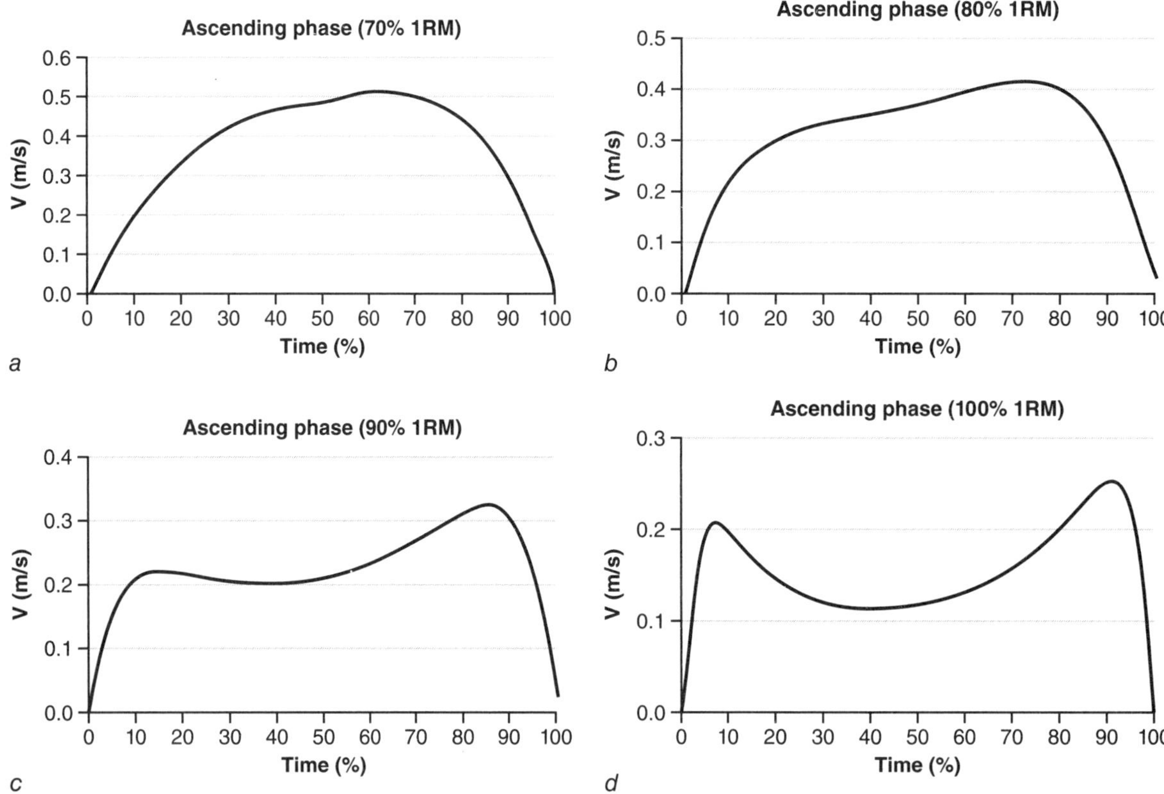

FIGURE 4.5 Bar-speed differences can be noted as the weight gets heavier. Even around 80 percent of 1RM you can start to see two peak velocities appear.

The Phases of the Bench Press

Similar to the squat, the bench press is broken down into four distinct phases: the start position, the descent, at the chest, and the ascent. Each phase sets the next one up for success. Let's start with how to get set up and get into the start position.

Start Position

This is where the bench press is going to start. Setting a good foundation for the bench and mastering the start position is paramount for success with this lift. This start position is something we want to make repeatable and predictable so that the rest of the bench press can be as well. We will dive into that here.

Set Up the Bar

The first thing you need to do to set up for the bench press is to get the bar at the proper height. Some benches may have only two options, and others may have a lot of options (see figure 4.6). It's always great to have flexibility in the bench setup, but not all benches are created equal, and I'd rather you be prepared.

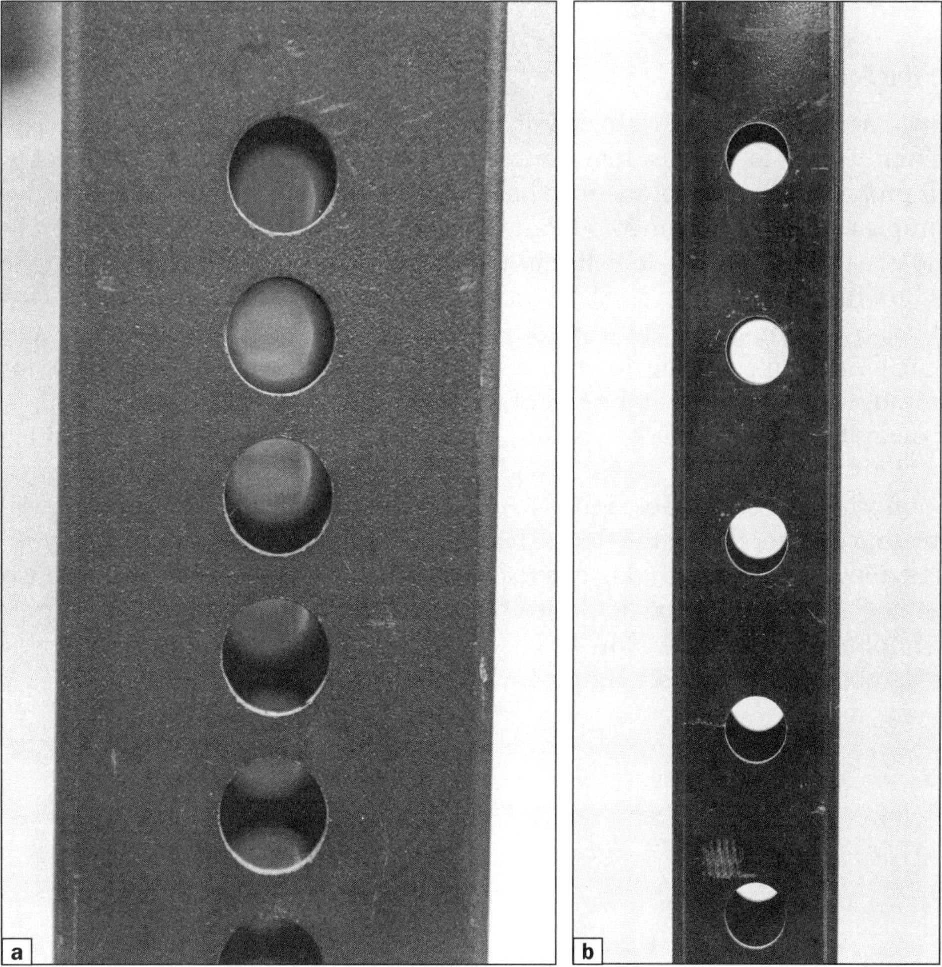

FIGURE 4.6 Two common rack types: *(a)* Westside and *(b)* two-option.

Start by lying on the bench and finding the bar height at which your elbows are slightly bent. You don't want fully locked-out elbows at the start, because you won't be able to get the bar out of the hooks. You also don't want to have to do a half rep to get the bar out, because that's just a waste of energy. The bar should be just high enough that when you grab it and extend your arms, you have one to two inches of clearance between the bar and the hooks so that you can cleanly unrack it.

Note that the bar height isn't the only important height to find. If you are using a full power rack, there should be bars, pins, or big heavy-looking platform arms that you can set up to catch the bar if you miss a lift and the bar comes crashing down. We want these safeties set up just under where the bar is when you are in the bottom position of the lift. For a squat, that's one or two pin holes down from where the bar is when you are all the way in the bottom. For the bench, it's one or two holes down from where the bar is at your chest. The safeties should be low enough to catch the bar if you were to relax underneath it but high enough that the bar doesn't smack into the safeties when you are at the bottom. Set these up *every single time.* Lifting is a safe activity, but things can happen. You can lose your balance, you can get distracted, you can misload a plate, or any number of other things can occur. Be prepared, and set this up so you can walk away from those mishaps to train another day.

Set the Feet

Now that the bar is at the right height, it's time to get into the start position. There are many ways to get this done, and if you ever watch a powerlifting meet you will probably see most of them. What I want to do here is get you started with a simple and repeatable method that will put you at a solid starting point. Over time you can change this to better fit your needs, but I recommend learning this method first.

Start by sitting about halfway to two-thirds of the way down the bench (see figure 4.7*a*). Don't even lie down yet. The first thing is to set is the feet. You don't want to start all the way at the end of the bench, because that will set you up too far away from the bar. Once you are sitting on the bench, place your feet at or just slightly wider than shoulder width apart, with the feet angled outward in a comfortable position (see figure 4.7*b*). For most, that's 10 to 30 degrees. Make sure your feet are flat on the floor. Then, without lifting your legs, I want you to think about doing a slight leg extension as if you were using the leg-extension machine at the gym. You should feel your quads flex and your feet get tight to the floor (see figure 4.7*c*). Now lie back, and be mindful to not hit your head on the barbell behind you (see figure 4.7*d*).

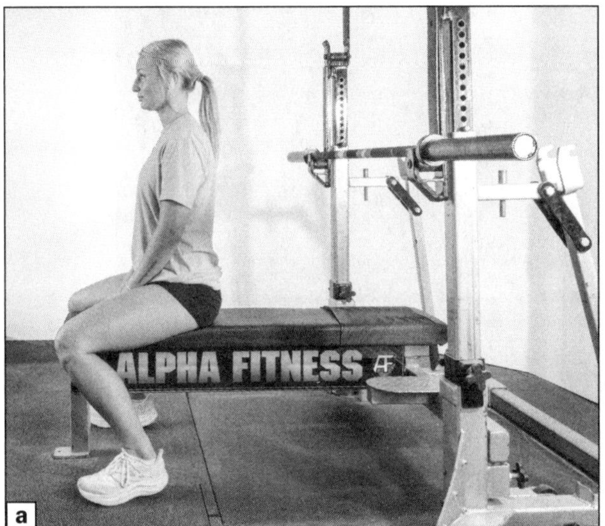

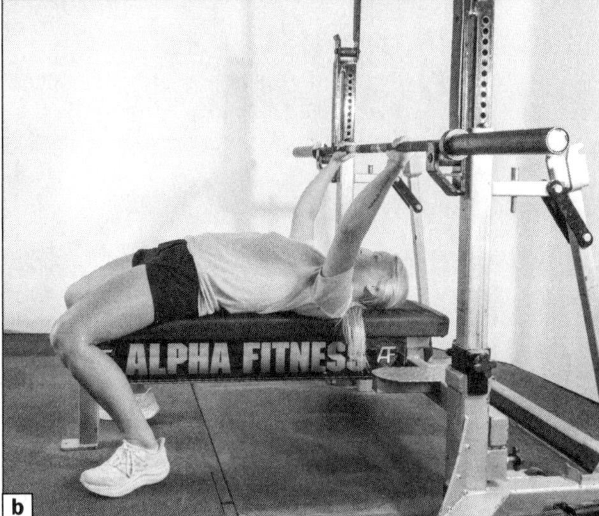

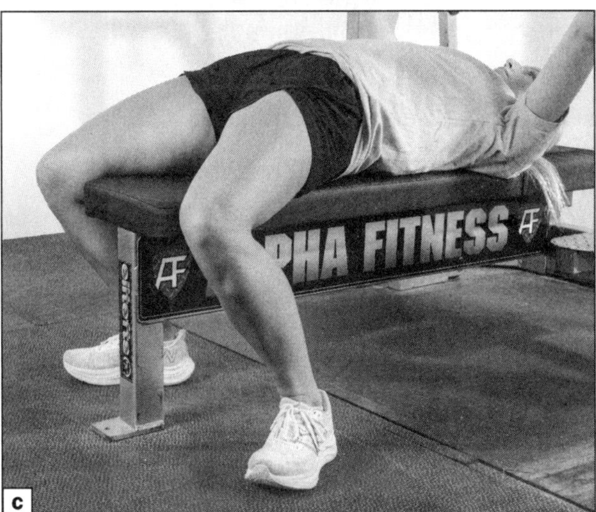

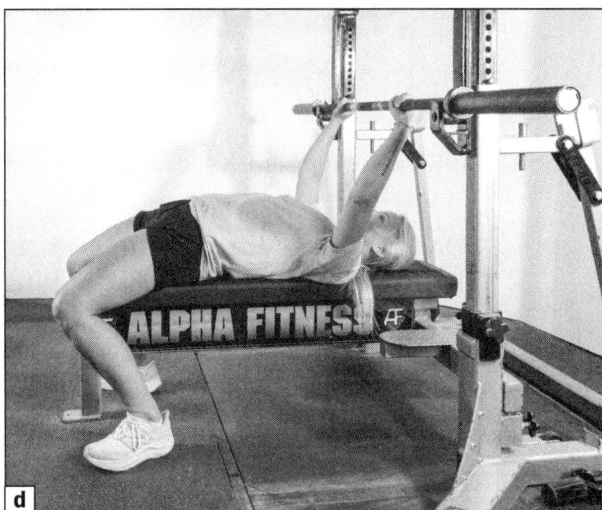

FIGURE 4.7 These are good examples of where to sit on the bench, where to place your feet, the foot angle to use, and how to create drive with the feet into the floor when setting up for the bench press. This may vary slightly depending on your height, but these are good starting points for most.

Position the Hands

Now that the feet are set and you are lying down, continue with the leg extension and position your hands on the bar. We are going to use the same landmarks on the bar that we used with the squat. That first ring, or the power ring, is going to be your frame of reference here. Grab the bar so that your pinky is right on that ring. You want your grip on the barbell to be deep in your hands so the bar is closer to your wrists than your knuckles (see figure 4.8). This grip will make it easier to keep the wrists stacked during the lift. More on that later.

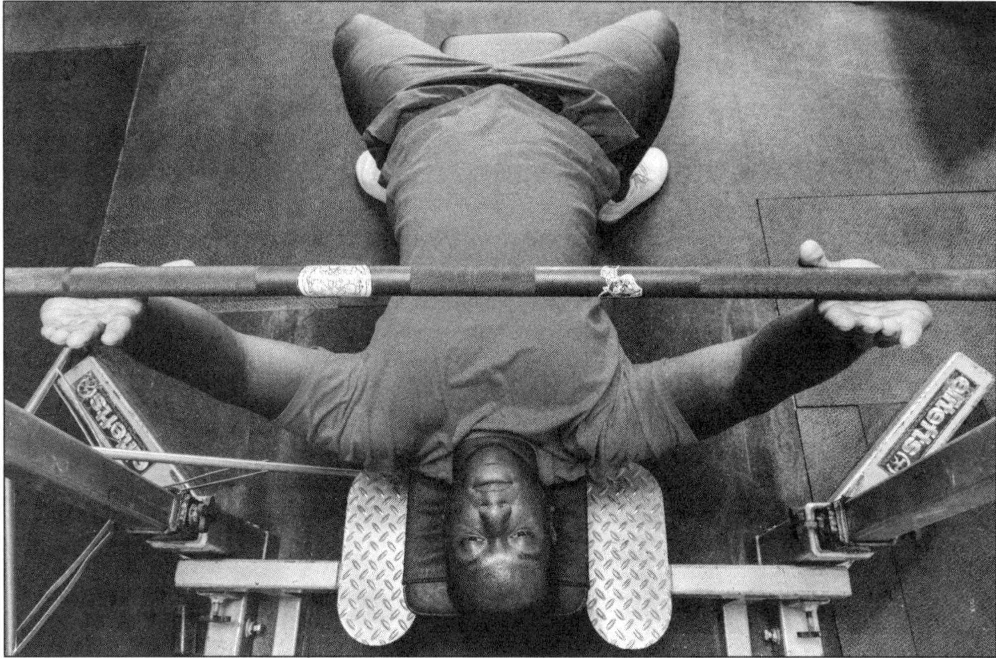

FIGURE 4.8 The barbell should sit deep in the hands when setting up for the bench press.

Once you have that grip in position, the next step is to tighten that grip as much as possible. Think about crushing the bar and pulling it apart at the same time (see figure 4.9). You should feel your forearms, shoulders, and upper back get tight at this point, all while you continue the slight leg extension. That's what we want as we build tension from here.

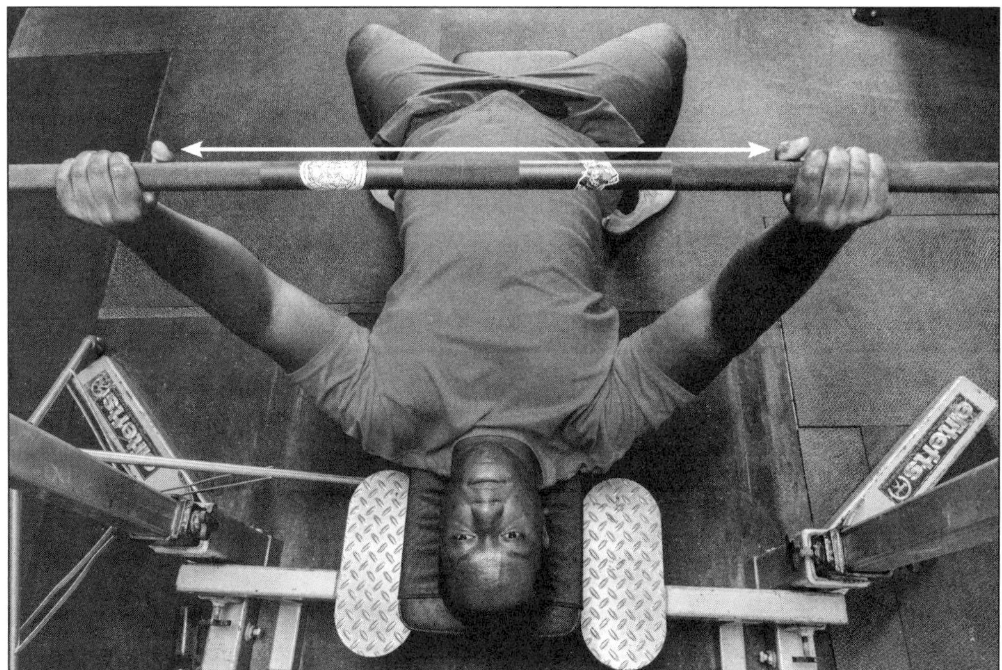

FIGURE 4.9 Pulling the bar apart creates more tension and will set up the rest of the bench press to keep better positions.

Get Under the Bar

Finally, you need to get your entire body under the bar and into the right position. Depending on how tall you are and how long your torso is, the bar may be anywhere from just above your neck to all the way down at your rib cage. To bench well, you should set up with your eyes directly under the bar when you are in the start position. To get there, you are going to keep that tight grip on the bar and do a slight row to lift your upper body off the bench. Then slide down the bench until your eyes are right underneath the bar. As you slide down, you should feel your legs get even tighter as you keep that leg extension into the ground. During this slide down, your hips may come off the bench slightly, and that's fine. Just make sure to get them back down onto the bench once you are fully in position.

Just like with the squat, as you approach getting all the way into the start position, you should try to take your shoulder blades and put them in your back pockets again. Once you are at eye level with the bar, this will drive your upper-back and trapezius muscles directly into the bench. At this point, your feet should still be flat on the ground with the tops of your knees below the top of your hips so that the body is locked in. Your butt should be in contact with the bench, and your shoulder blades should be pushing down into your back pockets. The bar should be at eye level, your head should be flat on the bench, and you should have a firm, deep grip on the bar.

There are two common errors, often seen later in the lift, that begin here with the setup. The first is running the bar into the rack, which happens when your eyes are not under the bar in the setup. Depending on the rack, even just having your chin under the rack can make this happen. To be fair, it's happened to all of us. But it happens more often when you are just starting out if you aren't diligent with the setup. Sometimes you may smack into the rack and power through it, but there are situations where this can become very dangerous.

We've talked about how skill can be limited with newer lifters, and this is the first situation where that can become a safety issue. The disruption of the bar hitting the rack can cause you to lose control of the bar and then get it stuck underneath the J-hook of the bench. If this happens, remember to stay tight, continue to grasp the bar, and drive into the rack until help arrives or you regain control of the bar (see figure 4.10).

The second potentially dangerous situation can happen with racks where the hooks are removed by pushing up on them. It's rare, but I've seen lifters hit these hooks and knock them completely out of the rack. If there are no hooks, there is no place to put the bar back. Yeah, I know. That's a scary situation. Eliminate risk by being deliberate with your setup, and if you are on a rack that is new to you, use your warm-up sets to make the needed adjustments to find your spot.

Another error that happens during the press is the hips rising off the bench and the feet moving. This is so common that it's comical. Two of the most prominent rules in powerlifting for the bench press are that the hips are not permitted to leave the bench and that the feet are not permitted to lift off the floor or slide while completing the lift. Here's the deal though: These errors are due to a lack of tension in the setup. The setup is the foundation for the lift. If you build your bench on a shaky foundation, something is going to move that isn't supposed to.

If I am working with a lifter who is experiencing either of these issues, we go back to drilling the setup and making sure each step is completed with maximal tension. If you are a beginner, this is going to happen more often as you learn

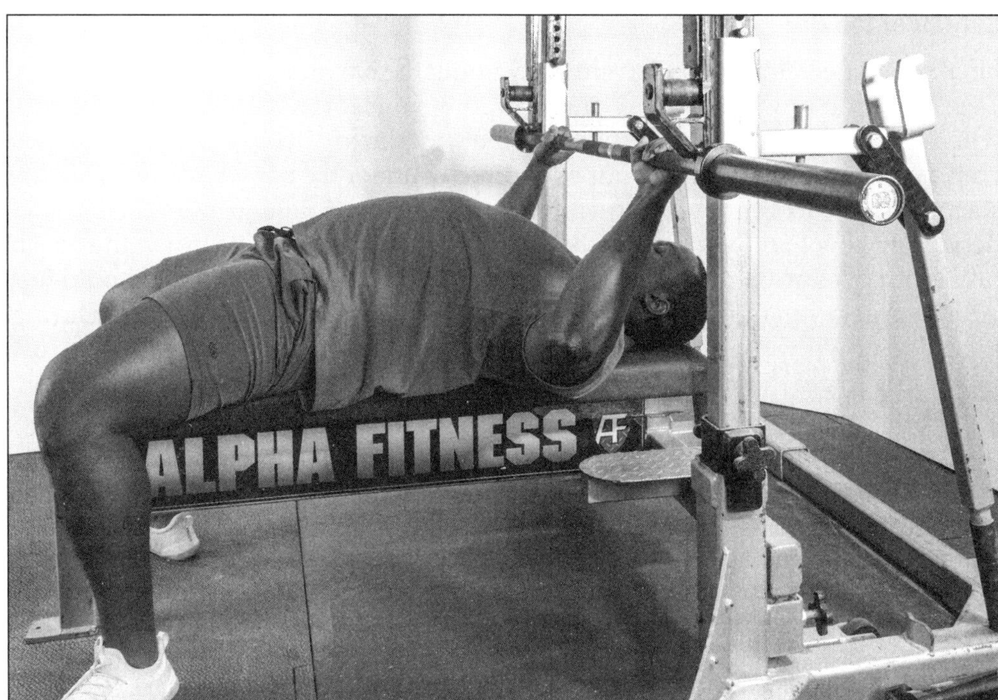

FIGURE 4.10 Example of what it looks like to have the bar stuck and wedged under a J-hook. In this situation, keep driving the bar into the hook, and start asking for help to get it unstuck and back in the rack.

and build your capacity to get tight. As you progress, you will get more and more comfortable with higher levels of tension in the setup, which will eliminate these errors.

Unrack the Bar

Now it's time to unrack the bar. If there is one error I see most often with beginning lifters, it's getting a great tight setup, as shown in figure 4.11, and then throwing it away when they unrack the bar. Whatever you do, keep that tension like it's a winning lottery ticket!

There are two ways to unrack the bar: by yourself or with a spotter. I always suggest using a spotter because it helps the unrack immensely while also keeping you safer. I know many people are nervous to ask for a spot. Many think that having a spotter means they are not doing as much work and are possibly missing out on gains. This couldn't be further from the truth. The unrack of a heavy bar in the bench press has no physical benefit. There is no hypertrophy or strength gain from it. It's simply an expenditure of energy that could have gone into the set itself. Anecdotally speaking, I have seen lifters get an extra rep in every set of a session simply by having a good spotter to hand the bar off to. One extra rep in every set, over multiple sessions, *adds up.* That spotter saves you energy and can also help you stay in position so that each setup prepares you for success. If you aren't sure how to ask for a spotter, check out the Working With a Spotter sidebar.

To Arch or Not to Arch?

A hotly debated topic with the bench press is the arch that some lifters set up with. My take is that it is within the rules of the sport of powerlifting to do this, so it's fine. What really bothers me is when people claim it will lead to higher injury rates. At this point, we have covered the SAID principle, and you know that the body will adapt to the load and stress put on it. There is no need to recap that point, but there are a few other factors that I want to touch on here.

The argument could be made that the spine's ability to support load is not optimal in full extension (i.e., an arched back). The problem is that the models that suggest that are based on axial loading, or the load pushing down on the spine vertically from the head like you would see in a standing position (Tungate 2019). That's not the case here where the lifter is lying down and the load is being applied horizontally. Additionally, from a physics and engineering standpoint, the shape of an arch is a massively stable structure to handle loads of this type and in this direction. Mimicking that shape to execute the lift should create greater stability and even protect against injury. The arch isn't inherently dangerous, so don't be afraid to utilize it in the bench.

So should you arch in the bench press? Ultimately, it's about your particular goals as a lifter. If you want a bigger chest, then going through a full stretch of the pecs at the bottom of the bench press is going to be more optimal for hypertrophy, so a less aggressive arch can be used here (Cudlip et al. 2022). That doesn't mean there is no arch, but it's just the natural one that presents with a good setup.

In the context of competitive powerlifting, optimizing the arch and maximizing the extent of the arch provide a competitive advantage and should absolutely be trained in those athletes. If you aren't going to compete, then working on creating a massive arch in the bench press is unnecessary. However, I would still encourage the natural arch that results from creating tension and stability through the entire body.

With or without a spotter, there are two simple phases to the unrack. Phase one is driving the bar straight up by extending your arms and stopping at the top for a second with your elbows locked out (see figure 4.12). Your shoulders should not move, and your legs should not relax. A spotter can help significantly in this phase by lifting the bar just enough to make this part really easy. They shouldn't do all of the work—just enough to get the bar moving upward in a controlled manner. You now have the bar high enough to move it out of the hooks, which is phase two. You are going to pull the bar out of the rack to where it is directly over your shoulder joints (see figure 4.13). I like to think of this movement as being like pulling an open window in your house down. The arms stay straight and pull the bar into position. This pulling movement is how you maintain tension in the setup because it won't allow the shoulders, lats, and upper back to relax. This is the start position, and you should feel locked in at this point.

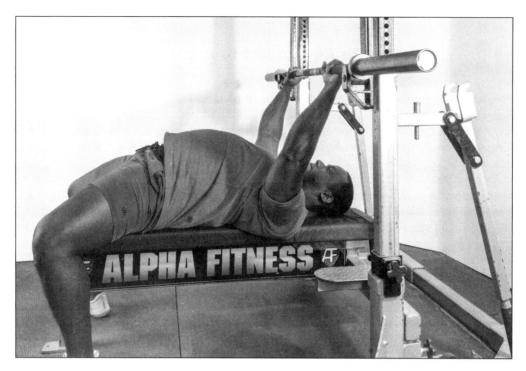

FIGURE 4.11 Start position of the bench press with the bar still loaded in the rack. Notice the feet haven't moved from where we initially put them, and note the amount of tension built in the setup.

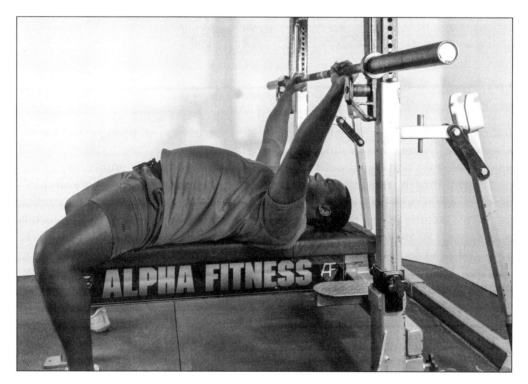

FIGURE 4.12 Bar out of the rack with elbows extended. Bar still over the hooks.

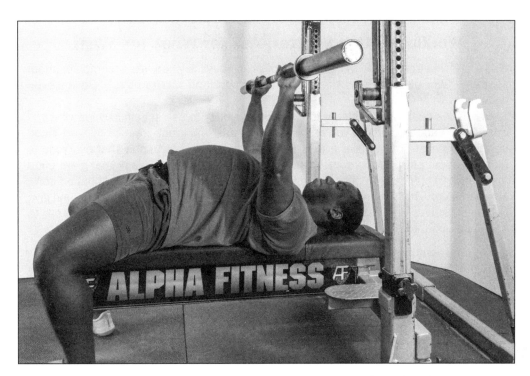

FIGURE 4.13 Bar pulled out and directly over the shoulders of the lifter. This is the start position to be ready to press.

The Descent

Now we get the bar moving. The descent of the bench press truly is the setup for the rest of the lift, and losing position here can lead to issues further down the line. The elbows should stay stacked under the wrists, and the wrists should stay stacked under the hands all the way down to the chest (see figure 4.14). This will lead to a straighter bar path and to more consistent touch points on your chest. From your tight starting position, bend your elbows while envisioning pulling the bar to your chest. This will help you keep your elbows stacked where we want them instead of tucking them too tight to the body or flaring them out too much. This pulling of the bar will also allow you to maintain more control over it. Going a step further, I also ask the lifters I work with to think about trying to pull their chest to the bar to meet it at the same time. This helps to keep their tension high.

Throughout the descent, your wrists should stay stacked in a strong neutral position under your hands. Not everyone will be able to maintain this position when first starting out, but it's the intent that matters the most here. I like to think of punching the ceiling or keeping my knuckles up. You should attempt, as best you can, to keep your wrists in this position instead of letting them passively bend backward (see figure 4.15). This passive position lacks the tension you need and can lead the bar moving out of position when you go to pause or press the weight, increasing the overall difficulty of the lift. As time goes on, you will get stronger and be able to handle heavier weights with your wrists stacked.

Working With a Spotter: Ask for What You Want

I have a few pet peeves in the gym. One of my biggest is when lifters complain about spotters. "Why did you touch the bar?" "Ugh, that lift-off was terrible." "Do you even know what you are doing?"

Here's the deal. As the lifter, it is your responsibility to ask specifically for what you want from a spotter. Even if you are brand new, this is a great practice to start incorporating because it will make everyone at the gym love you. I know that everyone is nervous about asking for a spot. I can assure you that when you ask that giant dude at the gym to help you out, the first thing that runs through his mind is "I hope I don't screw this up." That's human nature. So do yourself and everyone else a favor and give clear instructions on what you want. Here are some good examples of what to say to someone about to spot you so they are prepared:

1. "Start out by giving me enough space to set up."
2. "This is how and where I want your hands to be."
3. "This is the count I'm going to use to signal you to start helping me." (For example, "three, two, one," or "one, two, three," or "ready, set, go.")
4. "Give me just enough help to get my arms straight, and I'll start pulling the bar over my chest. Help me. Don't resist me."
5. "This is how many reps I have in the set."
6. "This is the safe word." (For example, "take it," "nope," or even "banana.")
7. "If I need help, don't snatch the bar. Give me enough help to get the bar moving again and stay with me."
8. "Thank you."

Here is exactly what I say to people in the gym, including the jokes I use (because I like to keep it light). I know it seems like a lot, but this little 30-second exchange can keep you healthy, lead to bigger lifts, and make you popular at the gym. Let's take a look:

> Okay. So first thing: Give me some space as I set up, because I bring my head all the way up to where you will eventually be standing. We want to avoid that awkward moment. Once I'm all set, I will tell you I'm ready out loud. My grip isn't super wide, but I'm most comfortable when you have your hands inside mine on the bar with an alternating grip. Plus, that will make you feel more comfortable lifting it out. Once you're set and comfortable, I will count down from "three," and we will lift on "one." So I'll say, "three, two, one," and I'll start on "one." All I need is a little help, like you're picking up a set of 20-pound dumbbells. Just enough so I can get my elbows locked. Once we are there, I will start to pull the bar over me. You can keep your hands on the bar, and it will feel like I'm trying to pull it away from you. Don't resist that. Just let it happen. Once I'm ready, I'll say "good," and then you can let go of the bar. I've got 5 reps to do here and I should be good, but if I need help I will specifically say "take it," and that's your cue to jump in and help out. Again, I only need enough help to keep the bar moving and to get it back to the rack. Any questions? I really appreciate you helping me out and keeping me safe.

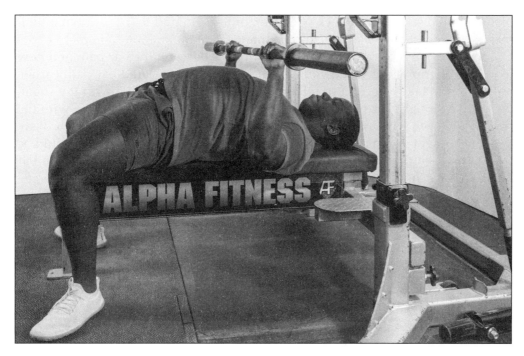

FIGURE 4.14 Proper vertical alignment of the elbows, wrists, and barbell in the descent of the bench press.

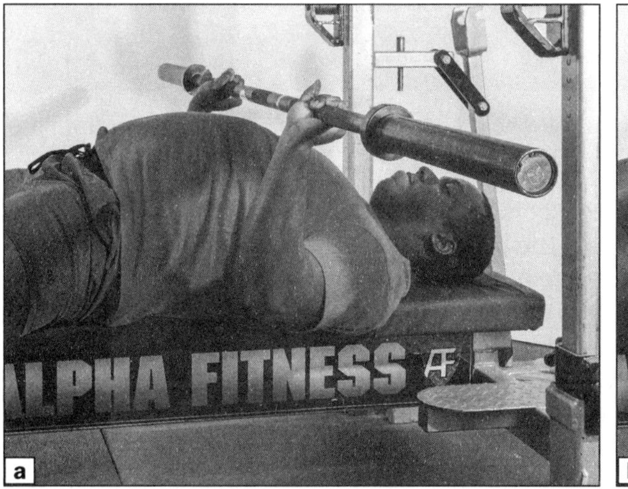

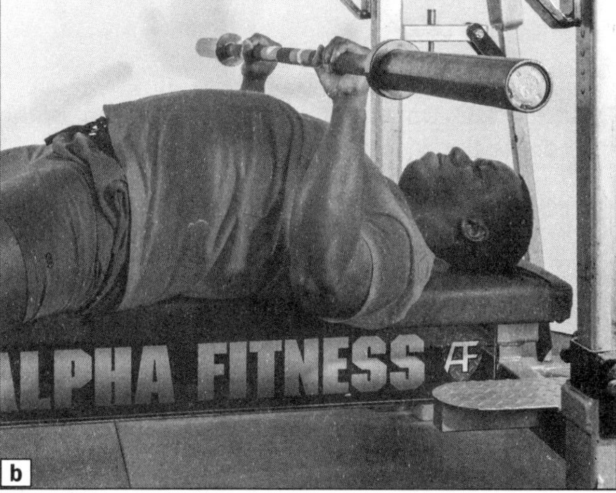

FIGURE 4.15 *(a)* Passive wrist extension can cause the bar to lose position. *(b)* A more optimal stacked-wrist position locks the bar into place.

So what is with all this stacking? Does this sound different from the squat? That's because it is. All lifts are about leverage, but the decreased range of motion and the lower margin for error on the bench make small position changes important. If the wrists break backward too much, the bar slots back toward the shoulders a bit more. If the elbows flare too much, the touch point can be too high. Stack the wrists and elbows for consistency, power, and leverage. And keep the rest of the body as tight as possible. The legs should continue to drive into that leg extension, the butt and head should remain on the bench, and the shoulder blades should stay in your back pockets. Continue to pull that bar down until it meets your chest just below the nipple line.

There are two more details to cover about the descent: the bar path and how to optimize grip width when you are starting out. We covered bar path earlier, but I want to take a second to reiterate here. In the bench, like with the squat, we want a straight bar path as it approaches the chest. The difference with the bench, however, is that it will be a straight line that is at an angle. If the bar were to come straight down from above the shoulder joint, the touch point would be far too high on the chest, compromising power and stability. Instead, the bar needs to travel horizontally on the descent so that it can touch the chest between the bottom of the sternum and the nipple line (see figure 4.16).

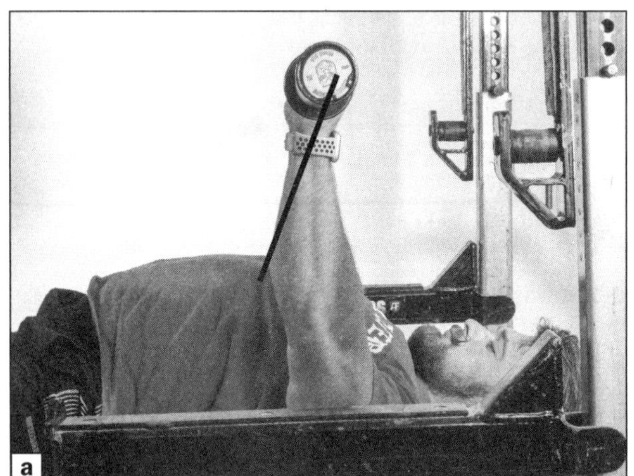

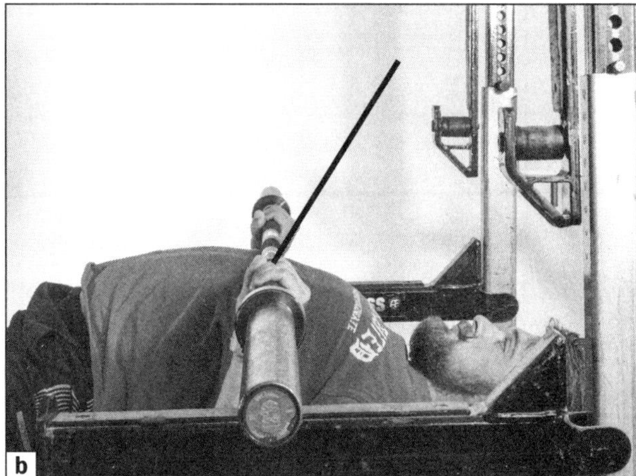

FIGURE 4.16 Optimal bar path in the descent of the bench should be a straight line angled down from the shoulder to the chest.

Lastly, how do you optimize your grip in the bench press as a beginner? Earlier in the chapter, I recommended placing the hands on the bar with the pinkies on the rings. This is a great starting position for most lifters. What if we want to dial this in more? That's when we start to look at where the elbows are when the bar is at the chest. When you're in this position, the elbows should be bent at 90 degrees and be aligned with the top of the bench pad (see figure 4.17). If the elbow angle is more acute than that, or if the elbows drop to below the top level of the pad, you can widen your grip one finger width at a time until you get into the correct position at the chest. Doing this can help you find your optimal grip width on the bench quickly and easily. Just remember to use the rings as a frame of reference for where your hand is for that grip. For example, for the longest time, my grip was with my ring finger on the ring. Find yours and remember it.

A common error that plagues the descent of a bench press is an inconsistent touch point. An inconsistent touch point can kill a bench-press set and your progress. For example, I have worked with an athlete who couldn't hit the same touch point in any rep of a 10-rep set. The bar was all over the place and, as you would expect, so was her performance. When the bar doesn't hit the same touch point each time, the descent is inconsistent and the jump-off point of the bar changes

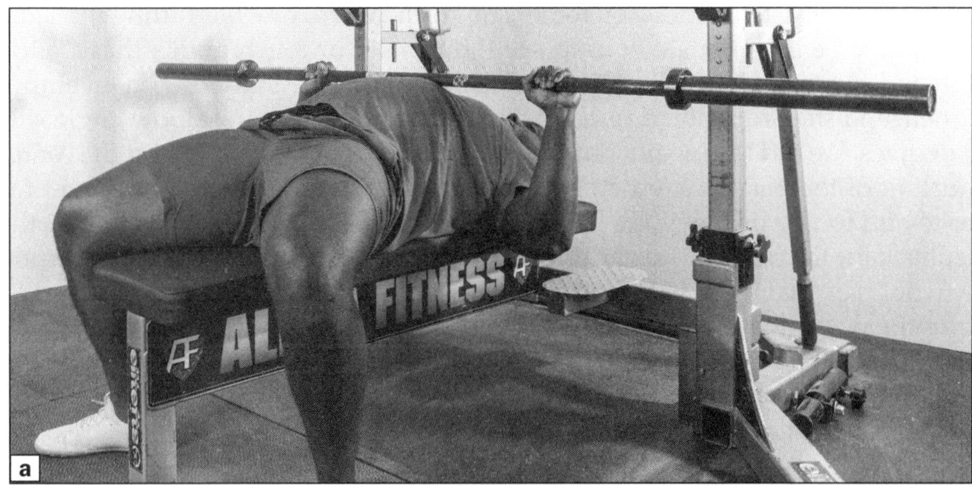

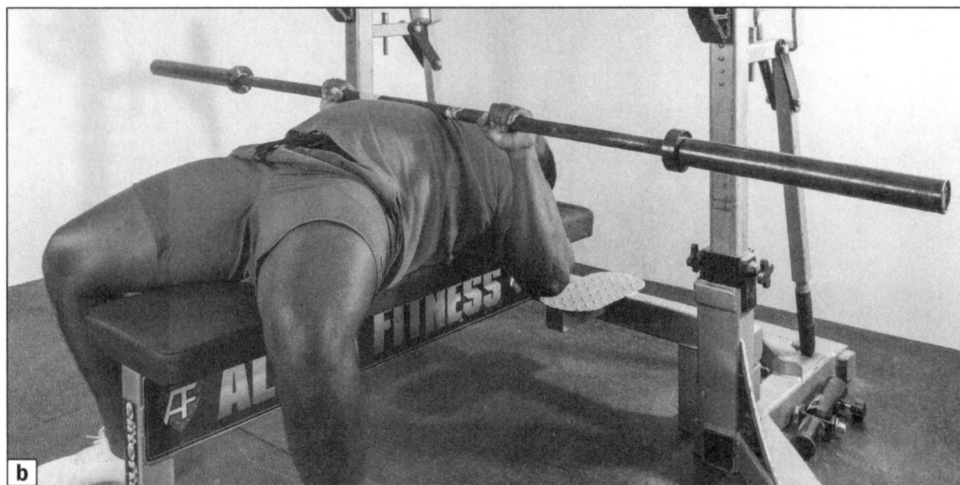

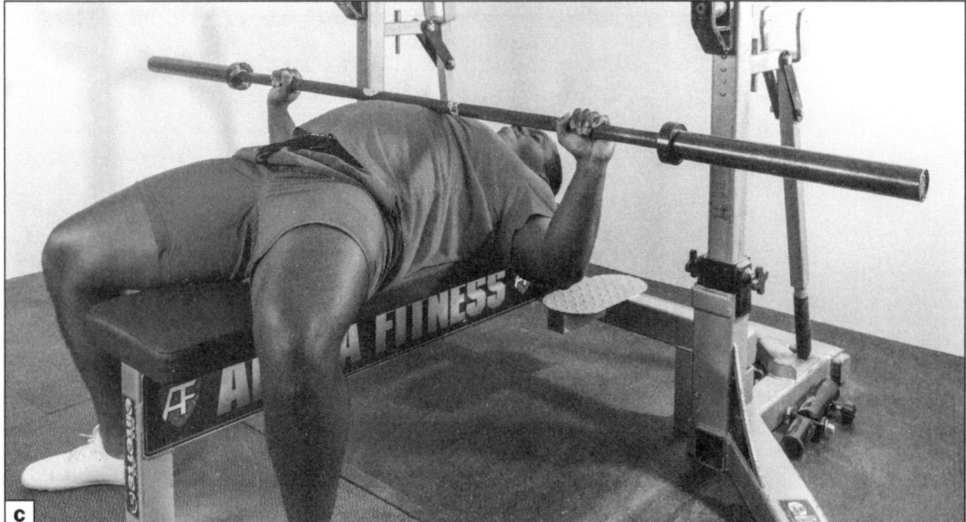

FIGURE 4.17 *(a)* Optimal grip-width starting point, with elbow angle at 90 degrees. Improper elbow angles: *(b)* less than 90 degrees, where the grip is too narrow, and *(c)* greater than 90 degrees, where the grip is too wide.

too often to consistently develop force. The key here is to practice hitting the same spot and to be intentional about it (see figure 4.18 for touch points that are too high and too low versus an optimal touch point). So we started with an empty barbell, and she brought it down to her chest, making sure the elbow angle was 90 degrees. We did that again, but this time we put a block of chalk on the center knurling of the bar. This left a chalk mark on her shirt, providing a target for her to aim for. By bringing the bar to that spot a few times, she got some tactile feedback for that spot. It was not my intent to have her look at the mark during the whole set; that would have thrown her completely out of position. However, it provided a visible frame of reference. She, or anyone working with her, could see whether she was hitting the chalk. After we did this, her maximum weight went from 165 pounds (73 kg) to 205 pounds (93 kg) in less than four weeks. Be consistent with the touch point.

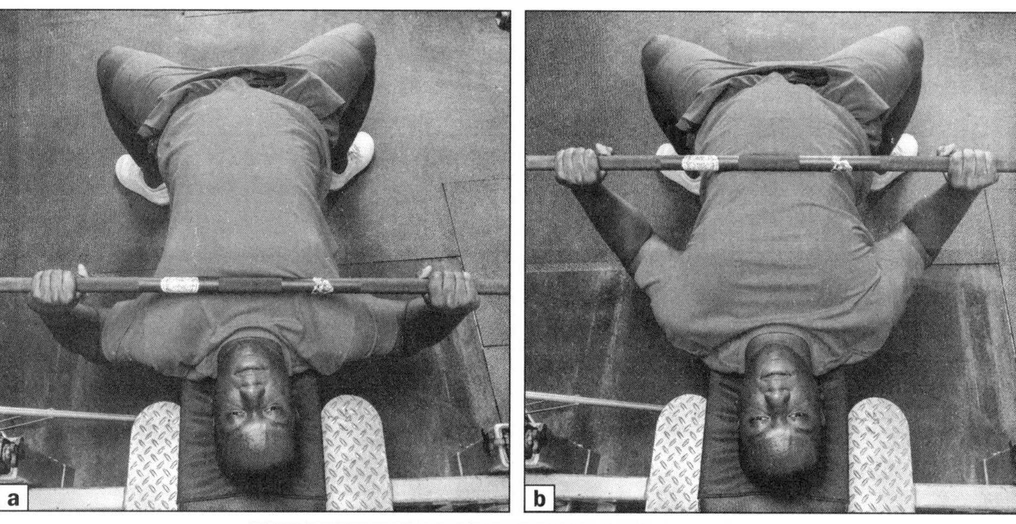

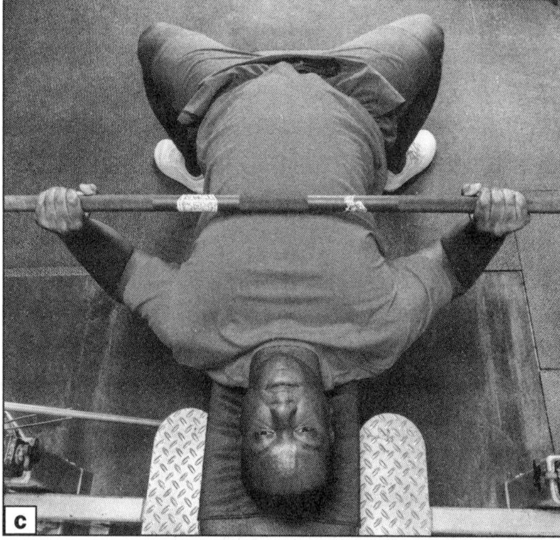

FIGURE 4.18 Touch point in the descent: *(a)* too high, with the elbow angle at less than 90 degrees; *(b)* too low, with the elbow angle greater than 90 degrees; versus *(c)* an optimal touch point for this athlete, with the elbow at 90 degrees.

At the Chest

This section is brief because very little movement happens when the bar is at the chest. However, this is the place where many lifters throw everything away. You are loading yourself like a spring during the whole descent. You are a bomb waiting to go off. You don't want to collapse, pour water on the fuse, and fizzle out right at the chest. The key is that you *must* stay tight here (see figure 4.19 for a comparison of proper tension and loss of tension). It will feel uncomfortable. It will feel like a lot of pressure. But that discomfort and pressure are what's going to help you lift the bar through the ceiling above you in the next phase: the ascent. Your grip should remain tight, and the bar should be at your chest. You don't want it hovering above you, and you don't want it sinking all of its weight into your body. Let it sink into your chest just enough to press into your shirt. Stay there as long as it takes to get the bar completely motionless and under control. In many cases, it's about a one-second pause.

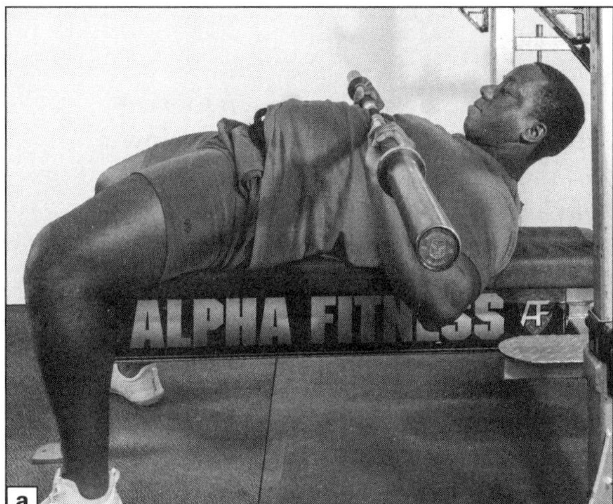

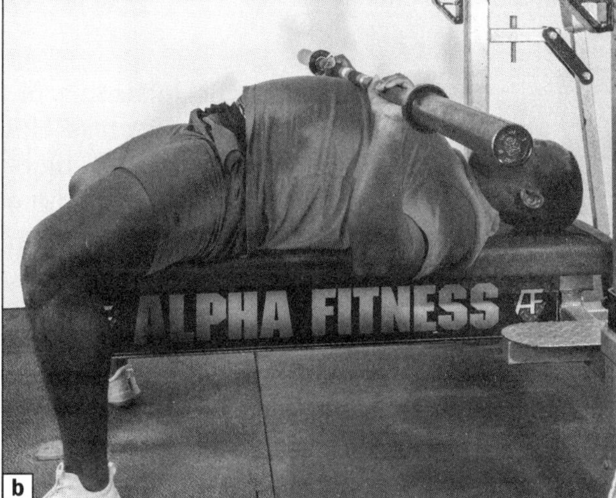

FIGURE 4.19 *(a)* Loss of tension with the bar at the chest with a collapse of the chest and arch as well as increased internal rotation at the shoulder. *(b)* Proper tension maintained at the chest.

The error I see most often at the chest is collapsing under the bar. I may sound like a broken record when it comes to staying tight, but there is a reason for it. Collapsing under the bar is when you lose all tension as the bar approaches the chest, and your torso flattens out on the bench underneath it. This affects a few things. First, it changes your shoulder position from a more externally rotated position to a more internally rotated one. The degree of this may be small, but the disruption in positioning changes the leverages and often results in a shrugging of the shoulders as well. Collapsing puts the bar higher on the chest and allows the elbows to get in front of the wrists. As a result, you lose leverage in the press (see figure 4.20).

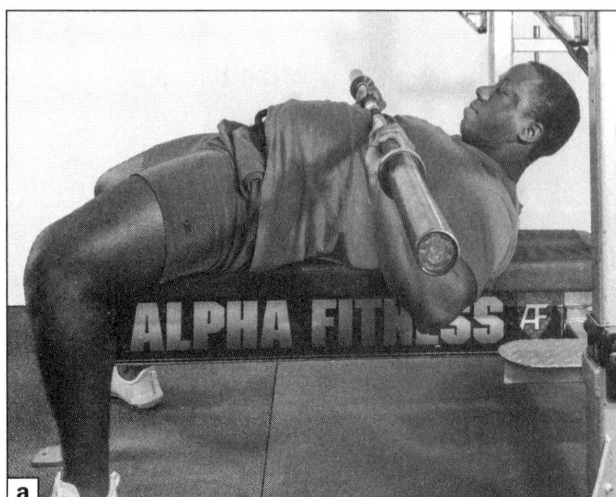

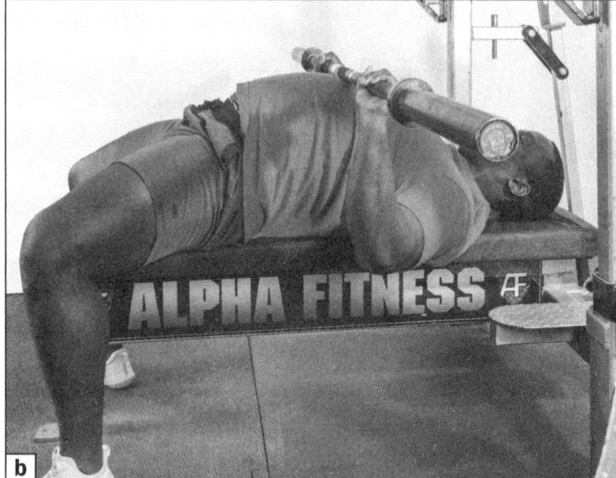

FIGURE 4.20 Examples of *(a)* collapsing under the bar with the arch lost, shoulders shrugged, and increased internal rotation of the shoulders compared to *(b)* where the bar should be at the chest.

Some people compensate for this, or try to, by pushing the bar down toward the feet when they initiate the press. However, this leads to the bar being too low at the chest and to the elbows flaring behind the wrists. You may be able to get away with this at lighter weights. But at heavier wights, you will never get the bar back into the position it needs to be in. Stay tight, pull your chest to the bar, and bench more weight.

The Ascent

The ascent should start with a quick pop off the chest like an explosion. As with all lifts, it has a sticking point, or a point of deceleration about halfway up, before hitting its second peak velocity. This is to be expected. Right off the chest though, it should look like that spring unloading. To achieve this, you don't just push the bar with your arms. This is when you draw on the energy that you've been holding in your lower body all this time. Your feet should still be firmly planted on the ground, so increase that leg-extension power and think about kicking so hard that you drive your whole body out of the top of the bench. The feet shouldn't go anywhere, but they will assist your upper body in producing force and help drive the bar back. A problem I see with beginners is that as they press the bar up, it starts to drift forward toward their feet. Once the bar goes in that direction, there's no getting it back. This big kick is known as *leg drive,* and it's one of the reasons I don't consider the bench to be only an upper-body tool. It's true that the primary movers are in the upper body. But once you've felt your legs and middle back cramp during a bench press, you'll understand how much the lower body contributes to power and stability in the lift.

Leg drive isn't the only thing that happens here though. At the same time that you kick your legs, you punch with your hands. Keep your shoulder blades in your back pockets and think about pushing yourself away from the bar, not just pushing the bar up. This will keep you locked in tighter and keep your elbows in a more optimal position as the bar rises. About one-third to halfway up, your elbows will begin to flare out as the bar elevates. It is at this transition that most hit their sticking point, and the key to overcoming it is to continue to push yourself away from the bar. The flaring of the elbows at this stage is normal and helps keeps them stacked under the wrists. Once you are past that sticking point, continue to extend the elbows until they are completely locked out and the bar is directly over the shoulders again. Now the rep is done. Figure 4.21 shows proper positioning of the bar throughout the movement.

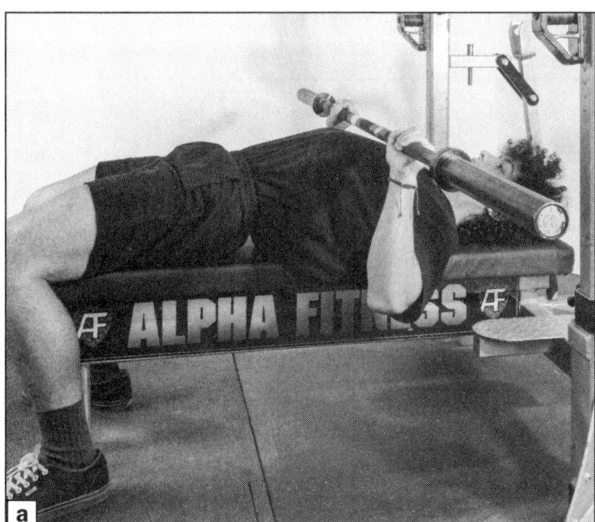

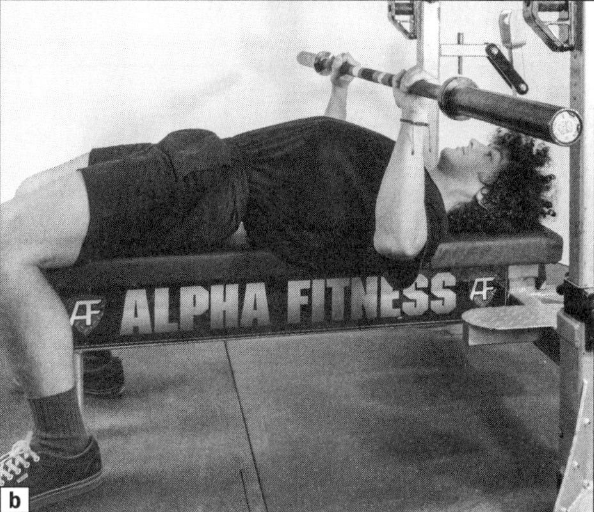

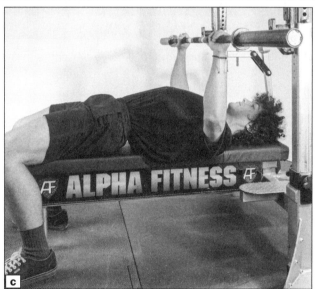

FIGURE 4.21 The ascent of the bench press *(a)* with the bar just off the chest, *(b)* with the bar at the common sticking point, and *(c)* just before lock-out where the bar accelerates again.

Bar path on the ascent is highly debated. I'm not going to be the one to set the record straight, but I will give you the information you need to analyze your bar path and get the most out of your lift. The bar path in the ascent of the bench can present in two different ways: in a straight line from the chest back up to the start position (see figure 4.22*a*) or in what looks more like a J-curve as the bar sweeps back toward the face while coming off the chest and then straightens out as it rises back to the starting position (see figure 4.22*b*). This J-curve tends to be more present with elite-level lifters working with maximal loads. The straighter bar path is seen with sub-maximal loads and with other elite-level lifters as well. Here is the big takeaway: As long as it doesn't go down toward your feet, go past the shoulder joints and too far over the face, or do a strange up-and-down dance during the lift, the bar path is in an acceptable range. Remember this when you are analyzing your bench bar path, and remember that there will always be some individual differences.

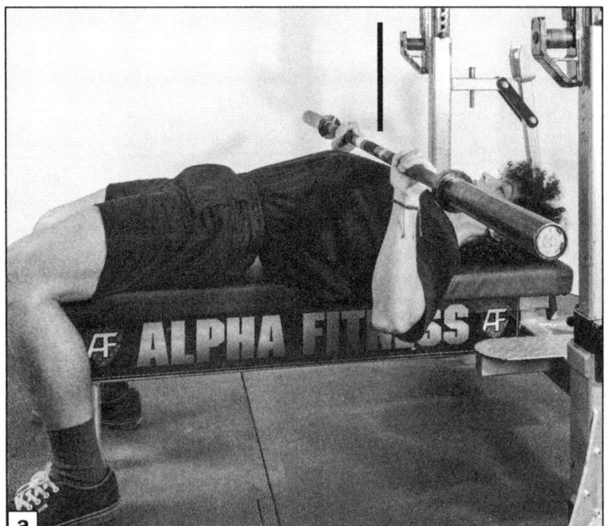

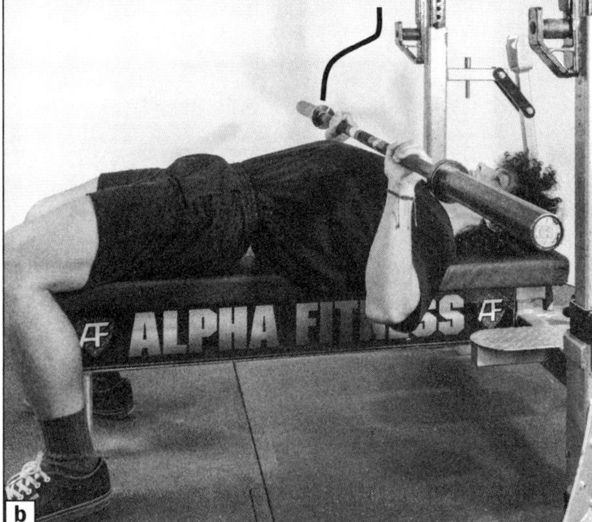

FIGURE 4.22 Comparison of the *(a)* straight-line and *(b)* J-curve bar paths in the bench press.

Bench-Press Variations

It's time to explore the close variations of the bench press. Whether you are working around an injury, you don't have the required equipment, or you have hit a plateau in your regular bench press, there will be something for you in this section. We will cover five of my top bench press variations to incorporate in your training so the progress can keep coming.

I want to save you time and frustration by pointing out a key aspect of the bench press in terms of progression and regression. As mentioned earlier in the chapter, the bench is the one lift where things can just stop when you add weight during a session. But why? The answer provides an important lesson in perspective. Here's a story I hear often in the gym: "Oh man, coach, I thought I had it today. Warm-ups were going well, and I felt really good. I got up to about 90 percent, and things were flying. I figured I could add just five more pounds to each side, right? Then I got stapled to the bench. Like, it just stopped. What do you think happened?" Here's the lesson I want you to learn: It's never "just" five pounds. Nothing in lifting is ever "just" anything. Be strategic with your weight increases.

Tempo Bench

It's helpful for new lifters to use tempo to learn how to maintain position before adding speed. If I am working with a lifter who lacks control in the bench press, using a tempo to add control is the first step I take. A 3-1-3 tempo, or a three-second descent, a one-second pause at the chest, and a three-second ascent, affords the lifter enough time under tension in each position to feel and control those spots, and it allows them to stack up some quality reps before we add speed to the movement.

This is also a great strategy for dealing with pain or injury during the bench press. A slower tempo tends to make the lift harder because of the time under tension, so we can use lighter weights without compromising effort. This tends to be less painful. The slower tempo also allows us to load the irritated tissues more gradually, which can help decrease pain and help in the healing process.

Floor Press or Board Presses

When it comes to developing lock-out power, the floor press and the board press are my go-tos. They are slightly different, and we will cover that here. First and foremost, I like to think of the floor press as being like the box squat but for the bench. This is because the contact between the floor and the elbows in the floor press mimics the contact between the box and the hips in a box squat. Similarly, a common error with the floor press is just tapping the elbow instead of allowing the entire upper arm to come into contact with the floor. (This makes it more like a touch-and-go bench, which doesn't have the same benefits.)

The limited range of motion of the floor press and the board press has two major benefits. First, you can typically overload these movements more to strengthen the upper portion of the lift and triceps more specifically. So if you notice that your lock-out is lacking or that you're getting stuck about halfway off the chest in your bench, this is a good way to address that. Second, the decreased range of motion is great in an injury scenario. The most common pain point for the bench press is close to the bottom of the range of motion. I will also note here that nearly everyone will experience this at some point in their bench-press journey. It's literally that common. Decreasing the range of motion can keep you out of that painful place and allow you the space to continue training, even at higher loads.

Floor Press

To execute the floor press, all you need to do is repeat your normal setup but while lying on the floor with the rack set where you can unrack the bar (see figure 4.23*a*). From here, nearly everything is the same as with a regular bench press except that as you come down, your upper arms will come in contact with the floor. Stay tight in this position, and control the weight by continuing to pull yourself to the bar as you normally would. You want to get the entire upper arm onto the floor. Depending on how short your arms are and how thick your torso is, the bar could be just at the chest, one to two inches off the chest, or anywhere in between. The key here is to get the upper arms all the way to the floor and to pause there for a second (see figure 4.23*b*). Then explode up to lock-out.

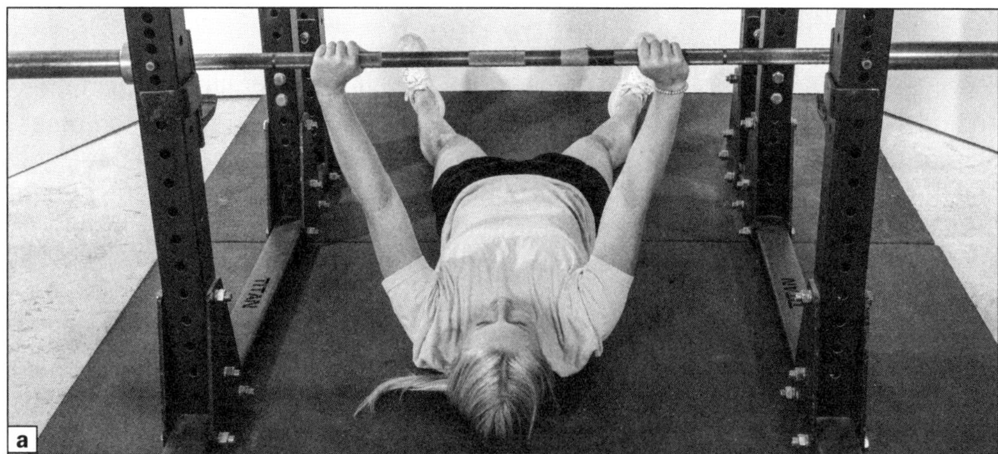

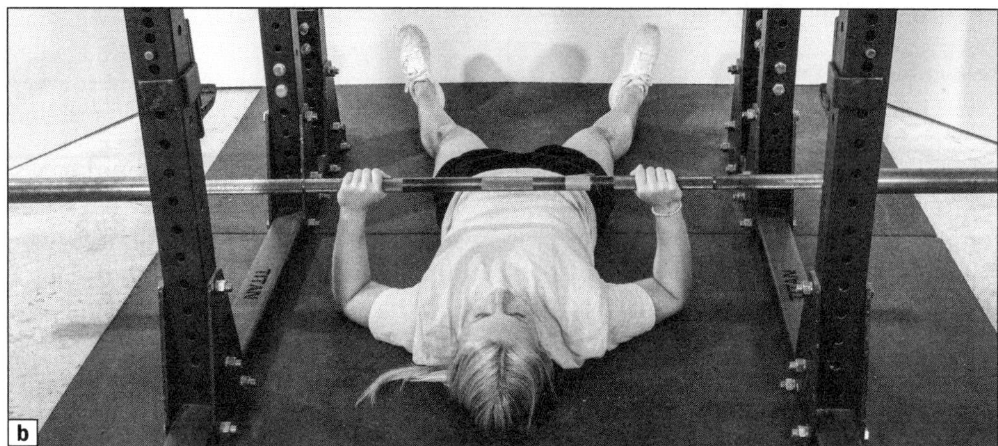

FIGURE 4.23 Floor press.

Board Press

The board press is slightly different because there's a board between you and the bar. There are two ways to accomplish this. The easiest way is with a piece of equipment called a *bench block*. There is no affiliation between myself and this company, but I can assure you that the Bench Block is a great tool to add to the tool kit. You simply attach it directly to the bar at the board height you want, and you are free to bench. The other way is to get a training partner to hold a board for you at your chest. A basic two-by-four plank of construction lumber from the hardware store is all you need, and you can nail several of them together to change the height. The setups I see most often use one, two, or three boards. I find these two setups to be the safest and most reliable ways to do a board press. Do not—I repeat, do not—shove a yoga block up your shirt and think it's going to stay there while you bench. Use the right tools to do this safely.

To execute the board press with the bench block, you unrack the bar as you normally would, and start to bring it down. The magic happens when the block touches your chest. At this point sink the bar down just enough into the block that you feel like it would create a little dent. You aren't trying to hover just above the block, and you aren't trying to break it with the bar. Place just enough weight on the block to create a dent, pause there, and then explode up (see figure 4.24). Do your reps according to your program, rack the bar, and watch your bench grow.

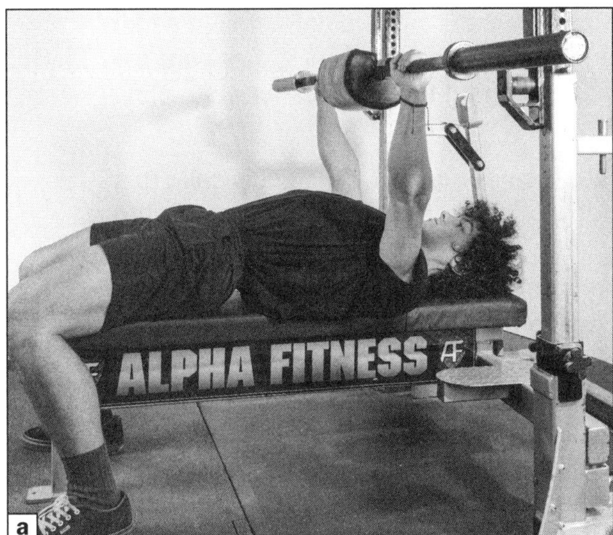

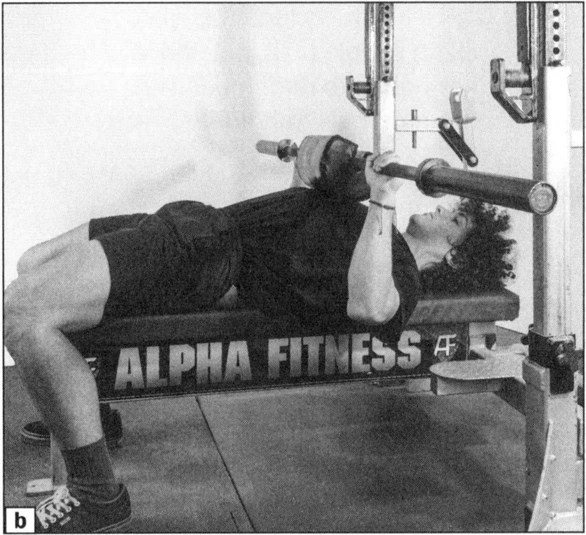

FIGURE 4.24 Board press with a bench block at *(a)* the start position and *(b)* the bottom position.

When a partner is holding the board for you, have them stand to the side while you get set up as you normally would. Once you are good and tight, your board holder should get into position and place the board on your chest as seen in the picture. This is when you are good to start your press, focusing on with the same goal as with the block press: Sink the weight down to the board just enough that you feel like it would create a little dent, pause there, and then explode up (see figure 4.25).

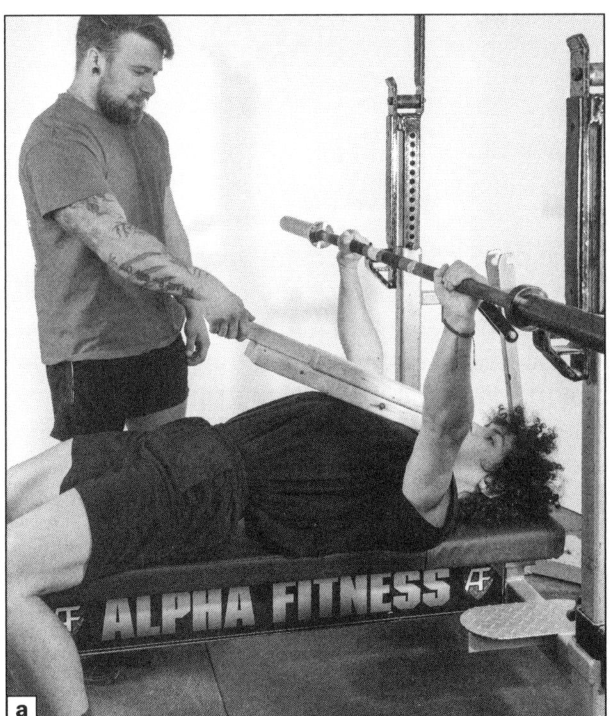

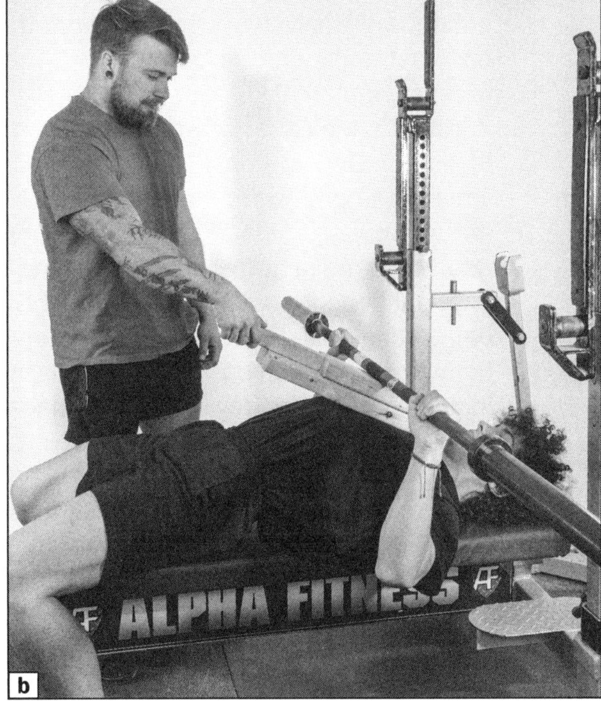

FIGURE 4.25 Board press with a partner holding a board at your chest at *(a)* the start position and *(b)* the bottom position.

I'd like to include a quick note on how to be a *great* board holder. It might seem like a simple task, but I have seen it done poorly far too many times. Here are the key points to remember when you're holding the board for someone or instructing them on how to hold it for you.

1. Give the lifter enough space to execute their setup and the lift. Typically, this means standing slightly off to the side of the lifter and extending the board over them from there.
2. Make sure the board is positioned right down the middle of the lifter's chest with the top end of the board being two to three inches from their chin.
3. Hold the board at an angle so that it lies flat on the lifter's upper chest but *not* flat across their entire body. This will ensure that the board doesn't move in any direction when the bar hits the board.
4. Hold on to the board tightly. Weight is going to come down on the board and may try to pull it out of your hands. Hold on to the handle tightly and keep the board stable.

Close-Wide-Grip Bench

Changing grips in the bench can have huge benefits over the long term. It can keep things from getting stale and can stoke continued progress. On my initial chase to a 440-pound bench (200 kg) I competed with three different grips and finally hit that number in a competition using close grip. At this point, I've hit 530 pounds (240 kg) with a pretty narrow grip considering my size, and I attribute that to training with so many different grip positions. From an anatomical standpoint, the rule of thumb is that wider grips elicit more pec and anterior shoulder contribution, while narrower grips are more triceps dominant. However, recent research has cast doubt on this assumption by revealing significant differences in only the triceps (Saeterbakken et al. 2017).

If that's the case, why do I bring up the issue of grip width at all? The answer is simple. Over the past 15 years, coaches, including myself, have observed that varying the grip width increases the bench press over time. How? I think there are a few ways. First and foremost, there's the psychological benefit: Varying the grip keeps training fresh by increasing buy-in and training enjoyment. As for the physical benefits, let's remember the two fail points I see most in the bench: the bar getting stuck at the chest (the weight is too heavy) and the bar getting stuck halfway up (the triceps aren't strong enough to lock it out). With the research indicating that a narrower grip increases triceps activity, it's only logical that using a narrower grip would be beneficial in building your lift.

There's another study that shows that for most powerlifters, a wider grip helps them to be more efficient and to be able to handle the most weight (Ferland et al. 2019). More than likely, this has to do with the decreased range of motion that comes with a wider grip, but overall, it does seem to be most people's stronger grip to take in the bench. So why not do some work with that wider grip and find out? That's the whole point of changing these grips: to find the strongest grip width that you have right now so you can perform at a high level while using other grips to supplement that as you build a monster bench.

To execute the lift with either of these grips, I like to keep things simple. From the unrack to the rerack, nothing changes except for the placement of your hands.

But I do have specific guidelines on where to start and the maximum distance you should go in either direction. For a wider grip, start at two finger widths wider than normal on each side (see figure 4.26). For many, that means moving out so that their middle fingers are on the rings instead of their pinkies. You can go all the way out to having your index fingers on the rings, but anything wider than that is outside powerlifting regulations and can start to create some discomfort. For a closer grip, move two finger widths in from your normal grip so that the pinkies are off the rings (see figure 4.27). Sometimes I switch the frame of reference and have lifters narrow their grip to where an extended thumb comes into contact with the smooth part of the bar. But don't go any narrower than having your hands right on the start of knurling. Anything more than that and it can be hard to get the bar to your chest.

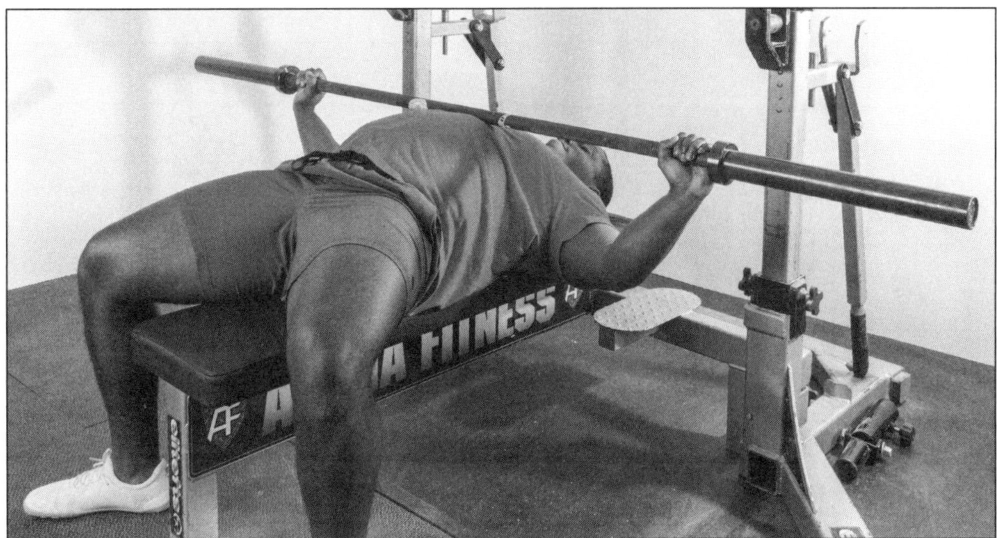

FIGURE 4.26 The wide-grip bench press will create an elbow angle of greater than 90 degrees at the chest which decreases total range of motion.

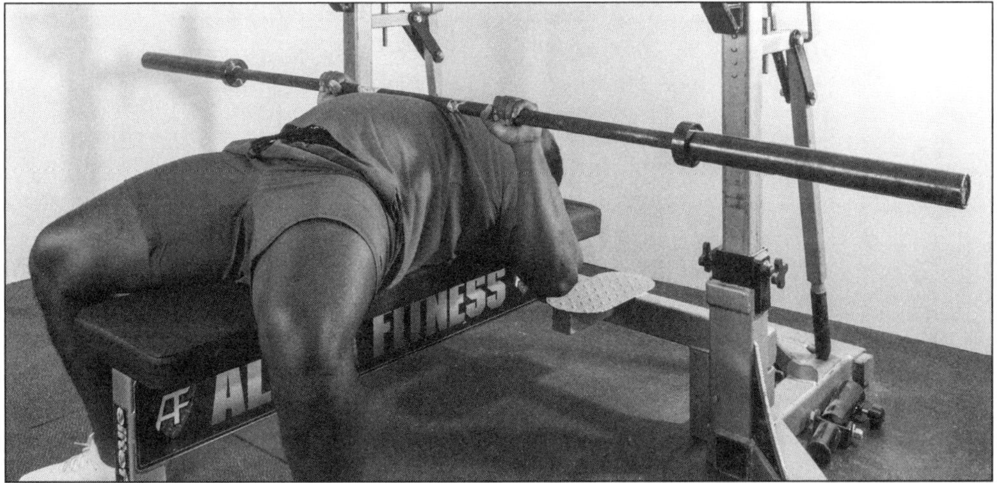

FIGURE 4.27 The close-grip bench press creates an elbow angle of less than 90 degrees with the bar at the chest.

The Double-Pause Bench Press

The double-pause bench press is a variation that taught me an incredibly valuable skill right when I needed it. When I was struggling with 440 pounds (181 kg), this is the lift that took me past the 500-pound (227 kg) barrier. It's a variation I still return to get my mojo back when I'm feeling weaker in bench. Essentially, it is a normally executed bench press with a pause at the chest and a pause halfway up to create two points where you have to accelerate the bar. As I mentioned earlier, the two common places I see people miss the bench press are at the chest and about halfway up. Forcing a pause in each of those positions teaches you to accelerate the bar through your weakest positions, which is a critical skill to learn.

I want you to think back to the velocity curves. We know that overcoming forces is necessary to increase the velocity past the sticking points. The double pause

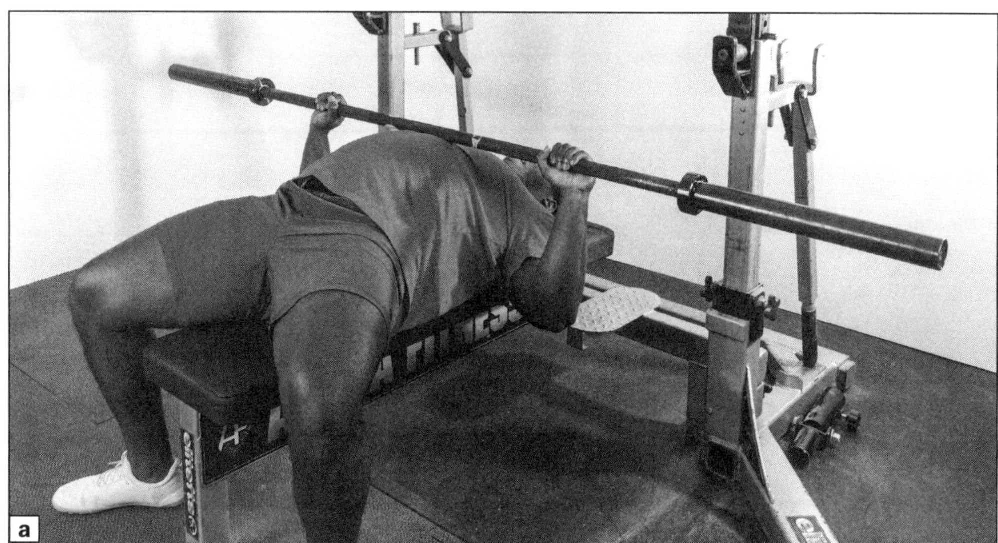

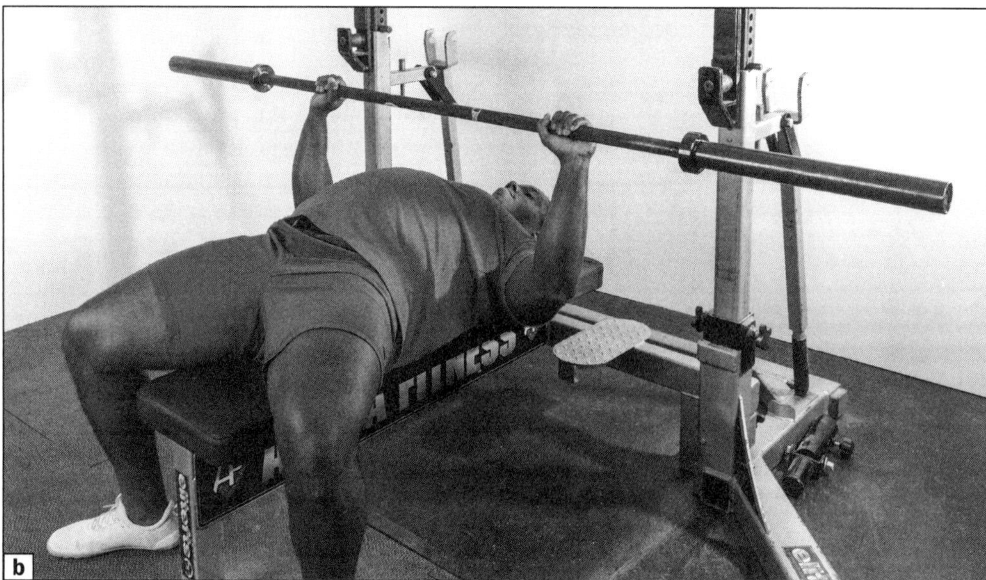

FIGURE 4.28 The two pause points in the double-pause bench press: *(a)* at the bottom and *(b)* on the way up. The key to the second pause point is to focus on it being at or close to your particular sticking point.

creates an acceleration off the chest, which teaches you how to use overcoming strength at the first sticking point. The stop halfway up, where the lift is the most difficult, teaches you how to drive through the sticking point when you're in your weakest position. The specific stopping point on the ascent will be slightly different for each person, but the key is to stop where it's the hardest to hit the brakes and then accelerate again after the pause.

To execute this, keep everything the same as with your normal-grip bench press. But when you bring the bar down to your chest, you're going to pause and be completely motionless for one to two seconds (see figure 4.28*a*). After that you're going to press. When you feel the bar getting to the portion of the lift that is more difficult, you're going to stop the bar again and make sure it stays completely motionless for one to two seconds (see figure 4.28*b*). Then reinitiate the press to get it to lock-out.

Dumbbell Bench Press

Last but not least, there is the dumbbell bench press. You're not always going to have access to a barbell, or there may be times when using a barbell for a normal bench may be uncomfortable and you've exhausted all the previous options. In those cases, I suggest a dumbbell bench press because it's more accessible, and it can be more tolerable for some individuals who are going through discomfort. This doesn't mean it's an easier variation.

With dumbbells, the weight is not connected the way it is on a barbell, so balancing the weight requires more stabilization strength. The dumbbell bench press also tends to have a greater range of motion because the dumbbells can break past the plane of your chest. If hypertrophy is the goal, the increased range of motion of the dumbbell bench is a huge benefit. When a muscle is under load, it's the end of the range of motion that determines the growth potential. The range of motion and the stretch of a dumbbell bench are much greater than they are with a barbell bench because the dumbbells don't run into your torso and cut off the range of motion.

From a safety perspective, the dumbbell bench press has an additional benefit. If you fail using a barbell, it's likely that the bar will end up pinned to your chest, even if you have a spotter. Whereas if you hit failure with the dumbbell bench press, you can just drop the dumbbells on the floor. As long as you don't drop them on anybody's feet, you're in a really good spot to stay safe. You should still use a spotter when you're dumbbell benching though, because you don't want to drop them on your face. So continue to use a spotter even though it's not a normal barbell.

There are a few key differences when it comes to setting up for a dumbbell bench press, and the first is how to get into the starting position. While seated on the bench, take the dumbbells and set them upright on the ends of your kneecaps just above where the teardrop muscle on your quads would be (see figure 4.29*a*). From here, kick one leg up and bring a dumbbell to your shoulder (see figure 4.29*b*). Then, as you kick the second one up toward your shoulder, lie back onto the bench and press both dumbbells up into the start position (see figure 4.29*c*). From here, set your shoulders and get into a tighter position just like you would for a normal bench press (see figure 4.29*d*).

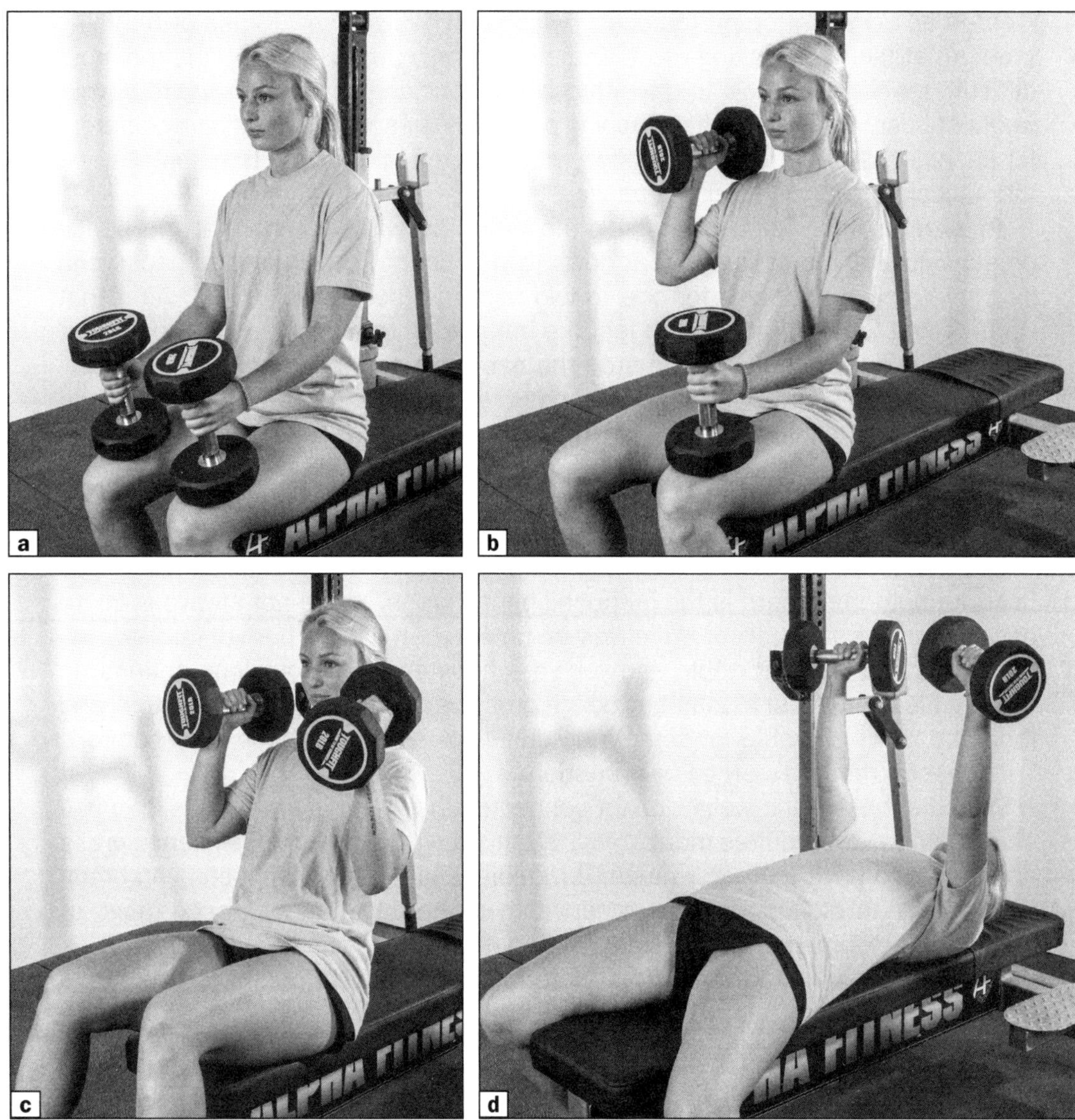

FIGURE 4.29 To set up for the dumbbell bench press, *(a)* put the dumbbells on the top surface of the knees, *(b)* kick one dumbbell up to your shoulder, *(c)* kick the second dumbbell up as you lie back, and *(d)* set your feet and shoulders and lock out the elbows.

Since dumbbells move more freely than a barbell, you can change the angle of your grip. I like to have people start off at a 45-degree angle (see figure 4.30*a*). Then you can change to a neutral grip, where your hands face each other (see figure 4.30*b*), or pronated grip, where your hands face down toward your feet. A pronated grip will naturally make the angle a bit wider and will feel more like a barbell-bench grip (see figure 4.30*c*).

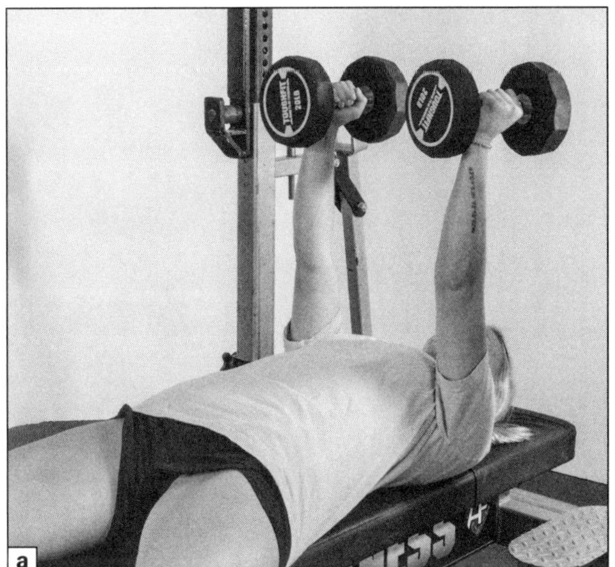

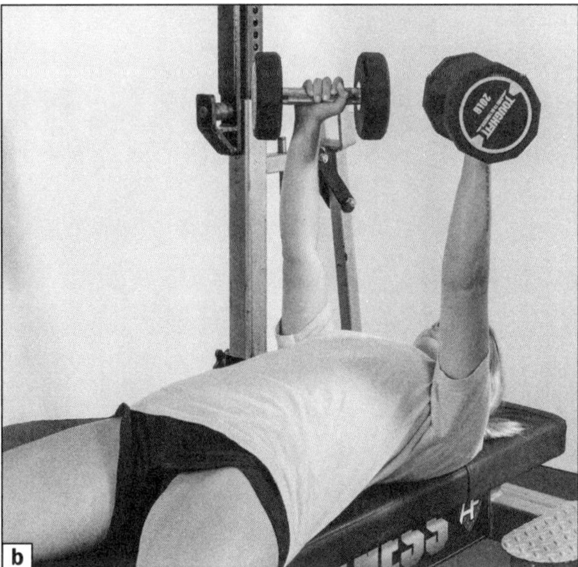

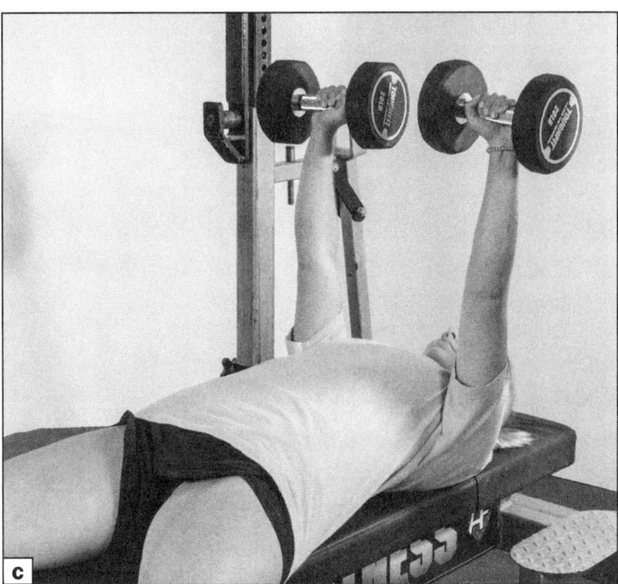

FIGURE 4.30 Three different grip types for the dumbbell bench: *(a)* neutral grip, *(b)* 45-degree grip, and *(c)* pronated grip.

Once you have the dumbbells in the start position (see figure 4.31*a*), everything remains the same as with a barbell bench. Your feet should be firmly planted on the floor, your glutes should be firmly planted on the bench, and your shoulder blades should be in your back pockets. Pull your elbows down and pull yourself toward the dumbbells (see figure 4.31*b*), and then explode off the chest as quickly as you can while keeping control of the dumbbells (see figure 4.31*c*).

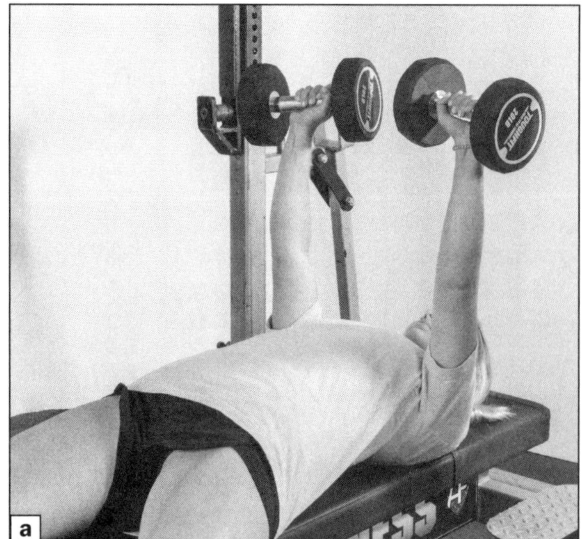

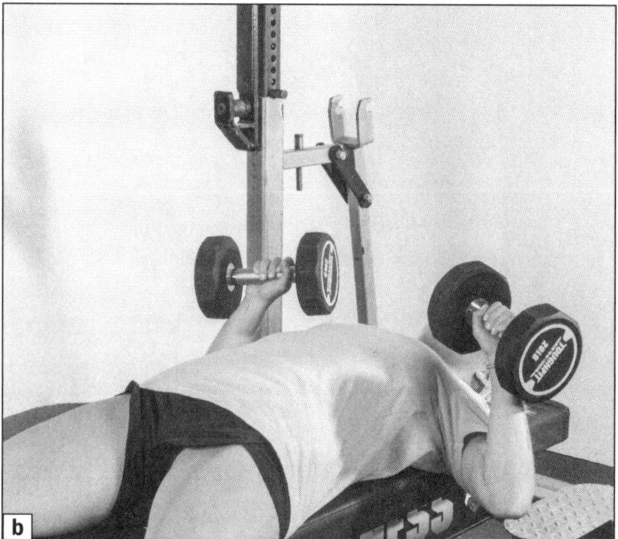

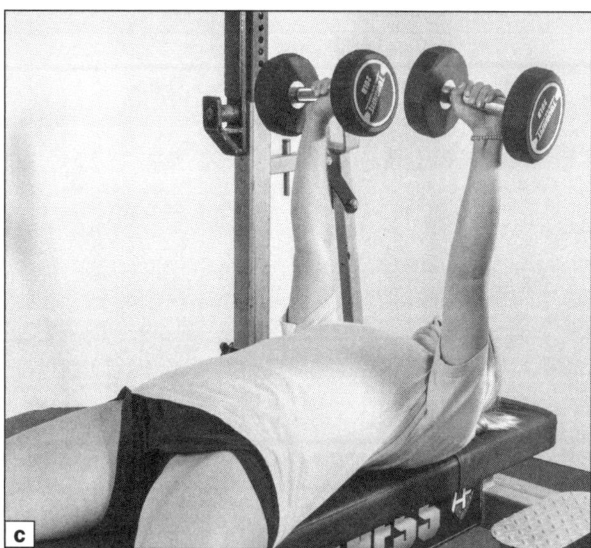

FIGURE 4.31 Each phase of the dumbbell bench press: *(a)* start position, *(b)* at the chest, and *(c)* lock-out.

Warming Up for the Bench Press

As with all the lifts, warming up for the bench will help your performance, but it doesn't have to take 30 minutes to get to your first working sets. Let's dive into the five exercises that I go to the most often for my athletes when warming up for the bench.

Push-Up

The push-up is a big go-to for beginners as a warm-up to the barbell, especially if their strength level isn't ready for 45 pounds (20 kg) yet. It's easily scalable, incredibly similar to the general movement of the bench press, and accessible because all you really need is the floor.

It's also great as a rehab tool for people with discomfort in the front of their shoulders or in their chest. Using the push-up, we can gauge the discomfort before we touch the bar to better determine the expectations for the session.

First, you need to pick the progression of the push-up you are going to do. There are many ways to progress and regress the push-up, from keeping your knees on the floor all the way to putting a plate on your back (known as a deficit push-up). You can find the right progression of a push-up by starting with the standard position on the floor with your knees off the ground. If you can do more than 10 reps here, then you can progress up to a more challenging position such as with your feet elevated. If you can do between 5 and 10, then this standard position is for you. If you can do fewer than 5, a regression would be helpful such as with your knees on the floor.

The next step is to set your hands. This is where we make it specific to your bench press. You want your hand width for the push-up to be the same width you are training for that day. So if you are training close-grip, make sure the width between your hands is the same as that grip. Same with wide-grip. The movement of the push-up itself isn't that much different than the movement in bench. Get into the position you selected from the progressions and brace the same way you would for a lift, filling your core with air and bracing down to keep your torso tight (see figure 4.32*a* for the top position for a standard push-up). Start to bend your elbows the same way you would for the bench, lower yourself until you can touch your chest to the ground (see figure 4.32*b* for the bottom position for a standard push-up), and then press back up. Your torso should not rock up and down, and your hips shouldn't reach the floor before your chest does. If that happens, the brace isn't tight enough, and I would regress the movement to where the brace can be maintained.

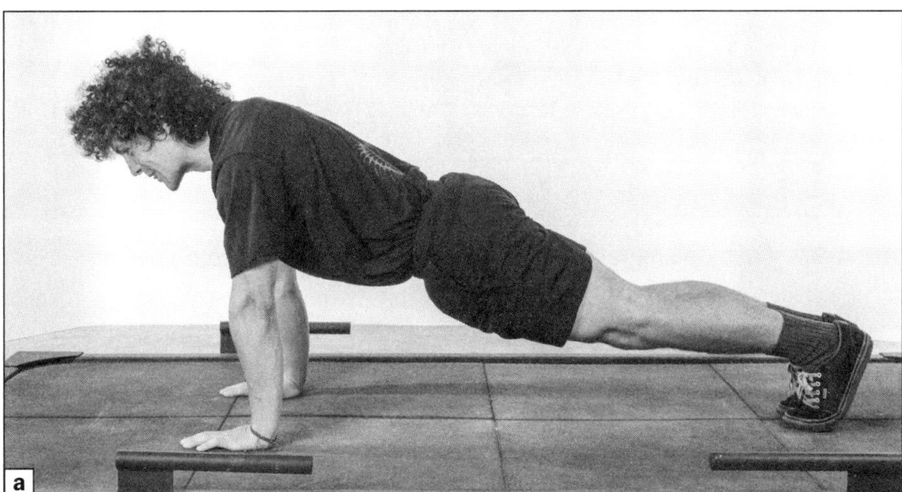

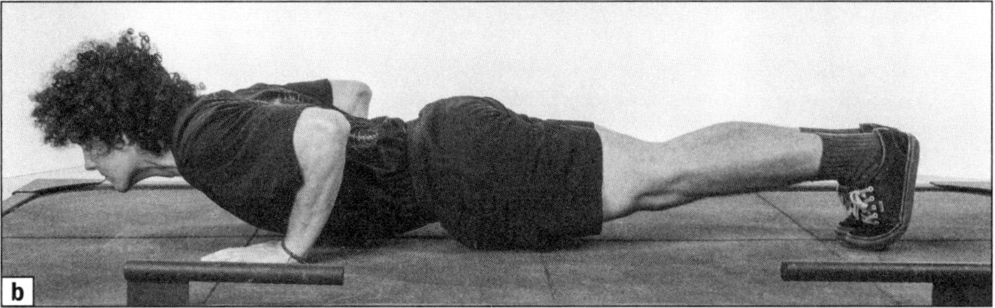

FIGURE 4.32 Standard push-up: *(a)* top position and *(b)* bottom position.

Sets of five to eight are good to get the blood flowing and to provide enough information to inform the session. There's no need to go to failure or to push these reps super high. If they are too easy, advance the progression (see figure 4.33). If they are too hard, regress the exercise (see figure 4.34). Remember: It's a warm-up, not a fitness test.

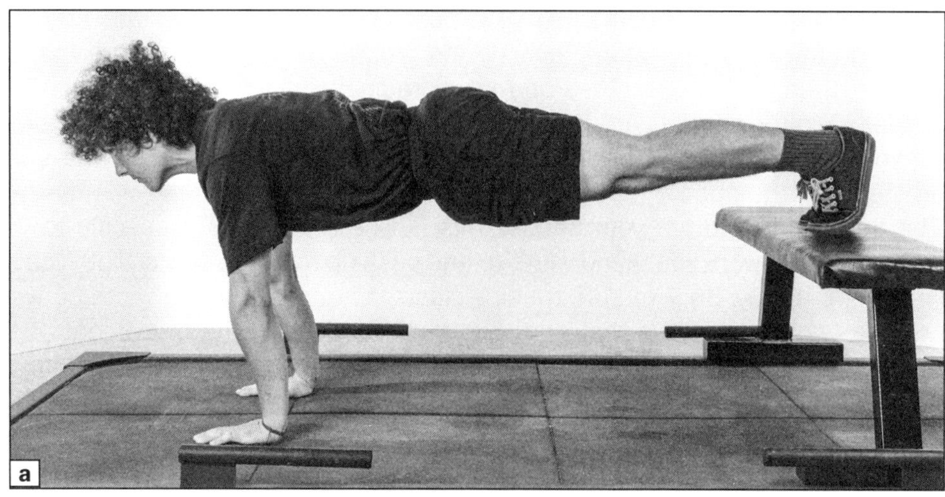

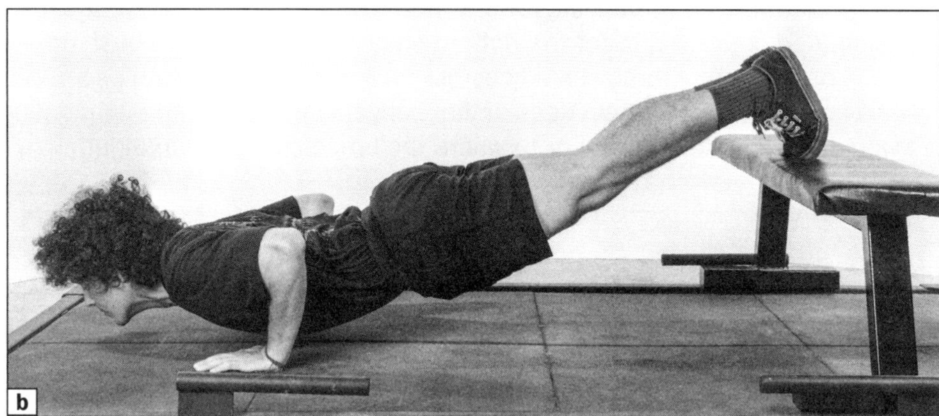

FIGURE 4.33 Push-up progression: *(a)* top position and *(b)* bottom position.

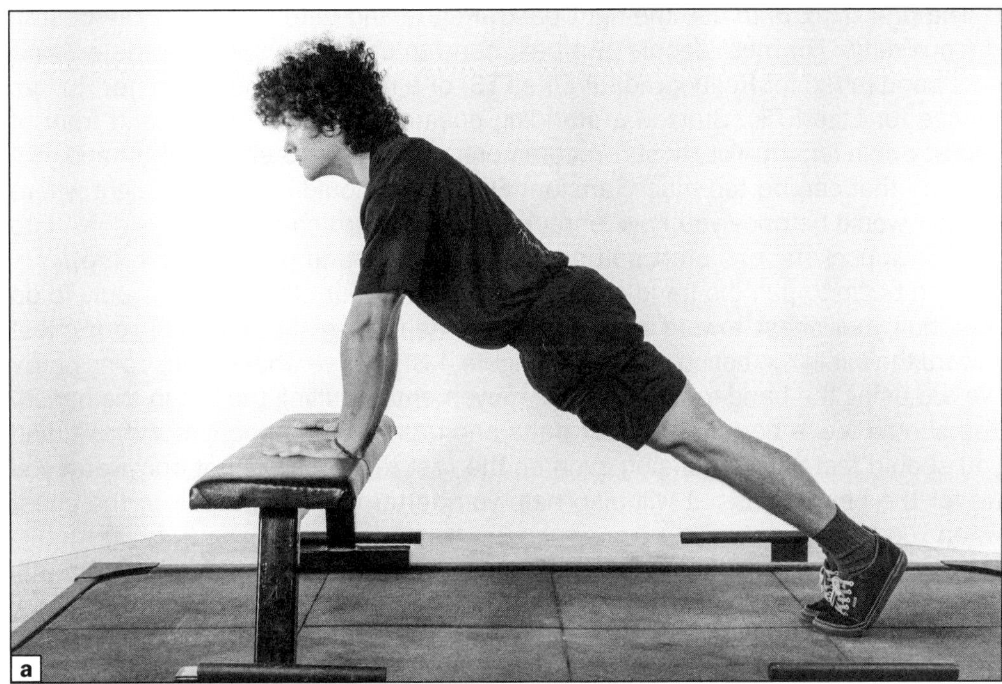

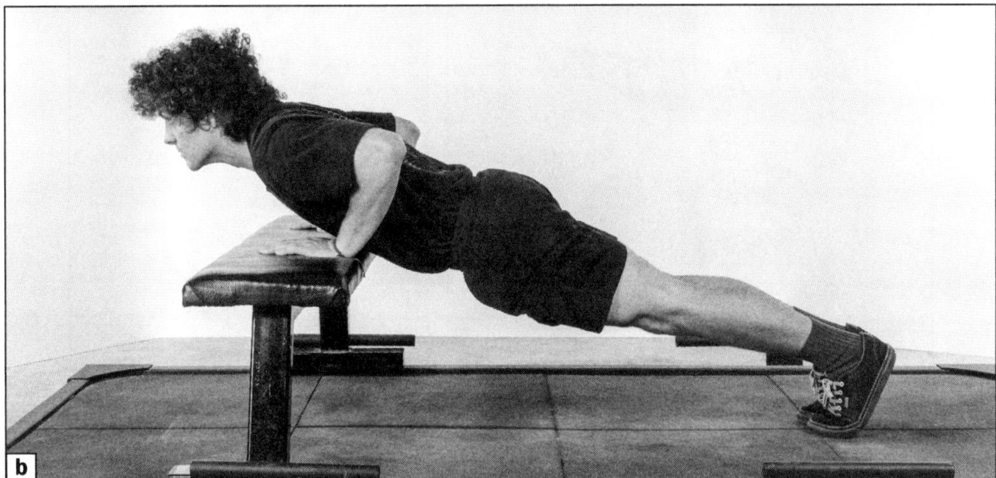

FIGURE 4.34 Push-up regression: *(a)* top position and *(b)* bottom position.

Banded Pull-Apart

The banded pull-apart is the exercise I see most butchered at the gym, so I am an absolute stickler when it comes to this exercise. While it doesn't work any of the primary movers, it does do two important things. First, it warms up the muscles responsible for stabilizing you and the bar during the lift (the upper back and also the lats if you do it right). It also teaches you the tension that you want on the bench (again, if you do it right). Seriously, the banded pull-apart is not only a warm-up but a teaching tool. If you don't know how to put your shoulder blades in your back pockets, or if you lose that position often, this is your exercise. So how do you do it right?

The first thing is to use the right band. Rogue and Elite FTS make the best in the business. For most people, the best band to use for this exercise is either a light band (a red for Rogue; red for Elite FTS) or a medium band (green for Rogue; orange for Elite FTS). Start in a standing position and hold the band in front of you at arm's length. For most, I recommend grabbing one side of the band, not both as that can be too much tension. The band should be at the height where the bar would be once you have unracked it. Set your shoulder blades down into your back pockets, and start putting tension in the band (see figure 4.35*a*).

Then begin to pull the band apart while keeping your elbows locked out. To do this, pull your chest toward the band in the same way that you pull your chest toward the bar in the bench press. (see figure 4.35*b*). See what we are doing here? We are using the band to simulate the movement of pulling the bar in the bench. You should feel a burn in your rear delts and lats if you do enough of these, and you should feel a lot of tension even on the first rep. This will not only warm you up for the bench press, it will also help you better control the pull to the chest when you bench.

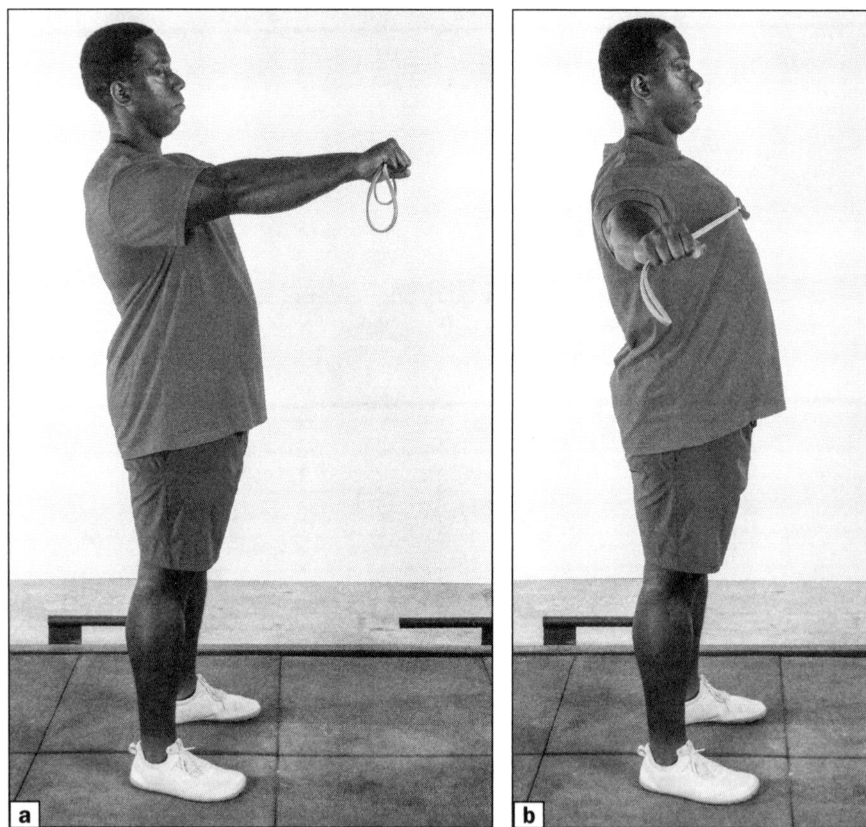

FIGURE 4.35 A banded pull-apart, keeping the arms straight and pulling the chest to the band similar to the bench press.

Half-Kneeling Arm Circles

If you do only one mobility exercise, it should be this one, which you may remember if you read the previous chapter. Common complaints during the bench are tightness or pain in the front of the shoulders and tightness in the front of the hips. Arm circles help with both of these problems and require nothing but you and a wall. I do suggest you use a smooth wall; I tried using a cinder-block wall and got my arm righteously chewed up.

To set this up, kneel down alongside a wall. Keep the knee closest to the wall on the ground, and bring your other knee up. Both knees should be bent at 90 degrees. You should be close enough to the wall that your shoulder is touching it, and you should be facing squarely in one direction (see figure 4.36*a*). Next, squeeze your glutes. You should feel a gentle stretch in the front of your hip and the down leg. Now extend the arm closest to the wall straight out in front of you with the palm facing away from the wall (see figure 4.36*b*). Keeping your hand in contact with the wall, start to circle your arm up and then back over your head (see figure 4.36*c*). As your hand gets higher, you'll feel it want to turn over (see figure 4.36*d*). Let this happen naturally. The key here is to try not to lean away from the wall; stay in that half-kneeling position while remaining as tall as possible. Keep circling your arm around behind you (see figure 4.36*e*) and then back toward your hip. When your hand feels like flipping back over, let it happen naturally. Keep circling the arm around until you get back to the start position, and that is one rep.

Since this is not a loaded exercise, you can keep doing reps on each side until you feel less of a stretch in the pecs, shoulders, and hips at the extreme positions. For the first set this could be eight reps, then five reps for the second set, and so on. Just remember to try and stay as square as possible through the movement. If you aren't able to stay square, and you find yourself bending your torso, move away from the wall enough to keep the movement smooth.

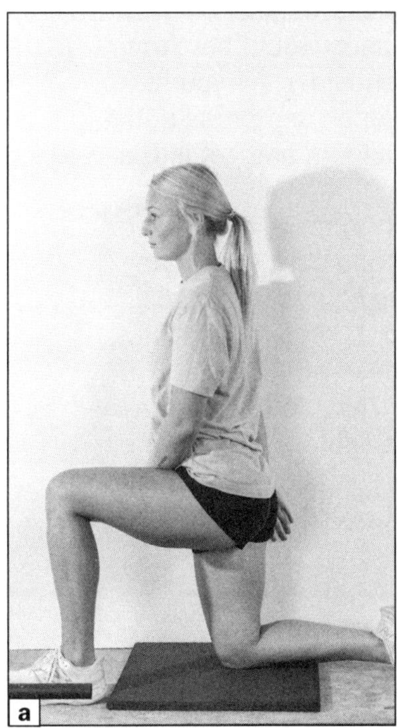

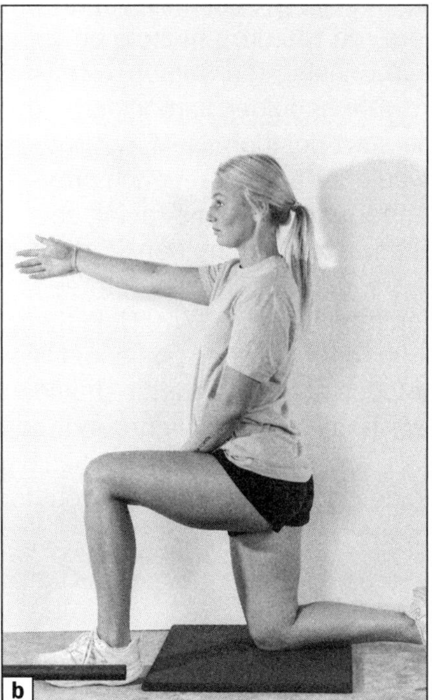

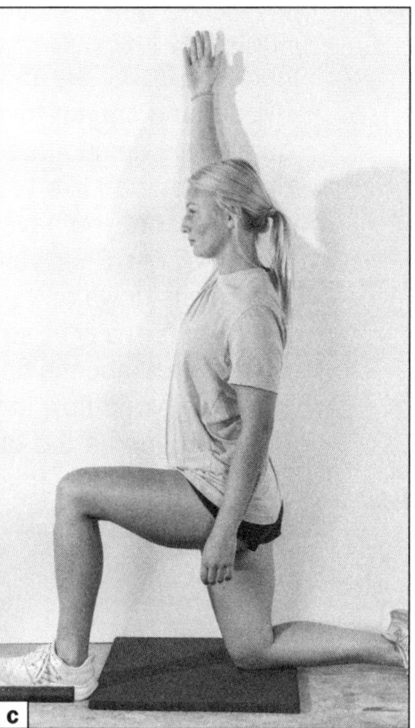

FIGURE 4.36 Half-kneeling arm circle.

(continued)

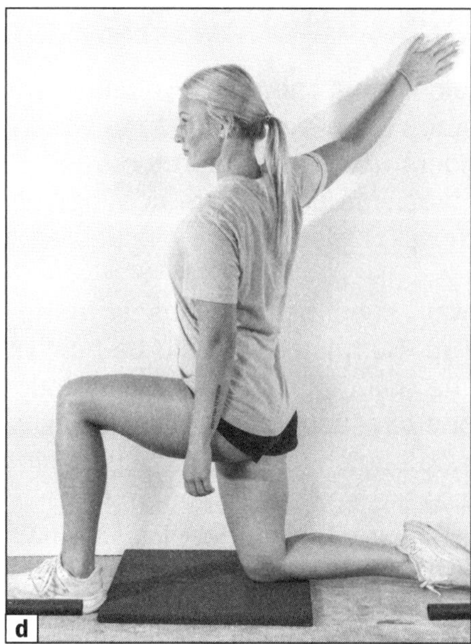

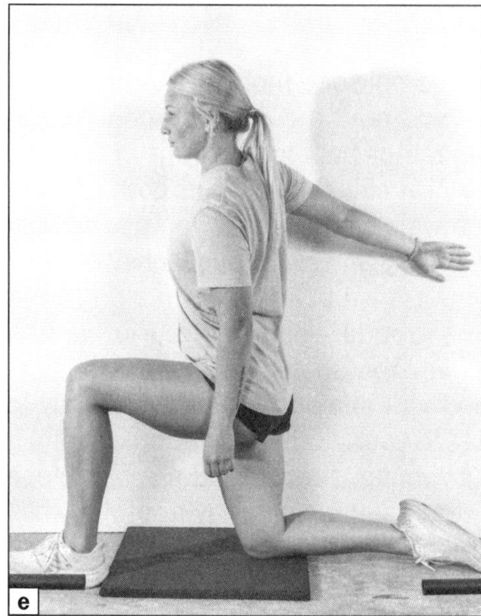

FIGURE 4.36 *(continued)*

Dumbbell Chest Fly

Have I already mentioned that a common complaint with lifters is pec tightness or pain? Well, it is. With the bench, the most common complaint I hear is of pain or the feeling of tightness in the chest near or in front of the shoulders. Using a simple chest fly can help address this problem very well, especially if we add tempo to it.

To get set up here, grab a set of dumbbells that you would consider to be on the lighter side. While seated on a bench, set the dumbbells upright on your kneecaps just above where the teardrop muscle on your quads would be. From here, kick one leg up while bringing the dumbbell to your shoulder. As you kick the second one up toward your shoulder, lie back onto the bench and press both dumbbells up and into the start position. Next, set your shoulders and get into a tighter position like you would for a normal bench press.

Make sure you have a neutral grip (palms facing each other) for this one (see figure 4.37*a*). Bend your elbows to no more than 15 degrees, and start to bring the dumbbells down to the side with a slow tempo of three to five counts. Keep going until you feel a light stretch (see figure 4.37*b*). Hold there for a second, and then bring the dumbbells back up to the starting position. I like these at higher reps to increase blood flow in the pecs and the anterior shoulders. They don't create as much fatigue as the others because the weight tends to be lighter. Plus, we are isolating particular muscles, so going to sets of 12 to 15 reps isn't that bad. Just keep it to three sets or under for your warm-up so you don't overtax your pecs.

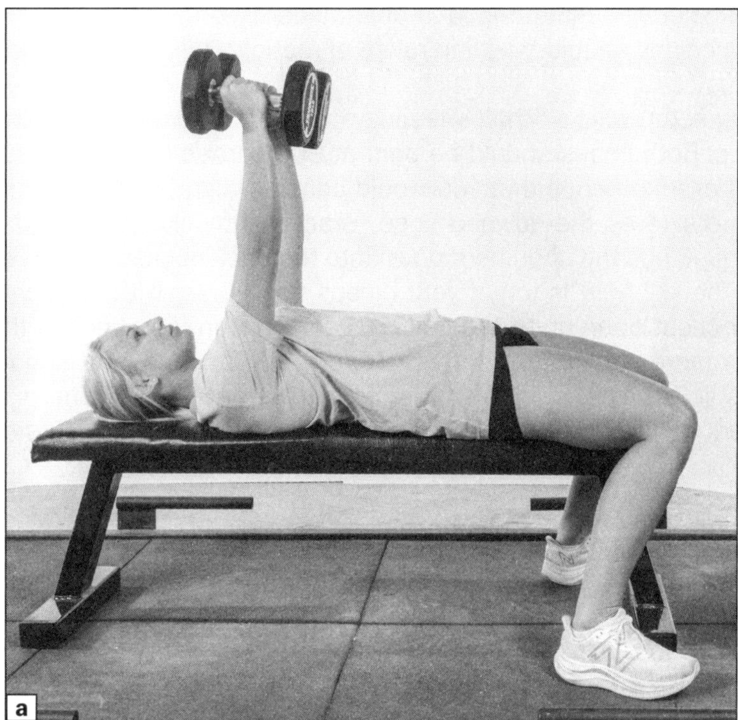

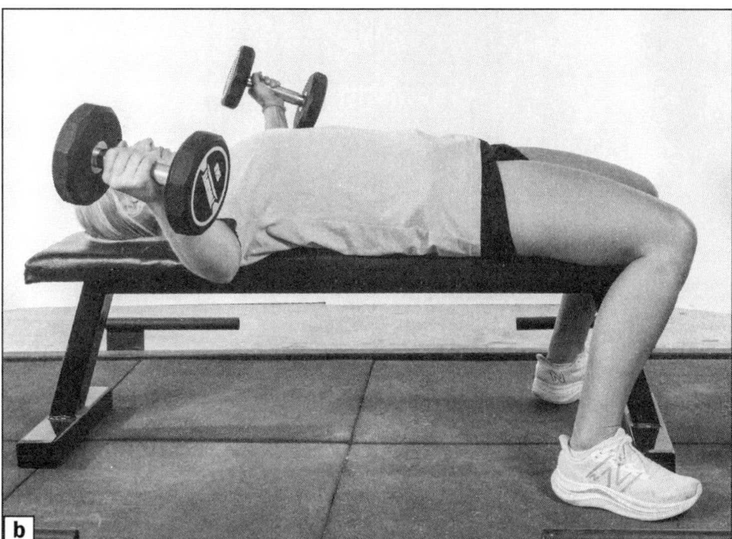

FIGURE 4.37 Examples of the different positions of the dumbbell chest fly: *(a)* the start position, with a slight elbow bend and *(b)* the bottom position.

Half-Kneeling Kettlebell Press

Yes, we are going to end with an overhead press. It may seem counterintuitive to use a vertical press for the shoulders to warm up for the horizontal press in the bench. However, there is evidence that a loss of shoulder flexion (the ability to bring your arm overhead by raising it in front of you) is a normal adaptation to the bench press. It's more common with elite-level lifters, but new lifters also complain of tightness in shoulder flexion as they learn the bench press. We aren't trying to completely negate this loss of shoulder flexion with this exercise, but it is great for keeping shoulder-flexion range of motion while also alleviating anterior hip tightness.

The initial setup will be a half-kneeling position with one knee on the floor and the other up. Both knees should be bent at 90 degrees (see figure 4.38*a*). Grab a dumbbell or a kettlebell that you would consider light, and hold it in the hand on the same side as the downed knee. Brace tightly like you would before you bench or squat, pull the shoulders down into the back pockets, and press the bell overhead. The key here is to get your biceps to your ear without leaning back or letting your chest open up to the ceiling. People often lean back in this position to try to get more shoulder flexion (see figure 4.38*b*). This isn't shoulder flexion though. It's spinal extension, which isn't what we are going for here. Three sets of eight work well here with a weight that is relatively light on both sides.

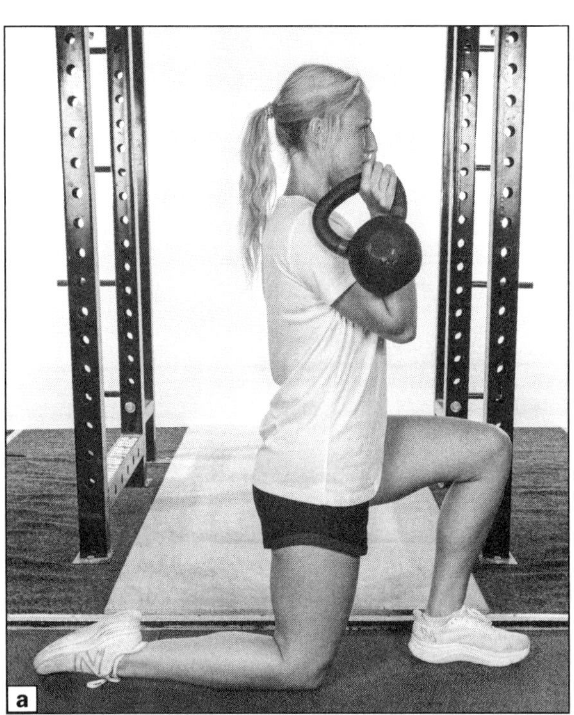

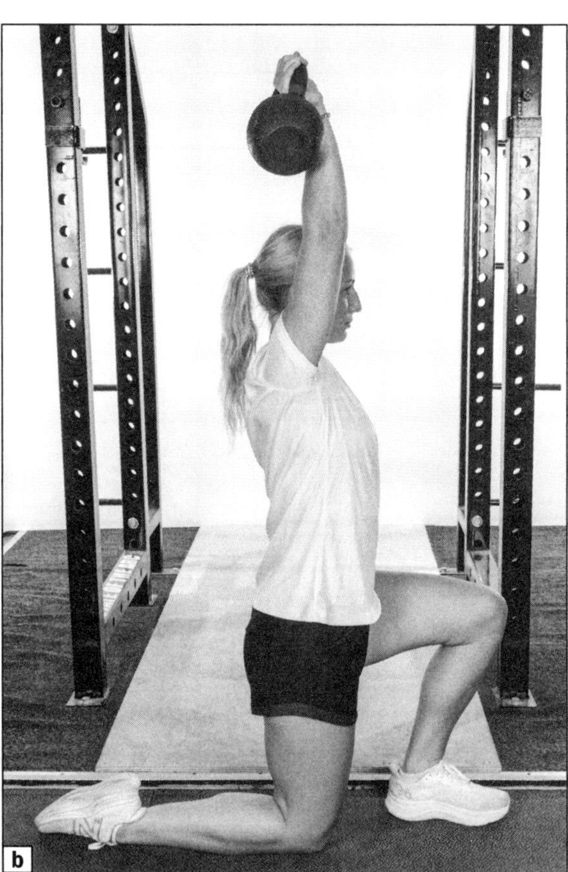

FIGURE 4.38 Proper position for the half-kneeling kettlebell press: *(a)* start position and *(b)* the top position.

What Is "Bench Press-itis," and Will It Happen to Me?

Bench press-itis is a common boogeyman that people talk about at gyms and at physical therapy clinics around the world. It's the idea that if you bench press often, eventually your shoulders will begin to round forward, creating an awkward and painful-looking posture.

The theory of how this happens goes like this: We know that muscle heals in a shortened state, and that bouts of lifting weights causes muscular damage. So if you're benching regularly, this cycle of muscular damage and healing eventually shortens the muscles to the point of negatively affecting shoulder position and posture. While the physiology here is true (muscle does heal in a shortened state), the application of it is wrong. In cases of massive muscular damage like a full rupture, cases of immobilization from an injury, or cases where there has been repeated trauma to a muscle with very limited recovery, we do see changes in muscle length that would cause postural changes. But to replicate that degree of damage in training, you would have to bench to or close to failure every day with zero recovery time in-between, and you'd have to do it over an extended period of time. Also of note: Very limited progress (if any) would occur over that span of time. In fact, there could be regression.

These scenarios just don't happen in a properly created and executed training program. The program and the executions of movement that we have outlined here in this book are built around full-range-of-motion training, responsible weight selection, and recovery time between sessions. Not only does something like bench press-itis *not* happen in a proper program, but good training actually helps increase available range of motion in the joints, decrease the risk of injury, and improve things like static posture. To wrap it up: Train to a full range of motion and make good decisions like the ones presented in this book, and bench press-itis will never be a concern for you.

You now know everything you need to know about the bench press. You know how to execute the lift step by step, from the setup all the way to the rerack, and what to look for in order to better understand the movement. You've learned additional variations of the lift to help you continue to progress as well as specific warm-up exercises to help construct your bench-specific warm-up. Now it's time to bring the bar to the floor and talk about the most feared lift of all: the deadlift.

Chapter 5

The Deadlift

I can already hear it. You opened to this chapter and somewhere in the background, "Danger Zone" by Kenny Loggins started playing. Welcome to the deadlift—the scary lift that everyone has heard about. There is a lot of noise out there about how dangerous the deadlift is and how it should only be performed by competitive strength athletes. For the record, though, this is patently false. When done correctly and programmed appropriately, the deadlift is a very safe and effective exercise for lifters of all levels. Not only is it safe and great in the gym, I would argue that it is the lift that can most positively affect your life outside of the gym. Everything gets easier with a good deadlift: yard work, playing with your kids, even cleaning the house. This chapter will explain how. You will also learn how to perform the two most common deadlift styles, how to use variations for the deadlift, and the best deadlift-specific warm-ups to get you ready to start pulling.

Reasons Why You Should Deadlift

While there are many claims that the deadlift has a higher rate of injury than the other lifts—especially of the lower back—this has not been found to be objectively true based on research. Among competitive powerlifters, however, strains of the pectoralis major during the bench press do occur at a higher rate (Bengtsson et al. 2018). Then again, competitive powerlifters, by definition, push their lifts to extremes, and that alone increases risk. With any physical endeavor, it's up to the participating individual to determine how much risk they're comfortable with. If you want to be an elite-level powerlifter, that is going to require training these lifts hard and often (even then the injury rate is lower than in other sports). But even if exploring that level of competition isn't your cup of tea, that doesn't mean you should never deadlift.

The reasons should be obvious, but let me explain them anyway. The movement of the deadlift is something you already do every single day every time you pick something up off the floor, whether it's a pencil, or your kids, or a puppy. The difference when you start deadlifting is the weight on the bar. The strength you develop from that weight adds up fast. My wife can deadlift over 300 pounds (136 kg) herself, and my best is well over 700 pounds (318 kg). On a regular basis, during yard work or while moving heavy things around the house like a couch, my wife and I ask each other, "What do people who don't lift do in these situations?"

So my first reason to deadlift is increased capability. Of all the lifts, the deadlift is the most applicable to daily living. Period. It sounds too simple to be true, but deadlifting and doing it well can improve your quality of life. It's been shown that weight training increases the quality of life in older adults, people with Parkinson's disease, breast cancer survivors, and many others (Nogueira et al. 2017 and Soriano-Maldonado et al. 2019). Excluding the deadlift as a foundational movement is a mistake.

The next reason to deadlift is its ability to decrease the risk of injury. That's right. The deadlift can actually help you stave off injury. What's more, it has been shown to be a necessary exercise in the rehabilitation of lower-back pain (Fischer et al. 2021 and Holmberg et al. 2012). How exactly does it help you stave off injury? In the same way that other lifts do. Strength training creates adaptations specific to the movements you are using. Deadlifts will help strengthen the lower back, the hamstrings, the upper back, and the grip among other things. Furthermore, it's been shown that individuals with lower-back pain move and lift differently during freestyle lifting tasks. Specifically, they move more slowly, more stiffly, and with a deeper knee bend than pain-free people do. This guarded behavior limits their movement options, and in order to recover from lower-back pain, you need to have as many movement options as possible.

Let's talk more about the lower back. The common advice to "lift with your legs, not with your back" may not be that accurate. You can't eliminate the lower back from movements, and what's more, you shouldn't. The lower back, the lumbar spine, and all the surrounding musculature are designed to stabilize you and to transfer force back and forth between upper and lower body. This area is the lynchpin of the entire body; force has no choice but to go through it. Given that fact, the best thing you can do for yourself is to progressively expose that area to those forces, and one of the simplest ways to do this is with the deadlift.

I don't mean to beat this to death. But it's inevitable that at some point, someone will come up to you at the gym and tell you that what you are doing is dangerous. Don't let that derail you or envelop you in fear. I am sure that person means well, but they are simply misinformed.

Elements of the Deadlift

In this section, we will cover all the elements that will help you learn and analyze your own deadlift. We will cover the bar-lifter unit, the bar path, and the bar velocity before heading into the phases of the deadlift. These details will give you the tools needed to learn the deadlift proficiently and build it to higher levels.

Before we begin, let's talk a little about the two most common types of deadlifts with a barbell—the *conventional* and the *sumo*. Throughout this chapter we will cover their similarities and differences. It's best to describe them here though, so you know what we are getting into.

The conventional deadlift stance is with the feet at or inside shoulder width apart and with the grip outside the width of the legs (see figure 5.1*a*). It's called the conventional deadlift because it is the most common one seen, especially in noncompetitive gym environments, and also because it most resembles how someone would typically pick something up off the ground. With the sumo deadlift however, the stance is with the feet wider than shoulder width apart—often much wider—and with the grip shoulder width apart (see figure 5.1*b*). This places the hands inside the width of the legs, more closely resembling the stance of a sumo wrestler. This stance is seen most often in competitive powerlifting, but it can also occasionally be seen in the gym. Neither one is right or wrong. One isn't inherently better than the other. I encourage you to train both on a regular basis to find the one that is most comfortable for you.

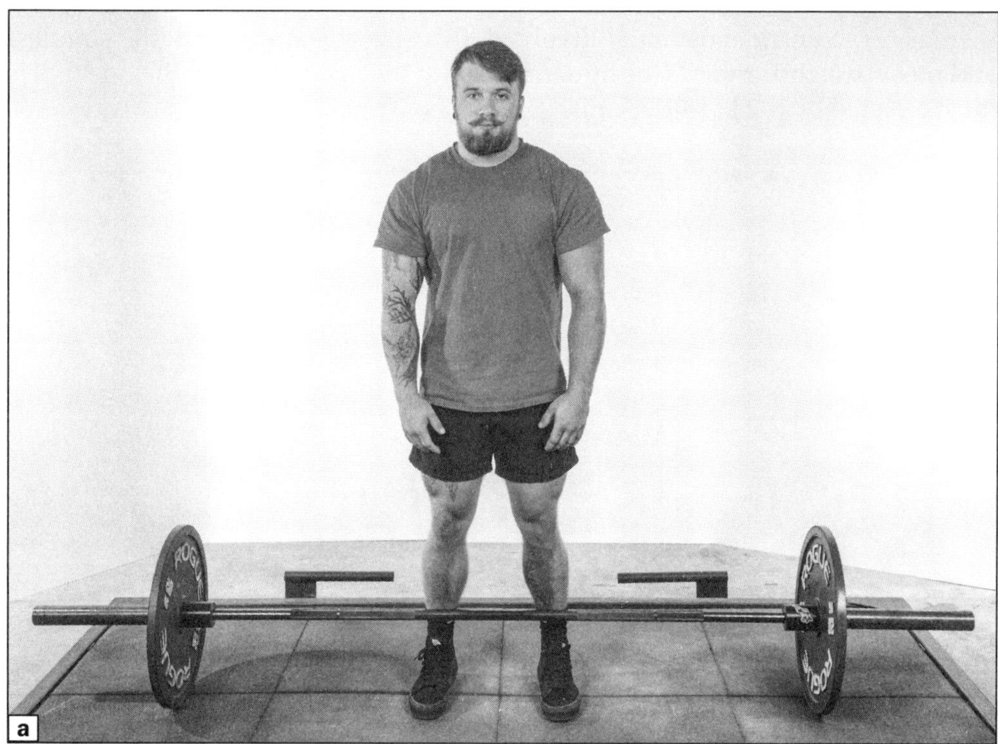

a

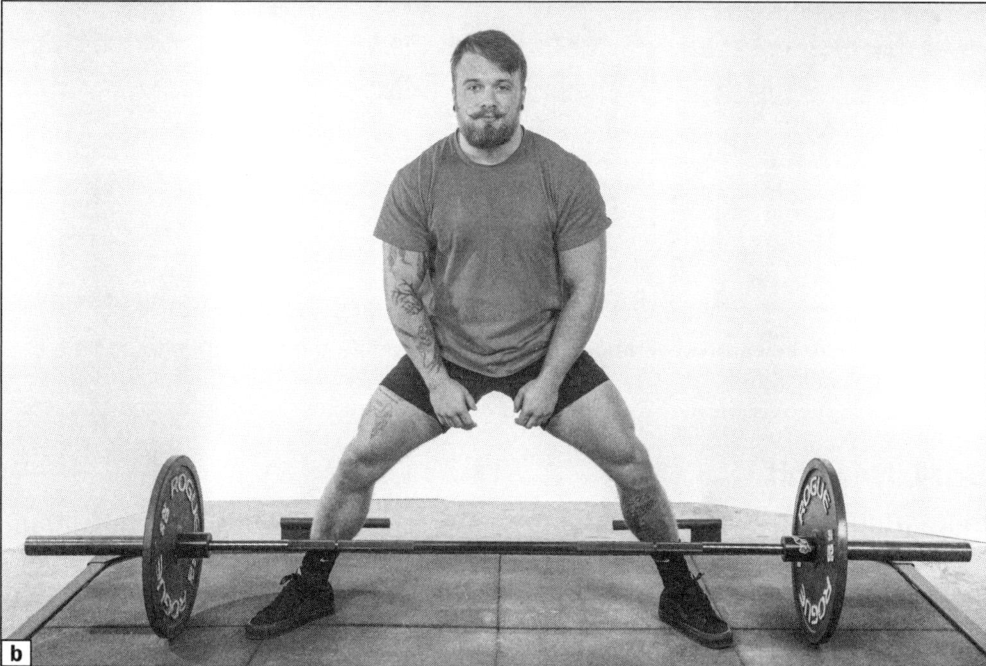

b

FIGURE 5.1 It's easy to see the differences in *(a)* the conventional and *(b)* the sumo deadlift stances. Just remember that one is not better than the other, and that training both is best.

Bar Path

The first thing to look at here is going to be the bar path. For the deadlift, the bar path should be a straight vertical line from the floor all the way to lock-out. That's the number one tenet for the bar path on the deadlift. If the bar path moves a little bit forward off the start, or if it comes a little bit back, then that is going to make the lift much harder to complete. Because the bar is starting on the floor, and there is no eccentric movement involved, this straight-line path is the simplest and most straightforward (see figure 5.2). With that said, it is also the one that is most affected by the bar-lifter unit.

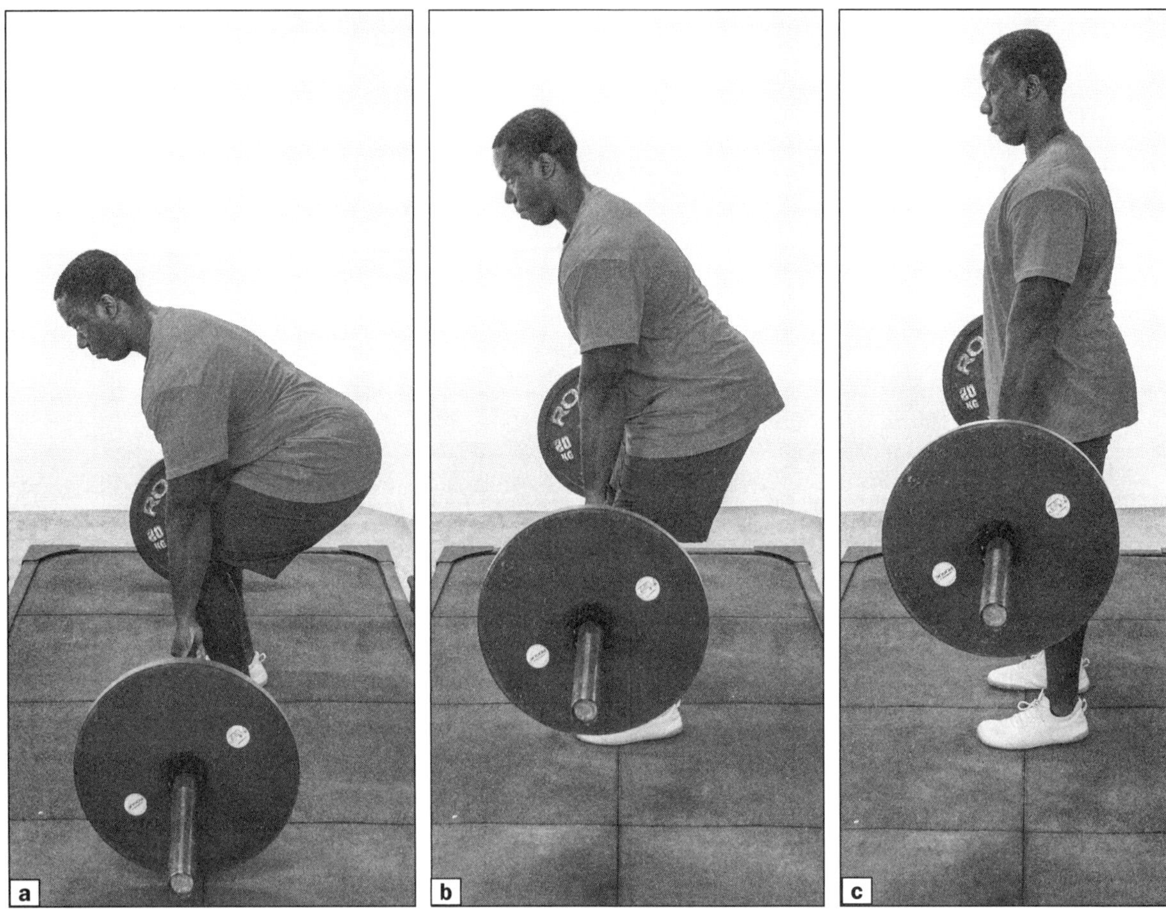

FIGURE 5.2 With there being no eccentric portion to the deadlift, the bar path should be a straight line from the floor to lock-out.

Bar-Lifter Unit

The bar-lifter unit for the deadlift differs quite a bit from the bar-lifter unit for the squat. In the squat, the bar is on your shoulders, and you are able to adjust your start position to make sure the bar is directly over your midfoot. This isn't the case for the deadlift. The deadlift will always be slightly in front of the midfoot because of your shins. The goal with the deadlift is to balance the bar-lifter unit by positioning the barbell in such a way that it leaves the floor in a perfectly vertical direction. As a starting point, position the barbell right over where the knots in your shoes would be if you were to tie them all the way at the top. Then you have to watch how the bar leaves the floor. If you are too close to the bar, the center of gravity for the bar-lifter unit will be out in front of you and the bar (see figure 5.3*a*). The result of this will be the bar swinging out away from you off the floor. If you are too far from the bar, the center of gravity will be closer to you than it is to the bar (see figure 5.3*b*). The result of this will be the bar swinging toward you and probably dragging up your shins. Any horizontal movement during the deadlift makes the lift harder, so find the position where when you start to pull, the bar comes straight up.

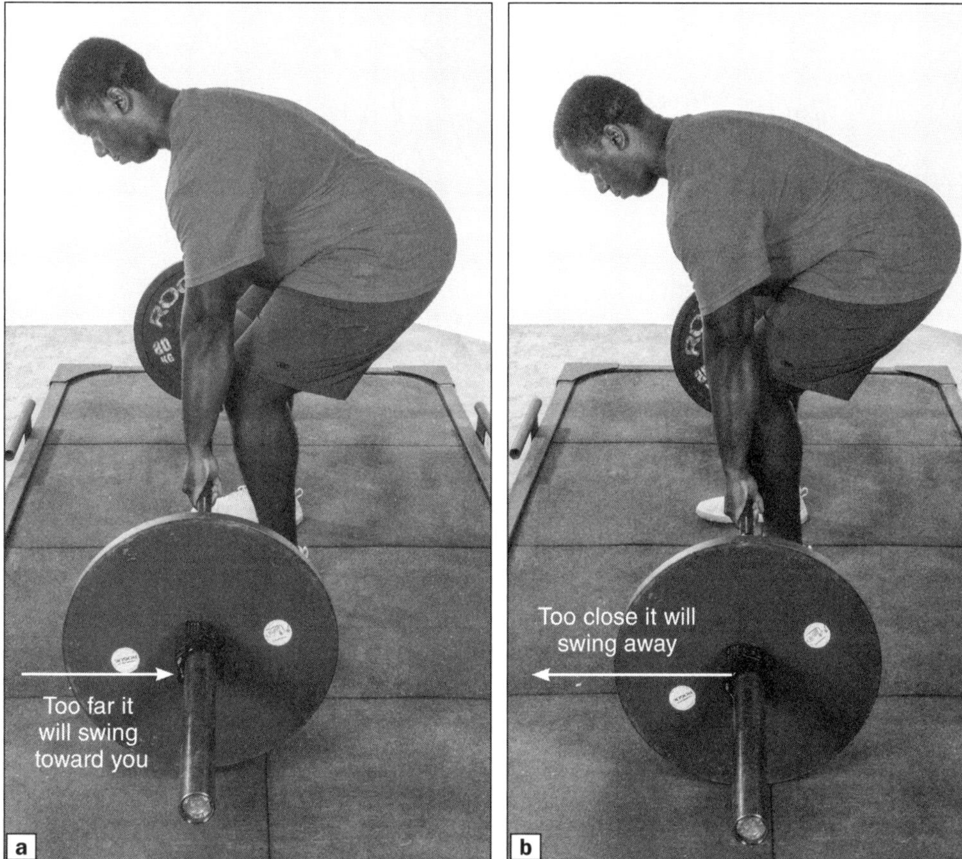

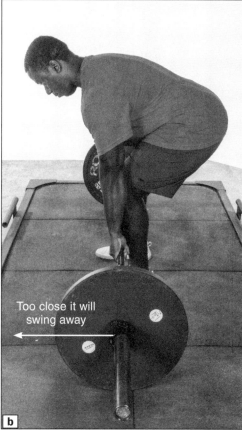

FIGURE 5.3 *(a)* If the bar is too far away, it will swing toward you. *(b)* If it is too close, it will swing away.

Bar Speed

This is where things get interesting with the deadlift. When it comes to the speed of the lift off the floor and near lock-out, the conventional and the sumo differ from each other, though they both have the same kind of trajectory and velocity patterns that you see in the bench press and in the squat. Because the deadlift has no eccentric portion (or lowering of the bar) preceding the concentric portion, there is no preloading of any of the musculature or any of the positions prior to the main movement (pulling and lifting the bar all the way up to lock-out). It's important to conceptualize this at the start and when your sticking points start to happen.

Take a look at figure 5.4. As you can see, the first peak velocity with the conventional deadlift is right off the floor, and then the first decrease in velocity is at the knees or just below the knees for most people. That's when the second overcoming force happens (the first overcoming force is to get it off the ground and moving). Then there's another peak velocity prior to coming to lock-out, and another slowdown on the way to the finish. Conventional deadlifters tend to have a harder time locking-out. Generally, the two sticking points are at the knees and just before the lock-out (see figure 5.5).

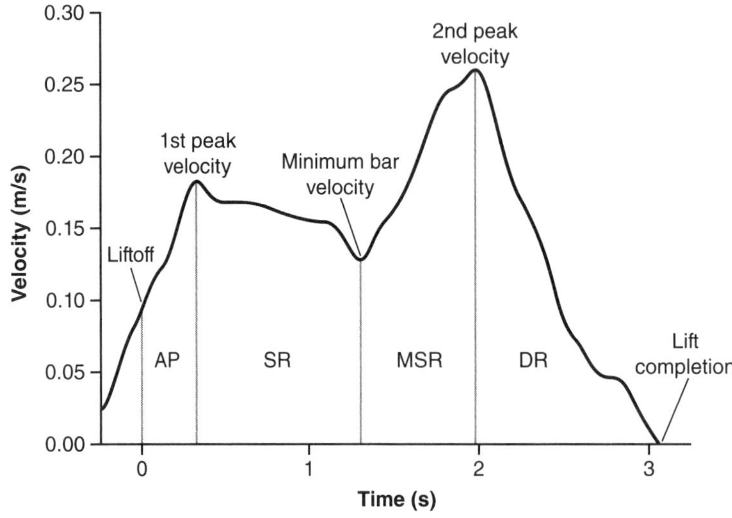

FIGURE 5.4 This is a good look at the vertical bar velocity during a conventional deadlift.

Reprinted by permission from R.F. Escamilla, A.C. Francisco, G.S. Fleisig, et al., "A Three-Dimensional Biomechanical Analysis of Sumo and Conventional Style Deadlifts," *Medicine & Science in Sports & Exercise* 32, no. 7 (2000): 1265-1275.

With the sumo, the bar velocity is flipped: While the bar flies off the floor with a lot of velocity with the conventional, that doesn't happened with the sumo. You'll often hear that sumo deadlifters must be more patient at the start of the lift so that they can be better off the floor and maintain position better. This patience off the floor is needed because the first sticking point in the sumo deadlift is right off the floor (see figure 5.6*a*). As a matter of fact, 10 percent more of the total lift is on the floor in the sumo deadlift compared to the conventional (Escamilla et al. 2000).

The next sticking point for the sumo is at the knees. There's a decrease in bar velocity as the bar approaches the knees and the lifter transitions into the lock-out (see figure 5.6*b*). The lock-out for the sumo is a short range of motion. It tends to be much faster and smoother than it is with the conventional, in addition to being less difficult. I don't want to paint with too broad a brush here—there are some sumo deadlifters who struggle with locking out, most often due to a loss of position. But generally speaking, lock-out for the sumo is easier.

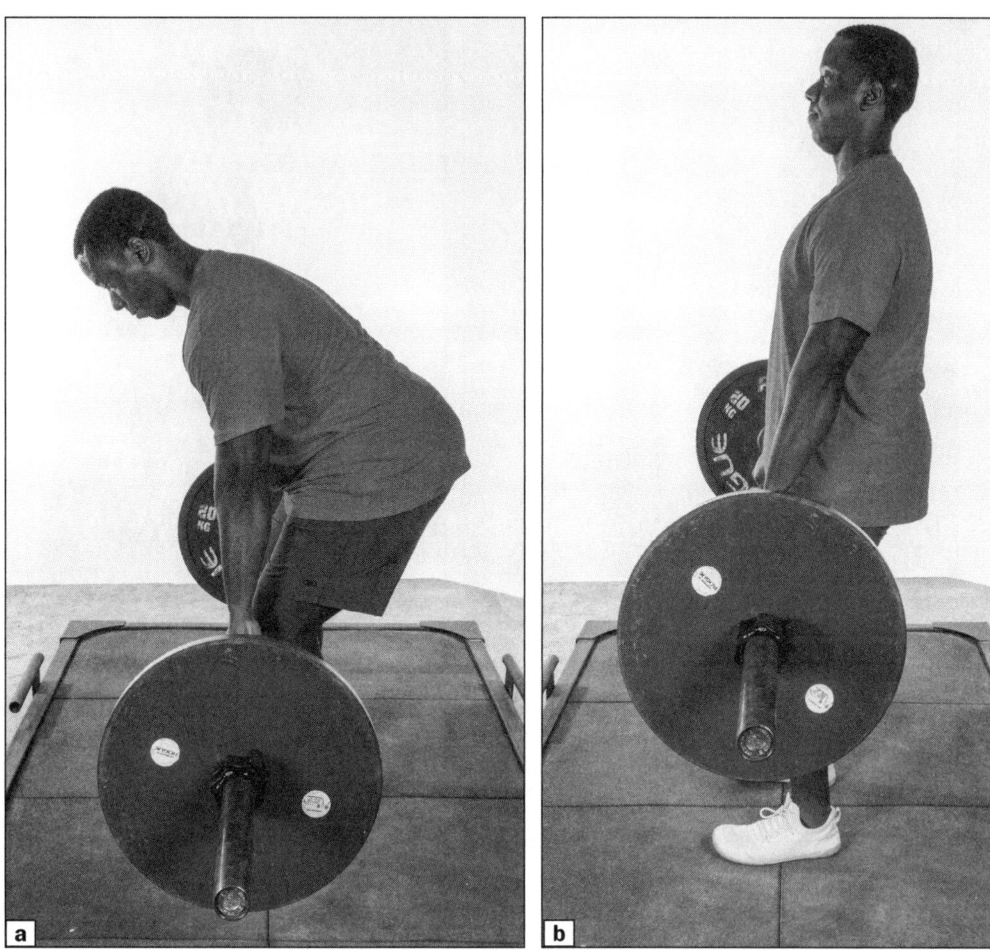

FIGURE 5.5 Two common sticking points in the conventional deadlift are *(a)* at the knees and *(b)* and just before full lock-out.

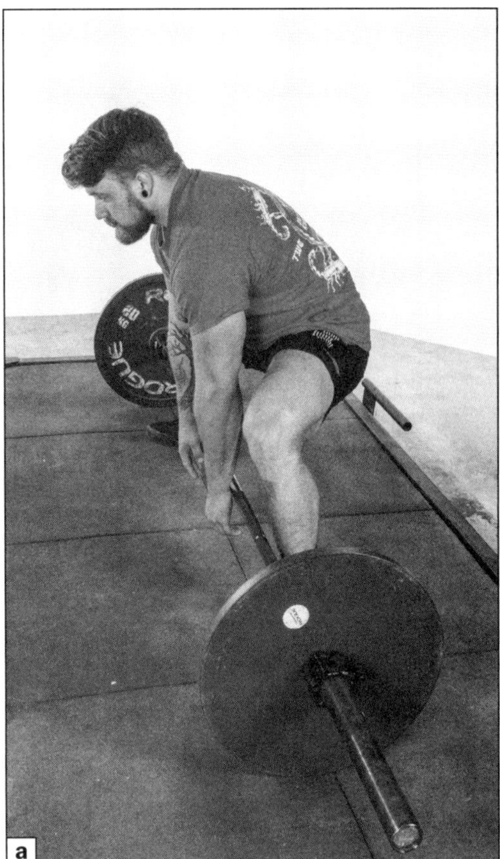
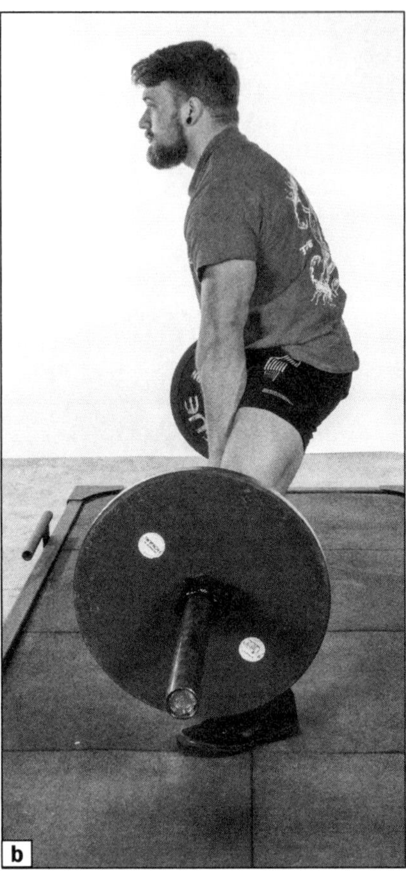

FIGURE 5.6 The two sticking points of the sumo deadlift are *(a)* right off the floor and *(b)* at the knees.

The Phases of the Deadlift

In this section, we will explore the phases of the deadlift: the start position, the ascent, the lock-out, and the descent. There are some distinctions between the conventional and sumo deadlift that I want to make sure we clear up, so we are going to split them up and walk through each of them separately.

Conventional Deadlift

The conventional deadlift is where most people start their deadlifting careers, and it's one of the most common styles that you'll see people using in the gym. It's characterized by the stance being just inside shoulder width apart with the hands grasping the bar outside the width of the legs. Here we will cover the phases of the conventional deadlift: the start position, the ascent, the lock-out, and the descent.

Start Position

First things first: Make sure the bar is at the right height. Adding a 45-pound plate (20 kg) on each end of the bar while it's on the ground just so happens to put the bar at the perfect height. However, the resulting 135 pounds (61 kg), may be too heavy for many to start. So how do you elevate the bar to the right height with the right amount of weight? The simplest solution is to use bumper plates, which are all the same size regardless of weight (see figure 5.7). If your gym doesn't have bumper plates, another solution is to stack plates on top of each other on the floor to create enough height (see figure 5.8). This will allow you to use an empty bar to start if that's a more appropriate starting place.

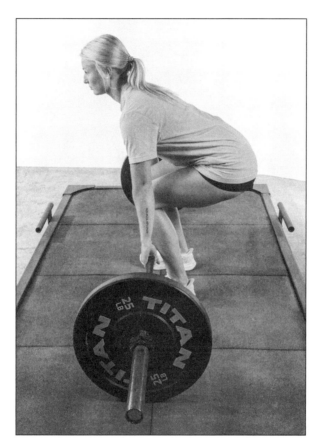

FIGURE 5.7 Bumper plates are the easiest solution for getting the bar to the proper height if you can't lift 135 pounds (61 kg) yet.

The last option is to use a power rack, like you did with squats, and to set the safety bars or pins at the same height as the 45-pound (20 kg) plates. This tends to be the loudest option; the bar will hit the pins when you put it down. You should check with your gym before doing this because some have rules against using the racks in this manner. I don't want you to spend the time setting that up just to get kicked out of the gym.

Now that the bar is at the right height, it's time to get into the starting position. Approach the bar, and position your feet underneath it just inside shoulder width apart. They should be turned out anywhere between 15 and 30 degrees (see figure 5.9). Once your feet are in this position, make sure that the barbell is over your midfoot. If you're in low-top shoes, this is going to be over where your shoes are tied. You should have about an inch of space between the barbell and your shin. That's the position for the barbell. Some people recommend having the bar right up against your shins—which isn't necessarily a bad thing—but that can lead to some bad positions later in the setup.

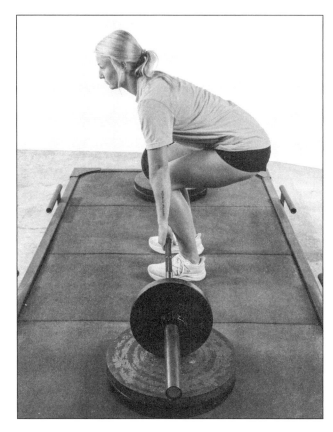

FIGURE 5.8 You can use 25-pound (11 kg) or 45-pound (20 kg) plates and stack them on top of each other to elevate the bar to the correct height.

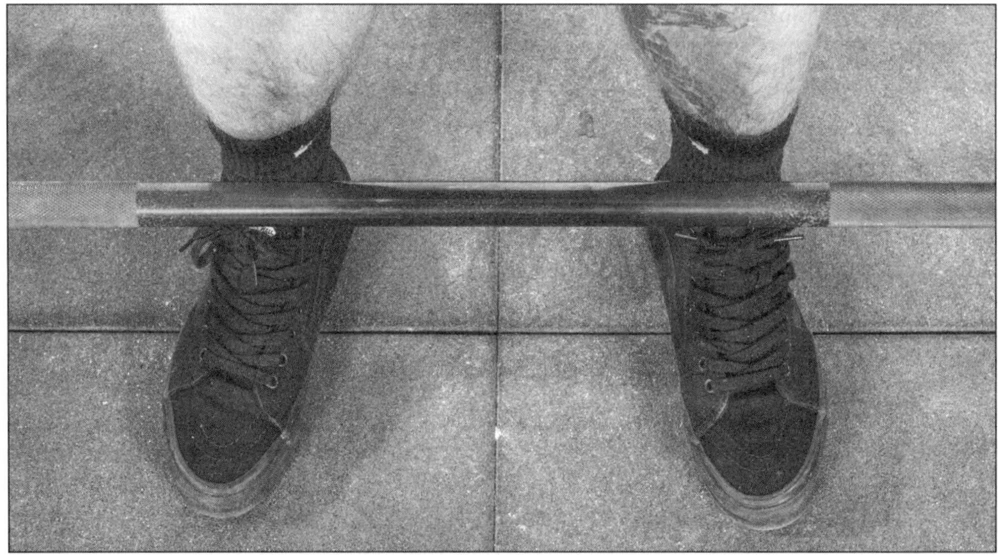

FIGURE 5.9 The foot angle and position with the feet turned slightly out and the shins roughly an inch from the bar is a good starting point for a solid deadlift.

Right now, your feet are underneath the barbell, your shins are about an inch away from the bar, and your toes are pointed out 15 to 30 degrees. It's time to start creating tension in the upper body. The cue that I like to use for the deadlift, and the way that I like to think about this, is to try to protect your armpits by "making your arms long" (see figure 5.10). Imagine that someone comes up behind you and tickles you under your arms. How do you react? You pin your arms down to your sides as hard as possible, keeping them as straight as rods. That's exactly what you should do here. Get your arms nice and straight, pin them down to your sides, and think about reaching your arms to the floor from that standing position. Try to make them as long as possible. This lengthened arm position will create scapular depression, which will pin your shoulder blades down and create tension. This is how you lock in the upper body to keep from losing position when you initiate the pull.

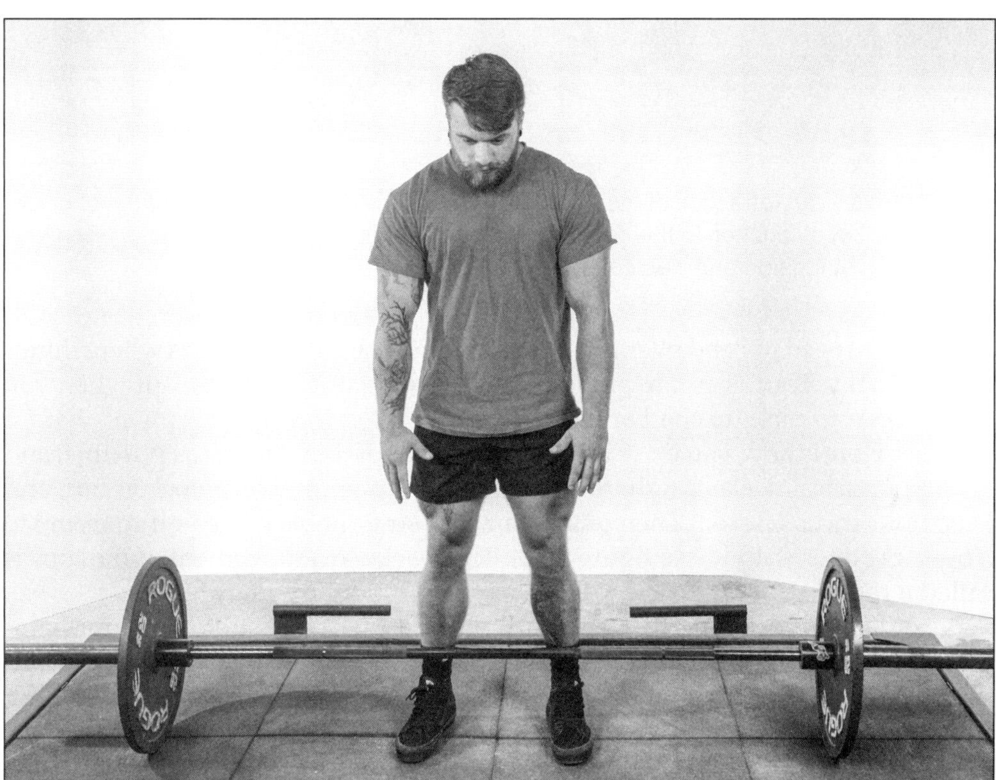

FIGURE 5.10 Making the arms long in the deadlift is a good cue to create upper-body tension.

A common error here is to retract the shoulder blades (see figure 5.11*a*). The problem with this is that it's not a sustainable position to maintain when you start to pull on the barbell. As soon as you start to pull, no matter how tight and strong you may be in that position, your upper back will still not be strong enough to withstand the weight that you're eventually going to lift in a deadlift. It will move those shoulder blades and create too much thoracic flexion. Once you lose that position, the bar will get in front of you a little bit, and it will be a much more difficult lift. Don't think about retraction of the shoulder blades, or trying to pull the shoulder blades together. You want to think about getting the arms long and down (see figure 5.11*b*).

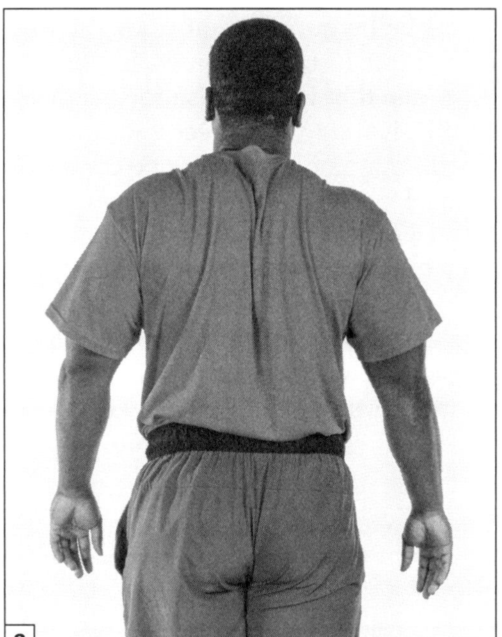

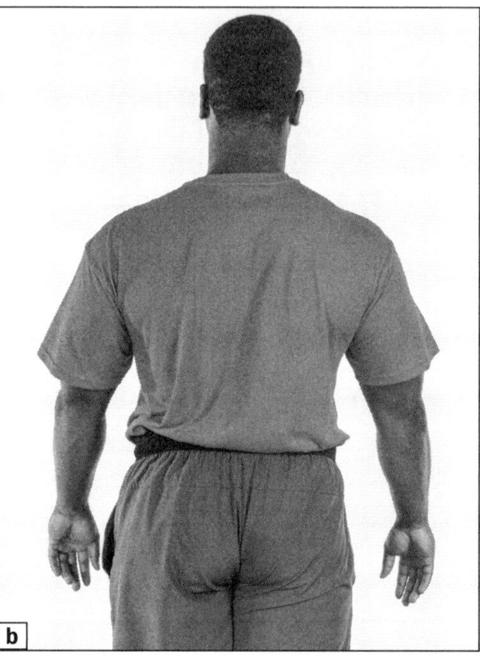

FIGURE 5.11 *(a)* Retraction of the shoulder blades versus *(b)* depression of the shoulder blades is a key distinction in the deadlift. When the ascent starts, retraction is often lost, leading to lost tension and wasted energy.

Now you need to bend over and get your hands on the bar. This is where things can get tricky: Your arms are pinned down straight at your sides, but when you bend down to pick up the barbell, you'll need to swing your arms forward a little bit. Here is how you do it: Maintain as much of that tension as possible, and keep your arms nice and tight to your sides. Keep your elbows locked out, and keep your triceps flexed. Then push your butt straight back like you're trying to close a car door with it (see figure 5.12). This backward movement of the hips is called a hinge.

Next, let yourself bend forward until you start to feel a stretch in your hamstrings. This is when you start flexing your knees and reaching down toward the bar. Get close enough to grasp the bar with your hands, being careful not to overshoot the bar (see figure 5.13). If your hands overshoot the bar, you risk losing tension. Focus on staying as tight as possible, not overshooting the bar, bending your knees, and pushing your hips back just enough to get within grasp of the barbell. I will talk about different grips that you can use in a little bit, but you should start with the double overhand. Grab the bar with both hands, and squeeze it as tightly as possible. Your hands should be directly underneath your shoulders—not a little wider and not a little narrower. If you're a bigger individual, however, you may have to widen the grip slightly so that your legs don't run into your arms during the pull.

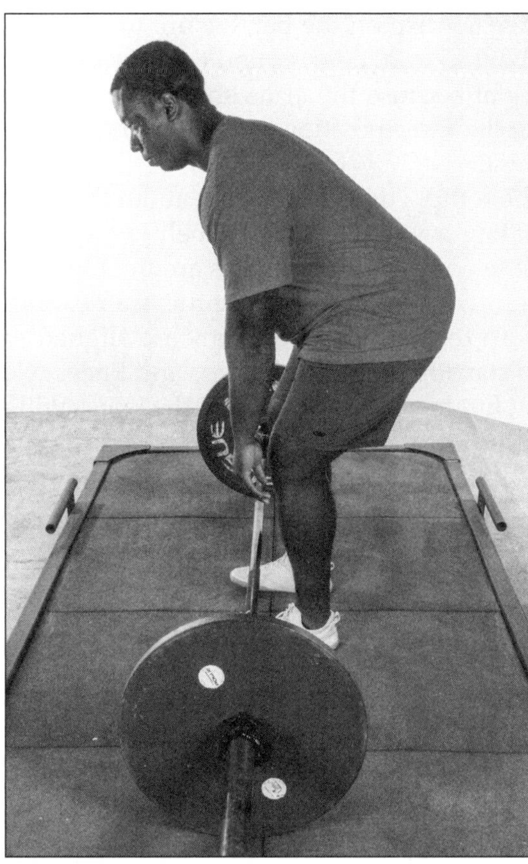

FIGURE 5.12 A proper hinge should look like you are trying to close your car door with your butt. It's a direct push back with hips as shown.

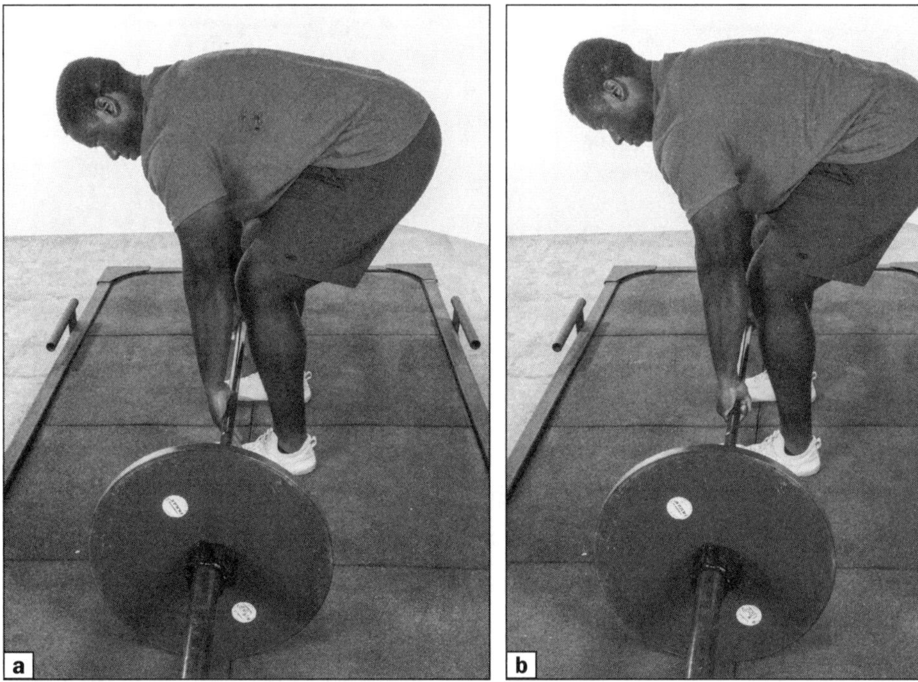

FIGURE 5.13 *(a)* Don't overshoot the bar with your hands, which risks losing the tension you've built. *(b)* You should be just within reach of the bar if you set up correctly.

Now that you have a grasp on the bar, ensure that your feet are underneath the bar and pointed out 15 to 30 degrees and that your knees are bent. Your back should be nice and flat because the arms should be locked in super tight. The bar should still be in the same position on the ground. That tension hasn't gone anywhere at this point.

At this point in the setup, you should think about the barbell, your arms, and your shoulders creating a window. The barbell is the bottom of the window, your arms are the sides, and your shoulders are the top. If you were looking at yourself in a mirror, it would be easy to see this frame. Shifting to a side view, the knees should push forward to where they are aligned with the front of the arms. This is a good starting point for the hips and knees to create a better push off the floor for most lifters. With taller lifters, the knees will come past the front of the arms, and with shorter lifters the knees stay behind the front of the arms. Wedge into the bar by sliding your hips forward toward the bar and letting your knees drift forward to the appropriate spot (see figure 5.14*a*). It's important to note that you're not bending the knees and squatting down to the bar which is a common error (see figure 5.14*b*).

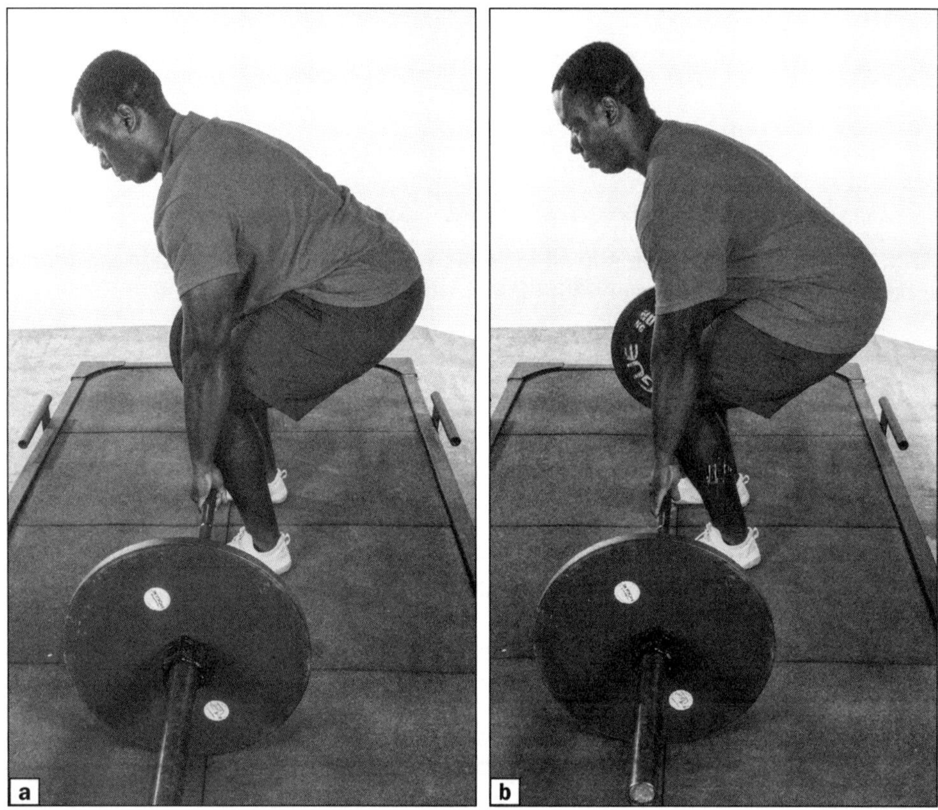

FIGURE 5.14 *(a)* Correct wedging into the bar by getting the knees through the window and *(b)* incorrect squatting to the bar.

You should feel like a loaded spring that's about to pop. Your eyes should be looking 10 to 15 feet out in front of you. Don't move your head in any direction; keeping it still is what will help keep you in a good solid position. As you stand up, keep your eyes looking 10 to 15 feet in front of you.

It's almost time to pull the bar off the floor, but we need to have a discussion about bracing first. Bracing is what helps you create as much tension as possible through your core and trunk. There are two different ways to brace in a deadlift: a top-down brace or a bottom brace. The top-down brace is the one that I personally use: I get my feet set up underneath the bar, I stack my shoulders down with long arms, and then I take a big breath in and tighten my core. Then I go through the rest of the setup sequence holding that brace. The bottom brace is the opposite of the top-down technique. You go through the entire setup sequence and then brace at the bottom just before you initiate the pull. I've also seen people get into the start position and roll the bar away from them to create space to get more air. This is known as a *dynamic start*, and I don't suggest it within the context of this book because it can create inconsistencies in start positions. Ultimately, the bracing technique you decide to employ in the deadlift is all going to come down to personal preference. Try both, and find the one that works best for you right now. Don't get married to just one approach though. Six months down the road it may become less effective, and you'll need to switch to the other one.

With your bracing locked in, you are now in the full start position (see figure 5.15). Let's be super clear: This is not a comfortable position, and you don't want to stay in it for an extended period of time. If you've done it correctly, you've created a lot of tension throughout your entire body, and now that tension wants to go somewhere. That "somewhere" is the barbell, so let's go ahead and start tugging.

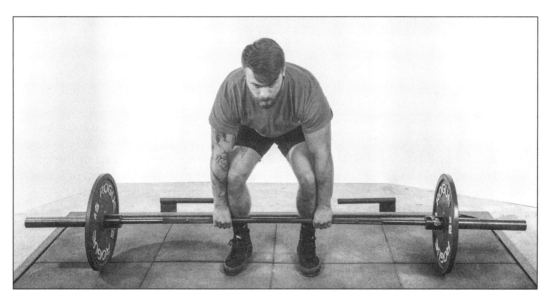

FIGURE 5.15 A proper deadlift start position with long arms creating scapular depression, feet turned out slightly, knees pushing "through the window" to wedge into the bar, core braced tightly, and hands gripped firmly around the bar.

Learn How to Brace

We covered this back in chapter 3, but it's important enough that I want to repeat it here. When it comes to bracing, the common advice to fill your belly with air is only one part of the puzzle. To have a strong, effective brace, you need to create 360 degrees of pressure around your torso. A way I love to teach this is by using a belt, and it doesn't have to be a lifting belt to start. You can use the one holding up your pants right now.

To begin, place the belt around your waist at belly-button height. You don't want it super tight. On the contrary, you want it loose, with a little wiggle room. Now take a big breath in—slowly—like we talked about in the setup to get ready to unrack for the squat. What you should feel is not just your stomach pushing out and into the belt but your whole abdomen and lower back beginning to push into the belt. Fill up the space between your torso and the belt so that your torso presses into the belt, locking it in place. If you need more feedback to feel this, grab a friend and have them put their hand inside the belt at your lower back. That tends to be the hardest place to feel this. Now hold that breath and bear down. Feel the pressure build up inside and the belt get even tighter. The last step is to top yourself off with a short, sharp breath through the nose. Then you'll feel what I'm talking about when it comes to tension and bracing. To learn this faster, do it a few times each day as part of your warm-up.

A word of caution: Some of you may get lightheaded when you first start doing this because you aren't used to the pressure you can create. There is no need to achieve that level of pressure early on, so scale it back if you feel this way. Also, over time you will adapt and be able to handle more and more pressure as you get stronger (Blazek et al. 2019). The human body is amazing and can adapt to nearly anything you throw at it, so keep practicing your bracing.

The Ascent

The ascent is when you start to move the bar off the floor, in that straight vertical line, all the way to lock-out. The number one thing to focus on when you initiate the pull is not pulling the bar itself but pulling the slack out of the bar. The intent here is to get as much of the tension into the barbell that you possibly can before you explode into it. Think of this as "getting the rattle out" of the bar. What does that mean? You have the barbell itself, and you have the sleeves on the ends. When the barbell is at rest, it sits at the bottom of those sleeves. When you pull on it slightly, you can hear it rattle at the ends as the bar rattles around in the sleeves. Initiate your pull by getting the rattle out of the bar first. Then as you get stronger and the weight gets heavier, this will help deflect the barbell because the barbell will bend. By getting the rattle out, you'll get all the slack out of the barbell before you pull so that all the force that you explode with goes into the weight itself and not into bending the barbell (see figure 5.16). We don't want to waste any of the energy needed to hit maximum loads, so get the slack out of the bar. That's step number one.

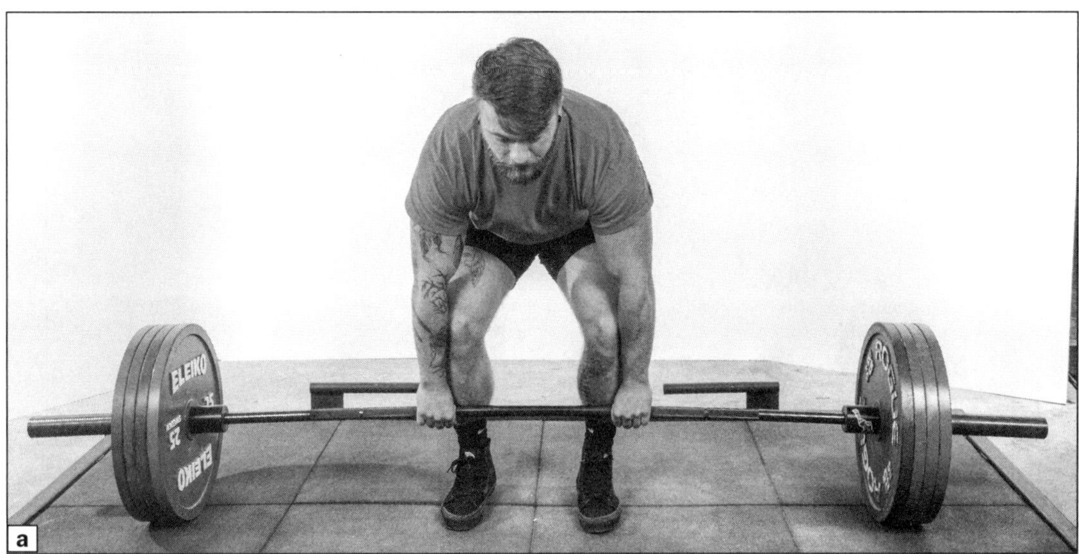

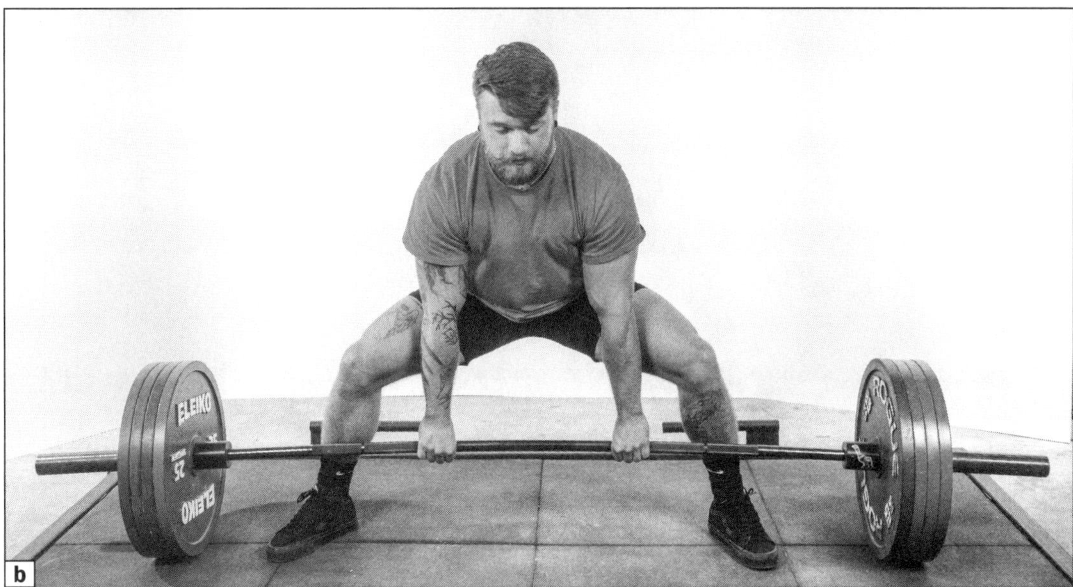

FIGURE 5.16 Heavy weights on a barbell will cause the bar to bend before the plates start to come off the ground. This bend, or slack, needs to be taken out of the bar as the first part of the ascent. You can see that here with *(a)* no tension on the bar and *(b)* with tension on the bar (sumo deadlift shown here for illustrative purposes since tension is easier to see in the sumo).

The last thing you want to do is to try to pull on the bar with your straight, long arms just to bend your elbows and throw away all the tension you created. Instead, wedge into the bar. Think about pushing your feet into the floor as hard as you can—almost like you're trying to do a leg press. Try to push the ground away from you, and drive your chest up. This should put you in position, and you should feel your arms get tighter. You should feel a rattle come out of the bar and feel all your tension ramp up even higher. Now you are like a loaded slingshot that's ready to fire. This is when you initiate the pull. If you are wondering what slack being pulled out of a bar looks like, see figure 5.17.

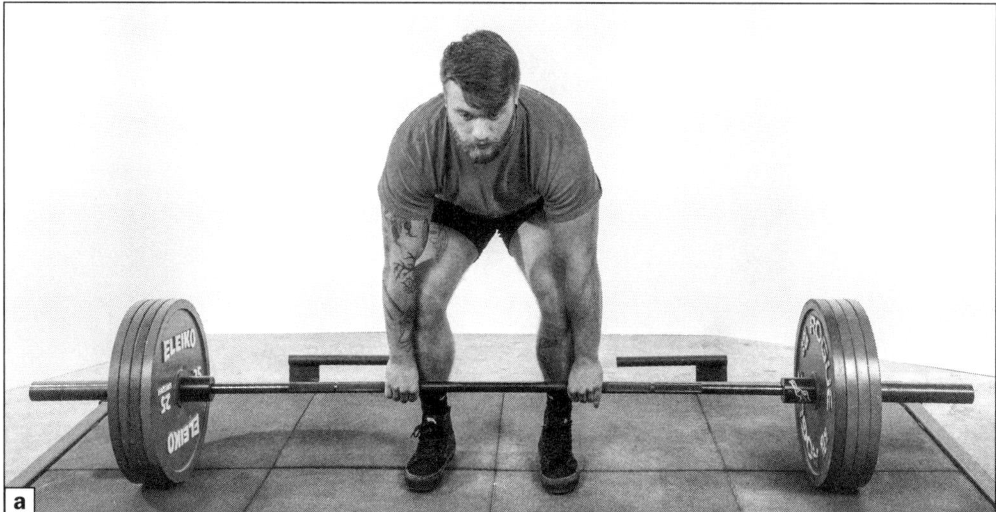

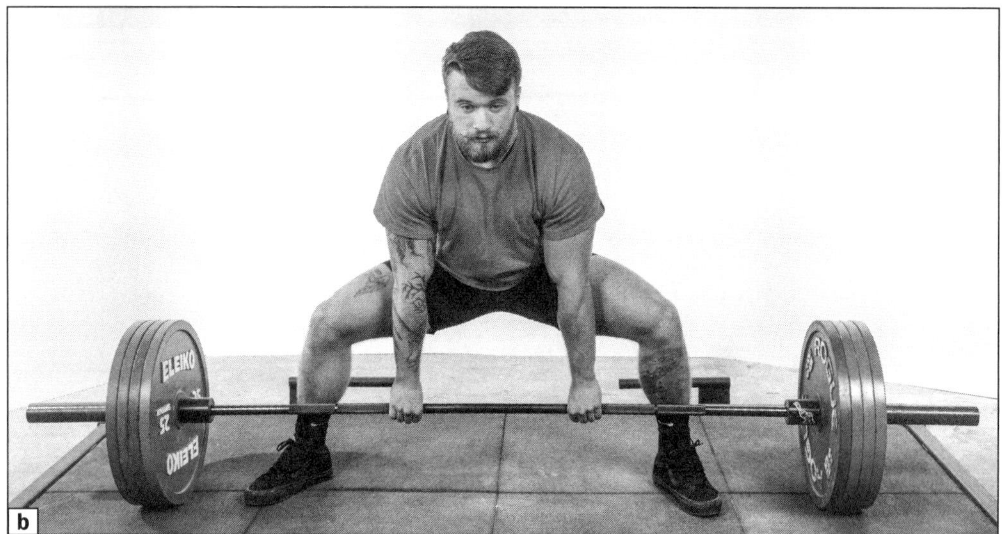

FIGURE 5.17 The start position *(a)* with no slack pulled out of the bar versus *(b)* where slack has been pulled out of the bar (sumo deadlift shown here for illustrative purposes since this is easier to see in the sumo). Notice how the position of the lifter changes.

Funnily enough, it's not a pull that you start with. It's a push. Keep pushing with the legs, driving as hard as you possibly can into the floor. This initial push will bring the barbell to just below your knees. This is where the transition happens. Ed Coan, one of the greatest powerlifters of all time (arguably *the* greatest), is responsible for one of the greatest cues I've ever heard: If you start thinking about bringing your hips to the bar when the bar is at or above your knees, it's far too late. You need to start thinking about that as the bar approaches the bottom of your knees because that is where the transition to a hip hinge truly happens. That's when the hips come very aggressively toward the barbell to get it to lock-out. To do this, you need to drive your chest up and your hips toward the barbell as hard and as fast as humanly possible (see figure 5.18). If you're doing this with lighter weight, it should be so fast, and the bar should stay so close to you, that you hit the barbell with your hips. That is what's going to get you to lock-out in a conventional deadlift.

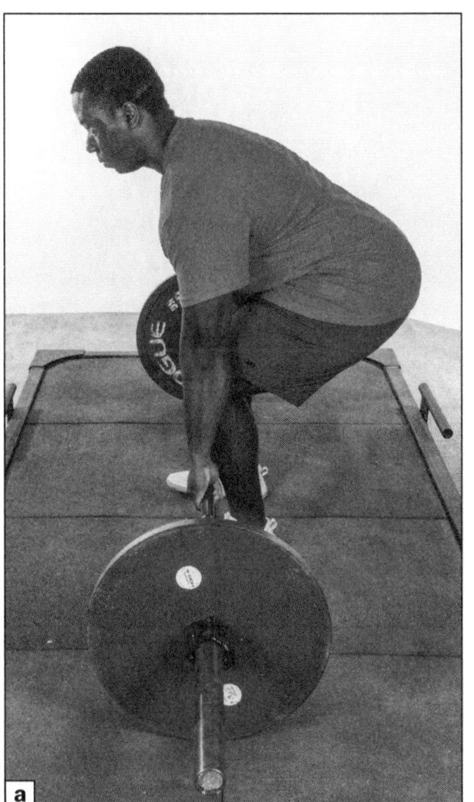

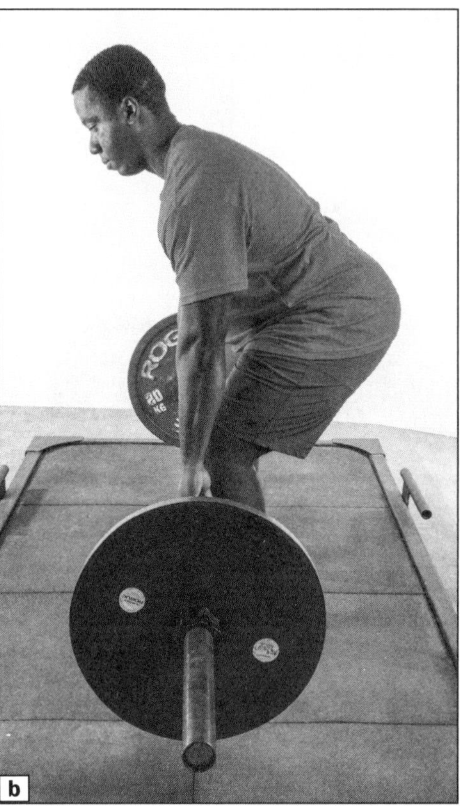

FIGURE 5.18 *(a)* The initial push off the floor shouldn't result in the hips going straight up. *(b)* The lifter should be in a position very similar to the start position but with the bar more elevated.

Old-school power lifters may talk about how bloody shins are the mark of a great deadlift. That's wrong. The bar should stay as close to your body as possible, but scraping your shins means the bar is too close. This tends to put you over top of the bar too much, causing you to lose leverage. Your knees will lock out early, and it'll put you in a position where lock-out becomes more difficult. Another common error is getting to lock-out and then leaning back super far (see figure 5.19*a*). When you lean back, your knees unlock. From a competitive standpoint, you must lock the legs for the lift to count. Additionally, it is wasted movement, making the lift less efficient and leading to poorer results over time. So when you get to lock-out, stand up straight, squeeze your glutes, and pull your shoulder back. That's how you finish a conventional deadlift. (see figure 5.19*b*). All that's left to do now is to put the bar down and celebrate.

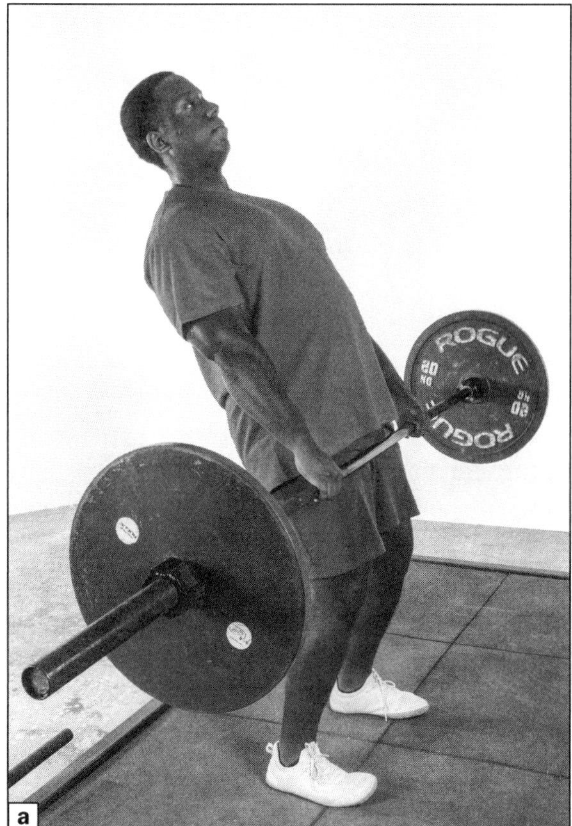

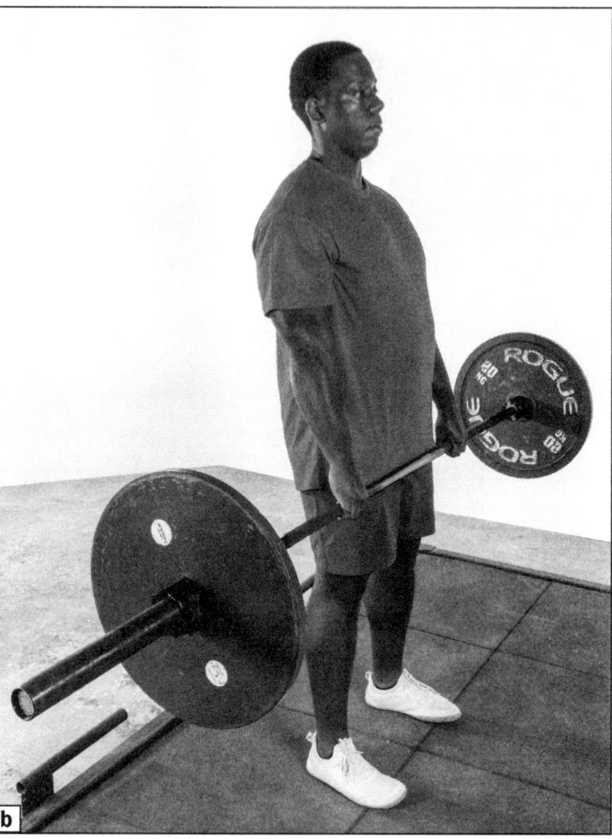

FIGURE 5.19 *(a)* An overextended lock-out with the shoulders extended past the hips, causing the knees to unlock versus *(b)* a complete lock-out with the shoulders hips and knees stacked on top of each other.

The Descent

There are two different ways to approach the descent of the conventional deadlift, and which one you choose depends on your goals. If hypertrophy, or an increase in muscle mass, is your main goal, a slower and controlled descent of the bar is best. The eccentric portion of lifts creates the largest hypertrophic stimulus to muscles, so controlling the weight down makes the most sense for that goal. If strength is the main goal, I suggest putting the bar down with little to no eccentric. Either way, the movement is going to stay the same.

To initiate the descent in the conventional deadlift, push your hips straight back just like you did to go from standing straight to the hinge in the starting position. Make sure you keep your breath in, and don't relax your brace. When you do this, the bar will start moving down past your thighs. As the bar begins to approach your knees, bend your knees while maintaining the tension in your core and trunk until the bar touches the floor (see figure 5.20). Whatever you do, don't open your hands and drop the bar from lock-out or try to accelerate the bar to the floor by pushing it down and slamming it. Both of those are poor gym etiquette and can get you kicked out of a lot of places. For the slower and more controlled descent that is good for hypertrophy, this phase lasts around two to three seconds and brings the bar back to the ground with exceptional control. The little to no eccentric takes under a second, and the bar descends at the speed of gravity.

Why do I differentiate these two styles of putting the bar down? When strength is the goal, the weight tends to be much heavier, and the eccentric portion of the lift creates a lot of fatigue. This fatigue, especially if you are going to be doing consecutive reps, can make maintaining positioning in the ascent on reps much harder. This variation in position can lead to less efficiency during the sets (and I would prefer to keep those reps as consistent as possible). Plus, there's no difference in terms of injury rates between the slow eccentric or little to no eccentric. As a coach, I am biased in favor of striving for as much quality as possible on the ascent in order to build as much strength there as possible—especially since competition in the deadlift is about how much you can pick up, not how much you can put down. I want as much energy going into the ascent as possible.

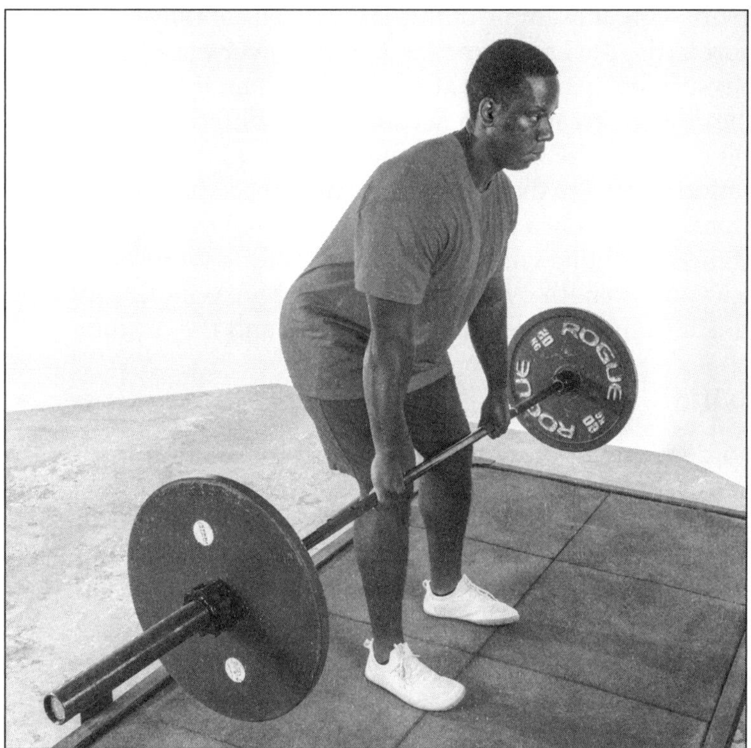

FIGURE 5.20 Putting the bar down in the deadlift is similar to getting into the start position. Hinge the hips back to start. As the bar approaches the knees, bend the knees until the bar is back on the ground.

Sumo Deadlift

Now it's time to learn how to cheat. That's right—according to the Internet, sumo deadlifting is cheating. In reality, the only time that it's cheating is during a Strongman competition (where it's not allowed). The sumo deadlift is characterized by a stance that is wider than shoulder width apart and by a grip on the bar that is inside the width of the legs. In some cases, the stance is so wide that the feet nearly touch the plates at the ends of the bar. This stance can greatly decrease the range of motion that's needed to get the barbell to lock-out. This is the main reason that people will claim that using this stance is cheating. However, a deadlift is simply lifting a barbell from the floor to lock-out. Whether it's sumo or conventional, it's all deadlifting as far as I'm concerned.

Cheating jokes aside, I'm going to teach you the sumo deadlift because I find it to be an incredibly valuable way to deadlift. I'm a firm believer that everyone should deadlift both conventional and sumo. Having both options is ideal for many reasons, but there are two that are the biggest to me. The first is that the conventional and sumo deadlift build each other. In the course of training, plateaus will occur where an increase in strength is harder to come by. By using both stances, when one plateaus, you can switch to the other and continue to build. Over the course of years of training, this can be very valuable to keep progress going and to help decrease the frustration of plateaus. The other reason I encourage people to learn both stances is so that they have options when aches and pains creep up. A great example of this is when a lifter may be experiencing pain or discomfort in the lower back or the knees. Lower-back discomfort can creep up with conventional deadlifting at times, and when this happens, switching to sumo for the day is a great option because of the different leverages the lift puts on the lower back. On the flip side, some sumo deadlifters can experience some knee discomfort similar to the pain you see with the squat. In this case, switching to conventional deadlift is a great option because of the way it loads the knees. Having options in training will increase your training longevity and that, in turn, will increase your strength over time. From here we will dive into the phases of the sumo deadlift: the start position, the ascent, and the descent.

Start Position

Great sumo deadlifters know the importance of a solid and repeatable start position for this lift. Your stance is going to be much, much wider, with your feet about twice shoulder width apart. To gauge the width here, I suggest using the rings on the barbell just like we did with grip on the squat and the bench press. Start with your shins aligned with the first ring and with the barbell the same distance from you as it was for the conventional deadlift. Turning your feet out at a greater degree (as much as 45 to 60 degrees for the sumo versus 15 to 30 degrees for the conventional) doesn't necessarily change the position of the bar over the foot. It should still be over your midfoot with the barbell roughly one inch away from your shins (see figure 5.21). You want that toe-out because it opens up the hips so they can function effectively in this position. Additionally, the hips are typically closer to the bar with the sumo deadlift, and the torso is more vertical—not completely vertical, but more so than with the conventional. Because of this, a lot of people have stated that the sumo deadlift is more quad dominant.

Now you need to create tension. The way to do this in the sumo deadlift is to envision yourself trying to rip the floor apart with your feet. Try to spread the floor or pull your heels apart, and try to rip the ground in half. Then set your shoulders nice and tight by making the arms long and pinning them down to your sides just like we did for the conventional deadlift. When you hinge back to bring your hands to the barbell, one thing to be aware of is that the stretch in the hamstrings typically comes on faster when your stance is wider (see figure 5.22). Once you feel that stretch, bend your knees just enough to get your hands on the bar.

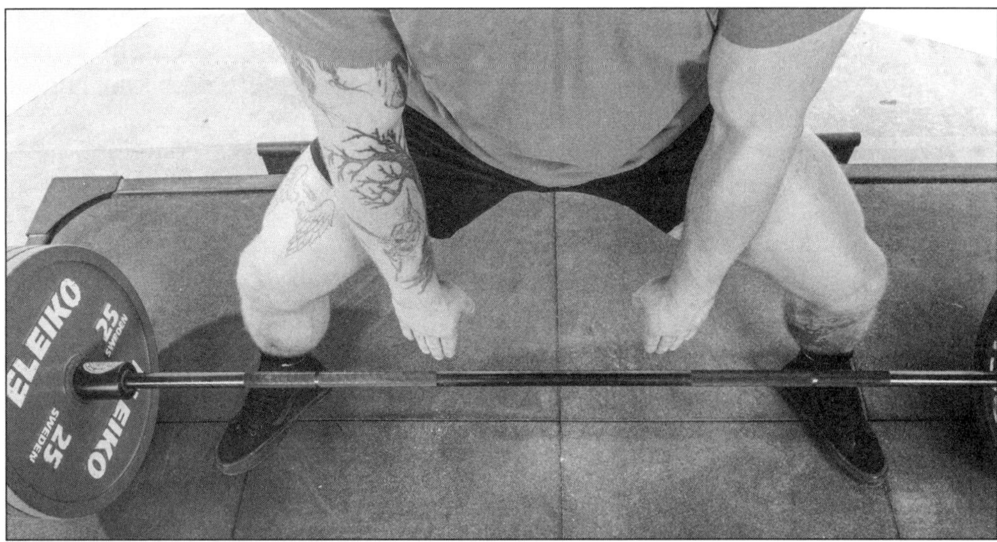

FIGURE 5.21 A wider stance creates a greater angle of the feet in the sumo deadlift.

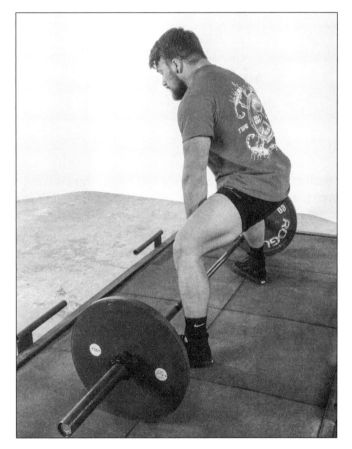

FIGURE 5.22 The initial hinge back to the barbell may cause the hamstring tension you are looking for to occur earlier in the sumo deadlift due to the widened stance and your hips being in closer proximity to the bar.

Your grip on the bar is inside the legs in the sumo stance, but the general guideline of keeping your hands directly underneath your shoulders still stands (see figure 5.23). I've seen beginners come in and grab the center knurling of the bar because they think they must have a much narrower grip. This isn't the case. You should be able to grab the barbell very easily with your hands straight down at your sides.

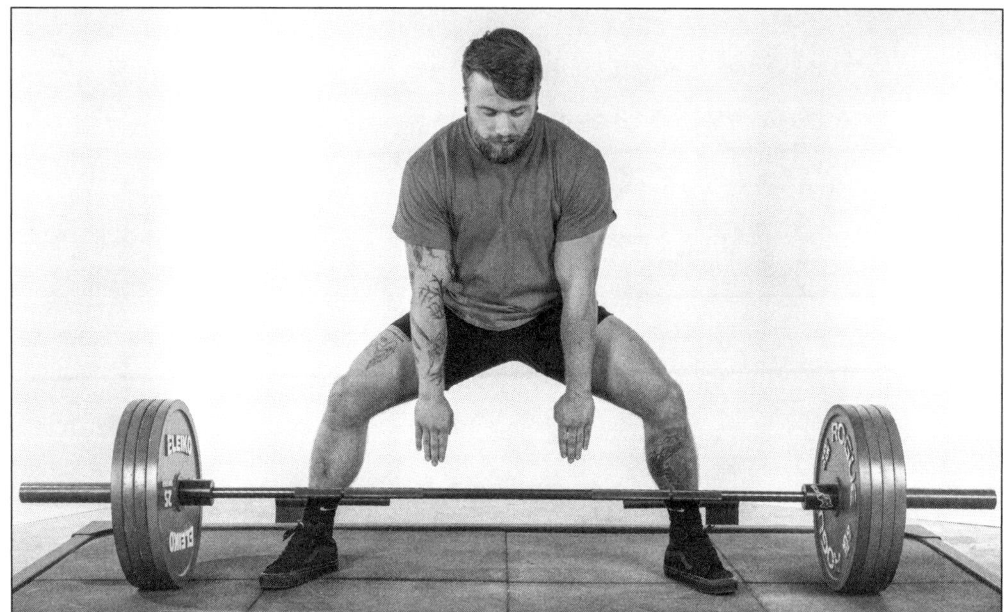

FIGURE 5.23 The hands in the sumo deadlift should be just underneath the shoulders.

Now you're ready to get the bar moving and begin the ascent. Don't skip your bracing! You have the same options here as with conventional: to brace from the top down or at the bottom of the start position. Either way, a firm brace is just as important with the sumo deadlift as it is with the other lifts. Take the time to lock in your bracing before you try to start moving the bar.

The Ascent

Now you are ready to pull the slack out of the bar. This is what is going to lock you in to a more vertical torso position and create more tension through the body (see figure 5.24). As with the conventional, keep your arms long and drive your chest up as you wedge your hips forward. One difference here for sumo is that you should also push your knees out as you wedge to create space for the hips. It's the same "knees through the window" concept but this time, the knees are outside the window. The key is to wedge into the bar by opening your hips. Just like with the conventional, this will improve your pull by bringing your hips closer to the bar and better balancing the bar-lifter unit.

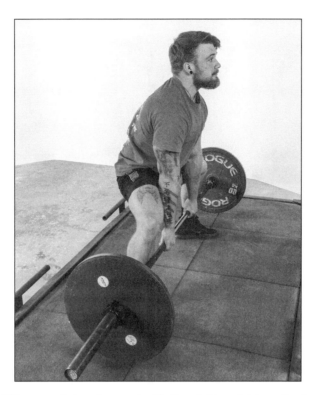

FIGURE 5.24 With enough tension and with the right weight on the bar, you should be tight enough to elevate the bar just slightly off the floor.

This is when you need to be patient because breaking the bar off the floor in sumo is the hardest part of the lift. It's still a push from the floor, but with the sumo, it's a push down and out (versus just pushing down like with a leg press). That "spread the floor" cue stands throughout the entire pull. This is the biggest difference between the sumo pull and the conventional pull. It's easy to tell if you aren't spreading the floor in this position because the deadlift will look like a conventional deadlift with a wide stance: The bar won't start moving until the hips rise too high, and the bar will get left out in front. For the sumo deadlift, you push down and out and drive the chest up. As you keep driving, the bar will start to move. Just like with the conventional, once the bar is moving, you need to keep pushing until it's approaching your knees. Remember that if you start thinking "hips to the bar" when it's at your knees, it's too late. As the bar approaches your knees, start driving your hips to the bar aggressively while you continue to stand up. A key thing to look for here is for the shins to be vertical just like with the conventional deadlift. This sets up an effective hinge to the bar and allows you to keep your balance through to lock-out (see figure 5.25). The shins should not be forward or inclined back but completely vertical.

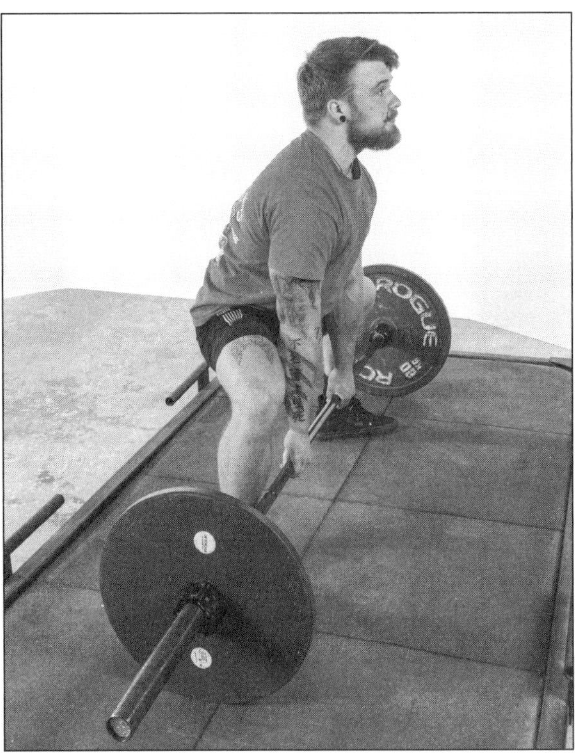

FIGURE 5.25 The vertical shin position in the sumo deadlift is key for keeping the bar-lifter unit in balance and setting up a successful hinge to lock-out.

With your shins vertical and the bar moving past your knees, you should already be starting to hinge, or bring your hips to the bar. Think of your hips like a door hinge in this instance. A door hinge can only move in one way, and that's to open and close. Your hips start off the lift "closed." Now you're going to forcefully open that hinge. This is a crucial balance point. With the wider stance, the balance from front to back is more difficult than with the conventional. It's important here to not lean back hard all the way at the top; this can cause you to stumble backward and lose balance. Stand tall, squeeze your glutes, let that big smile spread across your face, and then put the bar down.

The Descent

The descent of the sumo deadlift follows the same rules as the conventional deadlift with one added detail. With the wider stance, there is a risk of the feet sliding out slightly during the lift, leaving the pinky toes in a very precarious position for the descent (directly under the weights on the bar). If your stance is so wide that your feet start close to the plates, then once you have locked out the bar and are ready to put it down, turn your feet in slightly as you initiate your hip hinge back to bring the bar down. This will save those precious little pinky toes from getting smashed under the weight.

From here, the rest of the descent is the reverse of the ascent. Your hips hinge back, lowering the bar down your thighs until it hits knee level (see figure 5.26). Once it's there, bend your knees and bring the bar down to a stop back on the floor. Note that with the wider stance, the torso position stays more upright during this phase, with the last lowering portion to the floor looking very similar to a squat.

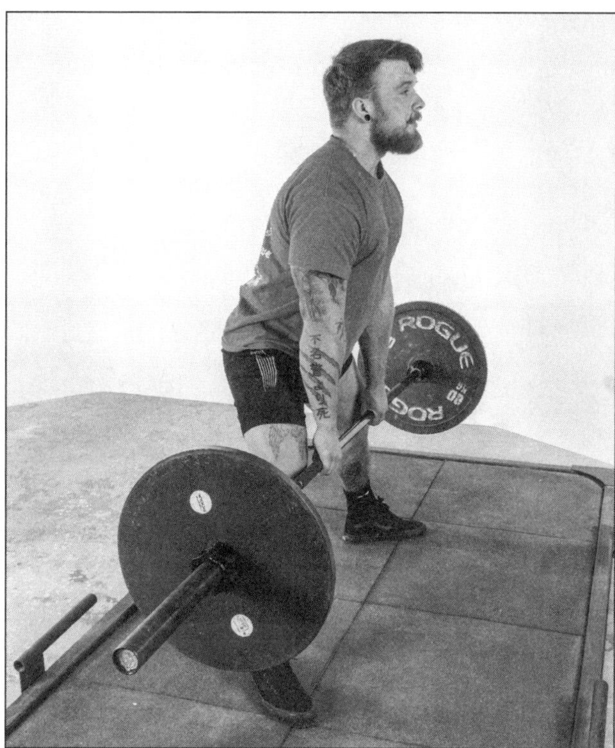

FIGURE 5.26 Initiating the return of the bar to the floor with a sumo deadlift requires a hinge back similar to a squat as shown.

Grips for the Deadlift

As you know, I teach the double overhand grip first because it is the easiest to incorporate. However, it is also the weakest grip, and it will very quickly become the limiting factor when lifting heavy weights due to the bar spinning out of the hands. In addition to the double overhand grip, there are two other grips that can be used for the deadlift: the alternating grip (or over–under grip), and the hook grip. There are pros and cons to each.

First, let's talk about grip in a general sense. The bar should be as deep in your hands as possible for the bench press, but that placement can weaken the grip in the deadlift. If you try to keep the bar high in the hand, it is going to drop down into the lowest part of the hand when you go to pull. Instead, start with the bar as low on the fingers as possible while still being able to get your fingers to connect with your thumb. It should look something like the grip position shown in figure 5.27. From this position, you must squeeze as tight as possible to maintain grip, but it is much more effective than smashing the bar high in the hand.

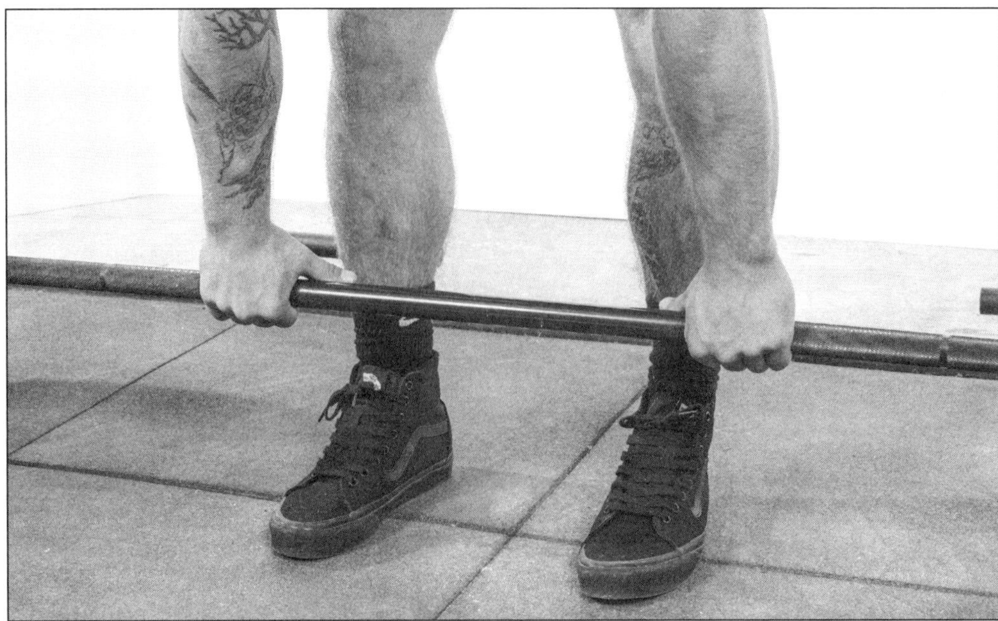

FIGURE 5.27 For the deadlift, the bar shouldn't be all the way in the palm of the hand. Instead, it should be lower into the fingers with the thumb still being able to overlap.

Alternating Grip

The first grip most people experience after the double overhand is the alternating grip. The limiting factor with a double overhand grip is that eventually the weight will be heavy enough to roll the bar out of your hand. Even a bar that doesn't spin well is still a cylindrical object, and it will eventually spin, opening your hand and making your grip less secure. The alternating grip counterbalances this spin. With one hand up and one hand down, the bar doesn't have a place to spin to, so it remains stable in the hand (see figure 5.28). It's a much more secure grip that will allow you to increase the weight you can deadlift. To pull it off, pick which hand to turn up, or supinate. For many, this is their dominant hand. Lock in the lats by making the arms long, but don't force the supinated arm to be even with the other arm. It will naturally be slightly farther away from your side and create a different carry angle. This is normal, and it will protect your arm.

One drawback with the alternating grip is that the side of the supinated hand tends to be more at risk for biceps injuries. This is often due to people pulling their arm in tighter to be even with their other arm, which forces slight flexion in the elbow. Once you start the pull, the biceps flex to try to prevent elbow extension. There is no way for it to overcome the load used in a deadlift, and it gets eccentrically loaded. If you do this with enough weight, the biceps can't handle it. The corrected carry angle helps with this by allowing the arm to stay completely straight while keeping the bar balanced.

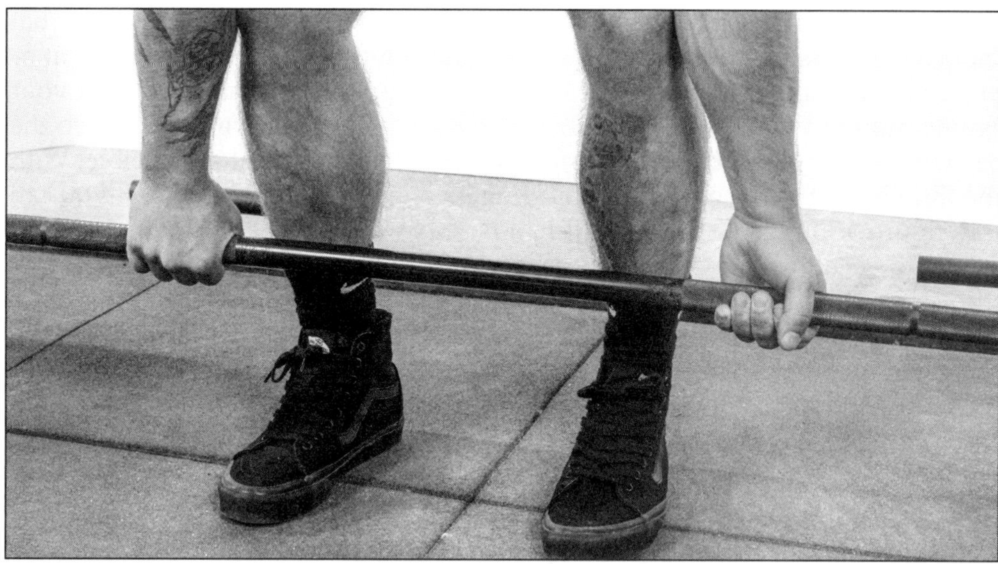

FIGURE 5.28 Having one hand pronated and one supinated will stop the bar from spinning. Note that the supinated hand is slightly wider out on the bar than the pronated hand.

Hook Grip

The next grip is the hook grip. It has one big downside: pain. That's not a joke either. I spent six months doing every pull exercise in the gym with a hook grip in order to build tolerance in it, and it never became comfortable. Basically, the tip of your thumb gets crushed against the bar with this grip. Instead of wrapping your thumb over your fingers, you tuck it under your fingers (see figure 5.29). This creates a fulcrum that the bar sits in, which keeps it from spinning in your hand. It also takes all the weight of the bar and drives it into the tips of your thumbs. The hook grip is an amazing grip though. It's secure and balanced. Since it's double overhand, there's a lower risk of the bar helicoptering. With both arms being straight, there is less strain on the biceps. It doesn't eliminate biceps injuries, but I would say the risk is smaller than with the alternating grip.

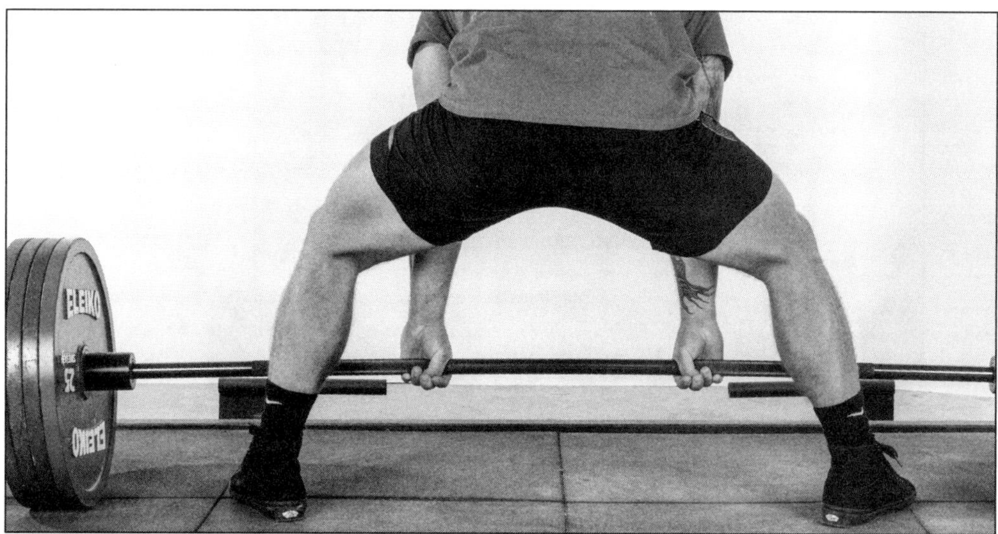

FIGURE 5.29 In the hook grip, the thumb is tucked underneath the fingers and pinned against the bar to secure the grip.

To set up for this, start by spreading your hand as much as you can so that the webbing of skin between your thumb and forefinger is stretched as tight as possible. Press that webbing directly into the bar. This will start to bend your thumb around the bar and set the angle for your thumb. From here, grasp the bar with just the thumb, clamping it down on the bar as tight as possible. With the thumb tight to the bar, wrap your fingers over your thumb the best you can (see figure 5.30). If you have small hands, this will be more difficult. The next step is to get all the way through the start position to the point where you pull the slack out of the bar. When you go to do this, the bar will set into your hand and pull itself deep into your fingers. You can't skip this step because it secures the grip and creates the fulcrum needed for the thumb to pin the bar in your hand. If you don't set the grip, the bar will spin out of your hands just like with a normal double overhand grip.

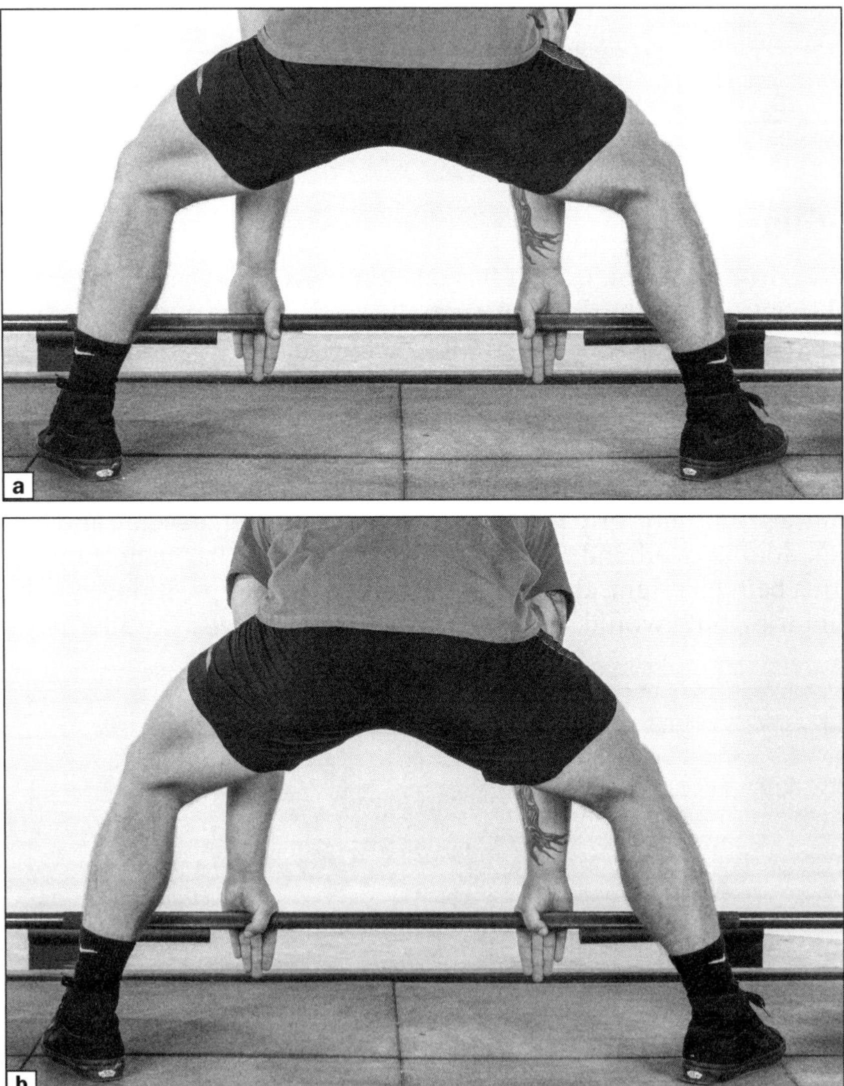

FIGURE 5.30 Setting the hook grip consists of *(a)* driving the hand into the bar, *(b)* looping the thumb around the bar, and *(c)* wrapping the fingers around the thumb.

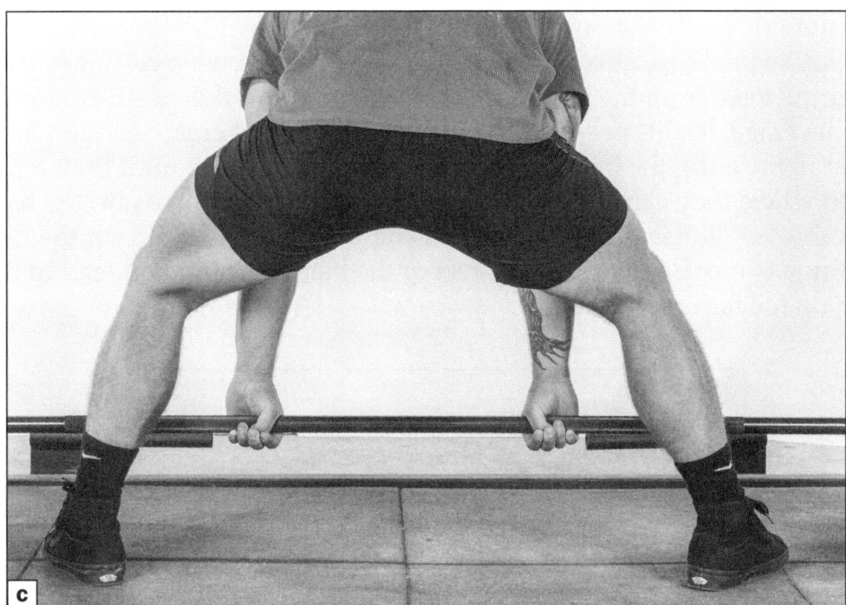

FIGURE 5.30 *(continued)*

Once that grip is set and the slack is out of the bar, you are ready to take that bar for a ride.

I can't skip something massively important here: Take care of your hands. Get a pumice stone and a callous shaver. Use lotion, and keep them from becoming a dry crusty mess. The fastest way to end a session is to rip off a callous and bleed all over the bar. Take care of your hands. Additionally, don't be afraid to use grip assistance like chalk. I know many gyms don't allow it, but with the invention of liquid chalk, it's becoming more of an option. Chalk will wick away the moisture in your hands and better secure your grip. Does it make you stronger? No, but it will keep you safer. That's right; I think chalk is a safety device. Use it if you can.

Wrist straps can also help, especially for high-rep sets, I like to use wrist straps to save my hands. I don't want to miss the shot at a heavy single because I tore my hands open on a set of 10. Don't believe the myth that using them will make you lose all grip strength. They have a very practical place in training, and having a set in your gym bag is a must. Chalk and straps are always in my gym bag.

Common Errors in the Deadlift

The common errors with the deadlift apply to both to the conventional and sumo deadlift. Similar fixes apply as well. The two most common errors in the deadlift are an early rising of the hips and a rounding of the back. Note that I did not specify the lower back. Rather, it's an error that leads to the appearance of the entire back rounding. We'll touch more on that later.

Hips Rising Early

There are two reasons for the hips rising early in the deadlift (see figure 5.31). The first is because the hips are too low in the start position, making the lifter look like they are the bottom of a squat. Many times, this is a result of athletes being told to not use their back during the lift, which is unavoidable because the back and all of its immense surrounding musculature must be involved in order to transfer the force from the legs to the bar. The problem this position creates is a lack of leverage. In this position, the hips are too low to create enough leverage to assist in breaking the bar off the floor, and they will rise until they reach the position where they can have the correct leverage to put force into the bar. Not only is this less efficient, but the hips rising before the bar can set the hips up to continue to move faster than the rest of the bar-lifter unit and lead to the bar ending up too far out in front.

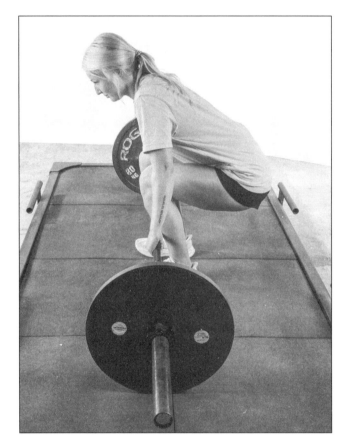

FIGURE 5.31 The hip position is too low and lacks the tension required to begin moving the bar off the floor.

The second circumstance where the hips rise early occurs when the start position is locked in and the bar breaks off the floor well, but then after the bar starts moving, the hips move back too fast and the knees lock out early (see figure 5.32). If you want to make your lock-out way harder than it needs to be, this is the position you want to be in. I am averse to using the words *weakness* and *imbalance*, but in this particular instance, the posterior chain gets overpowered by the leg drive off the floor. This tends to happen more with higher maximal loads of around 90 percent or more of 1RM.

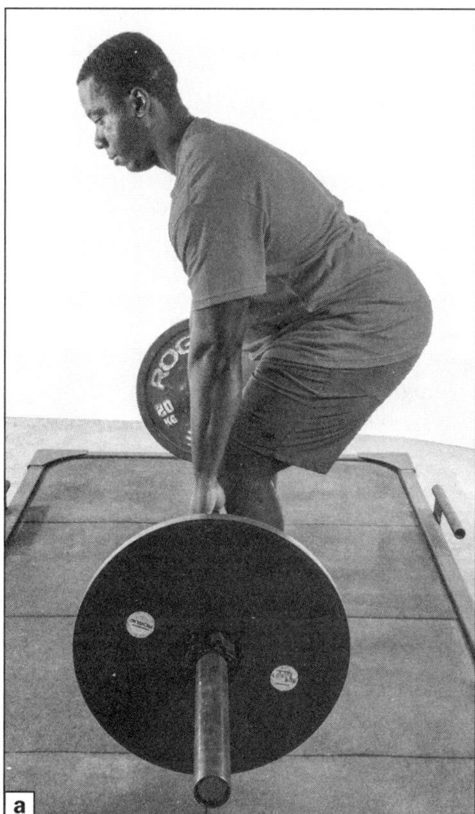

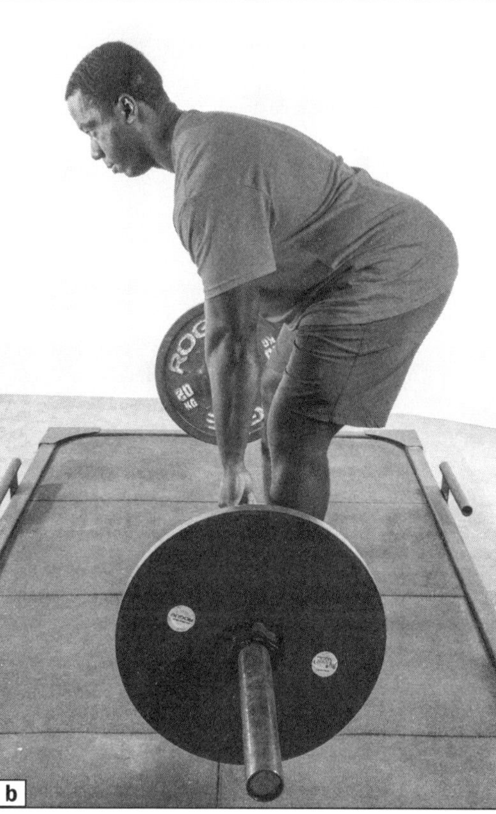

FIGURE 5.32 The hips and bar should rise at the same rate off the floor. If you notice that the hips have moved at a faster rate, like shown, the hips are rising too fast and too early.

The solution to both is a programming adjustment and a focus on the wedge during the lift. I like to start with variations like using a two-inch block pull to sure up the start position as the main work (this variation will be covered later in this chapter), trying to keep the intensity below the threshold where we see the breakdown, and adding in a lot of volume with exercises like Romanian deadlifts, good mornings, and other accessory lifts to bolster the strength of the posterior chain. The nice thing about the two-inch block pull is that it also elevates the bar enough so that the athlete can start with the better start position we are looking for. It's not a quick fix. Rather, it identifies a weak point in the lift that you can work on. This won't just improve your deadlift by the way. Your squat will love you for it too. Don't worry, there is a whole chapter on programming further along in the book. If you have a question here, it will be answered there.

Rounding the Back

Rounding can come from the lower back (lumbar spine) and the upper back (thoracic spine). We've addressed this before, but these positions aren't inherently injurious. They are, however, less efficient for the lift overall. It's also important to note that we are terrible at being able to see spinal movement with the naked eye. Some flexion of the spine is going to happen during the lift. Period. That's not the kind of flexion we are talking about here though. Take a look at figure 5.33; this is the kind of rounding we are talking about. This section will provide some more detail on what to look for and what to do about it.

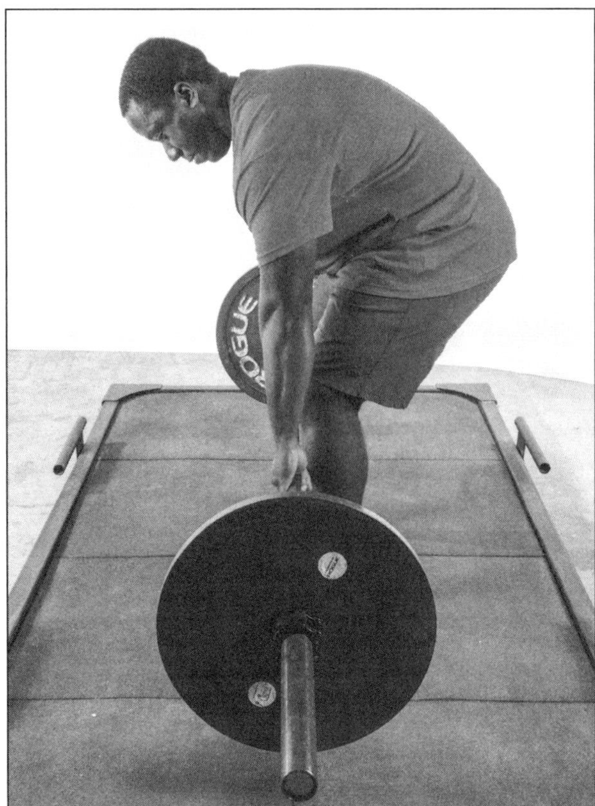

FIGURE 5.33 A large global rounding of the spine is what we want to avoid in the deadlift, especially if the lifter starts with the appearance of a flat back, and then it collapses into this type of position.

The first thing to look at is thoracic, or upper-back rounding, and when it happens. This is important because some taller lifters lock their upper back into flexion in their start position to make it tighter and to keep the bar closer. A great example of this is the elite Russian lifter, Konstantīn Konstantinovs. This guy is one of the best deadlifters ever to have walked the planet. The key to his success was that once he locked in and started pulling, nothing moved. He didn't go into more flexion beyond what he set up in his start position. It's that stability that is important in this context. The error occurs when the thoracic spine starts extended and then moves into flexion, creating what I call the *cascade.* This is when the thoracic spine begins to round, leading to the rest of the spine rounding throughout the movement as the inertia overcomes the ability of the muscles to stabilize (see figure 5.34*a*). It's the change in position that we want to avoid during the lift. These kinds of movements end up being inconsistent, leading to stagnation in progress over time. Positions should stay as consistent as possible, as shown in figure 5.34*b*, so that you can make the adjustments needed.

The other place for rounding is the lumbar spine, or lower back. When this area rounds early in the lift, it's often due to an incomplete brace with inadequate tension or the lifter not pushing well through the floor. It can also simply be that the weight is too heavy. That last one comes down to making good choices, but the other two we can address directly.

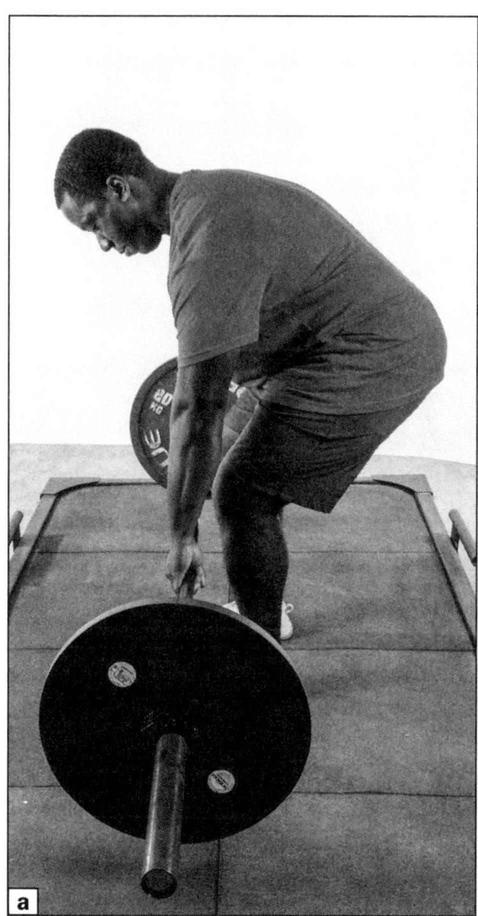

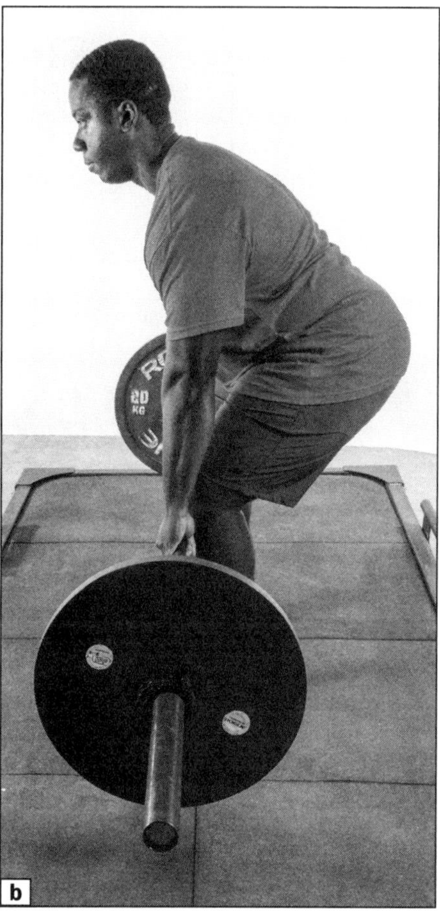

FIGURE 5.34 Notice the difference in bar position where *(a)* the back has rounded and the bar has drifted away from the body versus *(b)* the back stays locked in and the bar stays close.

Bracing is a skill, and there will be times when your strength level will start to exceed your skill level in certain aspects of the lift. Building tension is the foundation of a strong lift, so if you are deadlifting and starting to experience a rounding of the back during the lift, the first step should be to reevaluate your setup. Are you spreading the floor? Are your lats tight and your arms long? Are you breathing not just into your belly but into your back and a full 360 degrees around? Be deliberate. Become intentional with this. It won't be the last time this happens.

The other culprit can be an incomplete push into the floor during the initial phase of the lift. This is different than the hips rising back because in that scenario, the back and hips stay together as one unit, and we don't see as extreme of a position. With an incomplete push into the floor, it ends up looking like what my friend Quinn Henoch calls *the pooping-dog posture.* The lower back rounds, the hips tuck underneath, and the knees begin to lock prematurely (see figure 5.35). Also, the bar is typically about two inches away from the lifter. All in all, it's not the most efficient position for lifting weight.

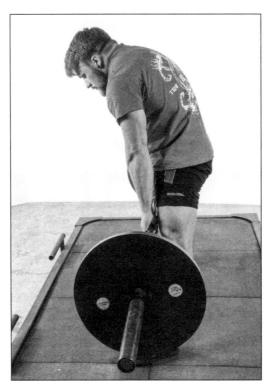

FIGURE 5.35 This is an example of the lower back rounding, the hips tucking under, and the knees locking prematurely, creating the "pooping-dog" posture and making for a much more difficult lock-out.

So how do we fix something like an insufficient leg drive in the deadlift? I like to use a deficit deadlift. This is a lot like the previous correction in that it's more of matter of programming intervention than anything else. It's important to note that a cue alone won't get you past this difficulty. You have to program intelligently to get the change you want. This builds on the concept that we talked about earlier: using movement variations to elicit a specific position change. This works by engaging the brain to learn the skill of lifting while still being able to lift hard. The deficit deadlift can help improve leg drive because in order to get the bar off the ground from a deficit, you must push with your legs more (we will cover this in detail in the next section). If you're not able to push well enough with your legs, your ability to use heavier weight or even to complete the lift becomes substantially compromised. The deficit deadlift will really attack these positions, especially if you're disciplined with the load.

I do want to add that many times, faults in the deadlift get attributed to a mobility problem. In my experience, this does not tend to be the case very often. In short, if someone can touch their toes, then they should be able to get down into the position for a deadlift. The sumo has a hip external-rotation component that can be limiting. However, it does allow most people to get into the positions they're going to need. If there is a mobility restriction, it's going to show up as the inability to bend forward and reach the knees. This is because the initial setup requires you to reach down toward the knees, and then once you start to feel the stretching of the hamstrings, you flex at the knees so that your hands can reach the barbell. If this happens to be a place of restriction, then there are ways to address it with positional drills and other variations of the lift, but often a mobility restriction is not the actual limitation with a deadlift.

Deadlift Variations

Just like with the other lifts, we can use variations of the deadlift to build the technique that you will use primarily. This is a great way to put yourself in different positions and strengthen other areas of the lift to be more successful. Here I'm going to address six of the variations that I really like to use for the deadlift.

Pause Deadlift

The pause deadlift is one of my favorite deadlift variations. It's a great way to spend some time in positions, especially if an athlete loses position at certain phases of the lift. This can challenge those positions and teach the lifter to better maintain those difficult positions. For the pause deadlift, you set up and execute the movement the same way you would for the type of deadlift you are training (see figure 5.36*a*), whether that's conventional or sumo, and then add at least one pause throughout the movement. My two favorite places to pause are two inches off the floor and right at the knees. As discussed earlier in the chapter, there are two positions where the barbell slows down—just off the floor and as the bar approaches the knees. Pausing in these positions for at least a second can strengthen those areas and help athletes feel more comfortable during the lift (see figure 5.36*b*). A general rule of thumb that I have is that if you're not good in a particular position, spend more time there, and that's really where the pause comes into play. Just like with the double-pause bench, these positions will self-select overtime as you find your difficult position, but I like to start at two inches from the ground or at the knees. After the pause, finish the lift all the way to lock-out as usual (see figure 5.36*c*).

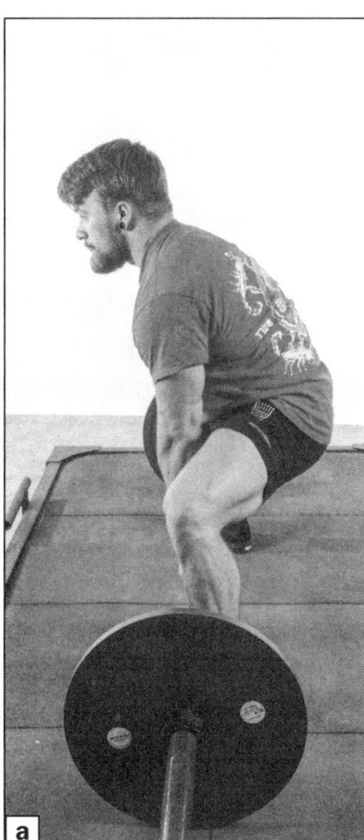

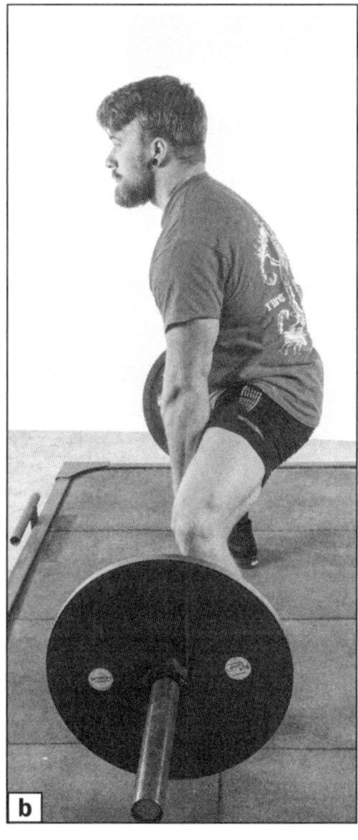

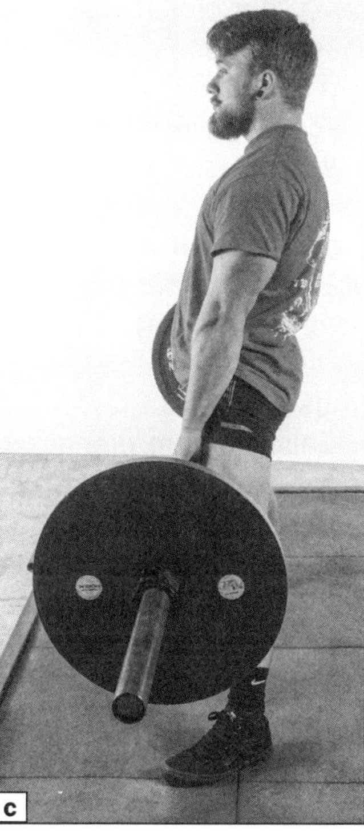

FIGURE 5.36 An example of a paused deadlift at the knees. The rest of the deadlift remains the same, but you pause right at the knees and hold there for a second once the bar comes to a complete stop. After the pause, reaccelerate the bar all the way to lock-out.

Chair Deadlift

I don't think there's a better variation to teach tension and start position for the deadlift than the chair deadlift. The chair here serves the same purpose as the box does in the box squat: It provides an external constraint to help build the position. Additionally, this can help reinforce the vertical shin position as the bar approaches the knees in both the sumo and the conventional deadlift.

To set up for the chair deadlift, you'll need a sturdy chair that's just about as high as where your hip start position is in the deadlift. You can also use a box if you don't have a chair available. First, get into your position underneath the bar with the same width and positioning that you would if you were setting up for your sumo or conventional deadlift. Then sit on the chair, but only sit on the edge of it; don't sit all the way back. This is the start position for where you are going to be on the chair.

Next, make your lats tight and your arms long the same way you would in your normal deadlift setup. Then hinge forward to grab the bar, keeping your butt and your weight on the chair. Remember that in this position, you should still have tension through your legs like you're driving into the floor (in a conventional deadlift) or spreading the floor apart (in a sumo stance). Once you've grasped the bar, drive your chest up, continue to push through your legs, and get the slack out of the barbell. This should feel like a very familiar position because this is your normal start position, but your weight should still be on the chair. It should feel like a 50/50 split. Fifty percent of your weight should be on the chair, and 50 percent of your body should be driving up into the barbell. This is where you start (see figure 5.37*a*).

The key to the chair deadlift is to slide off the chair. To initiate the movement, drive your hips toward the bar and wedge in. The chair is there to help you feel these positions, so as soon as you start to wedge into the bar and come off the chair, the bar should also start to move. If the hips rise early off the chair and the barbell is still on the floor, one of two things has happened: Either the chair is too low or you didn't wedge into the bar properly to get the effect of the exercise. The bar should elevate off the ground as your hips slide in toward the bar, wedging the way we've described before. Your shins should become vertical as the bar approaches your knees (see figure 5.37*b*). With the chair deadlift, make sure to finish all the way at lock-out and to maintain your balance (see figure 5.37*c*). If those positions tend to be difficult ones for you, the chair deadlift is the variation to use.

This is where programming for a chair deadlift is going to be different than it is for other variations. With the chair deadlift, I like to only do singles because resetting back and forth can be a little difficult. Singles allow you to reset each rep, and I like to do more sets. An example of this would be eight sets of single reps at 60 to 65 percent of your one-rep maximum. I have gone as far as to have maximum singles for this if the individual has a chair that's sturdy enough. This can challenge these positions a great deal and as well as teach maximum tension for maximum weights.

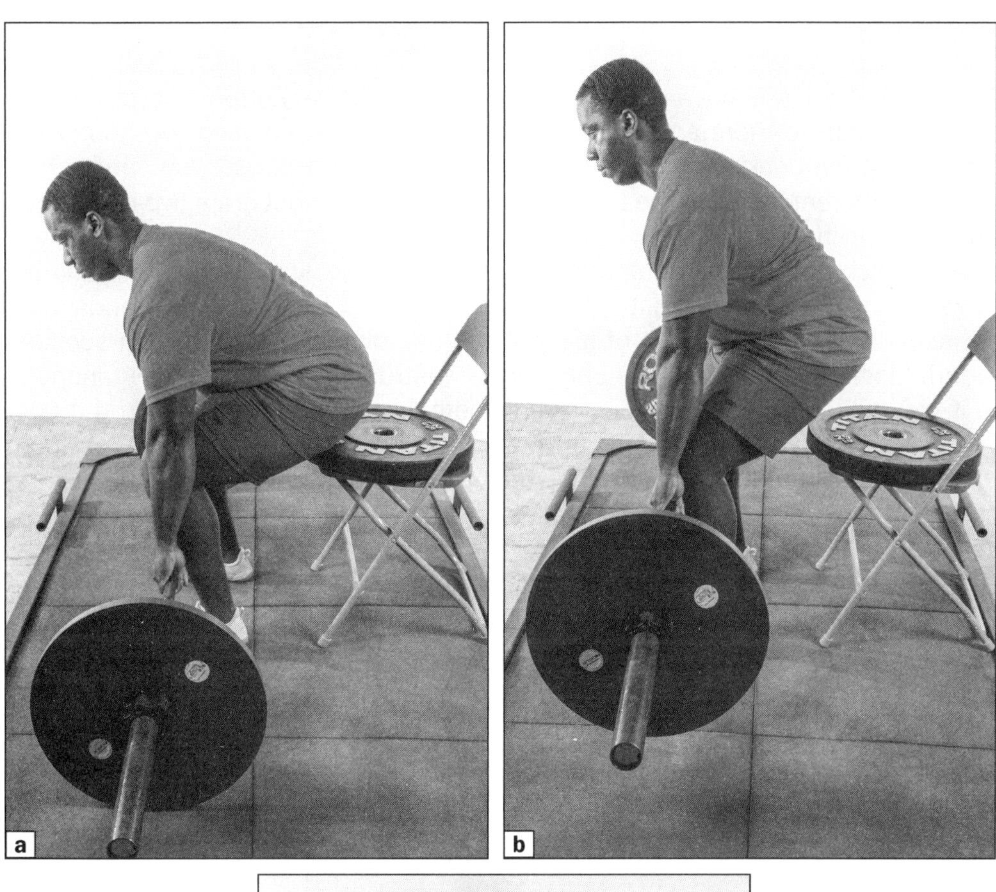

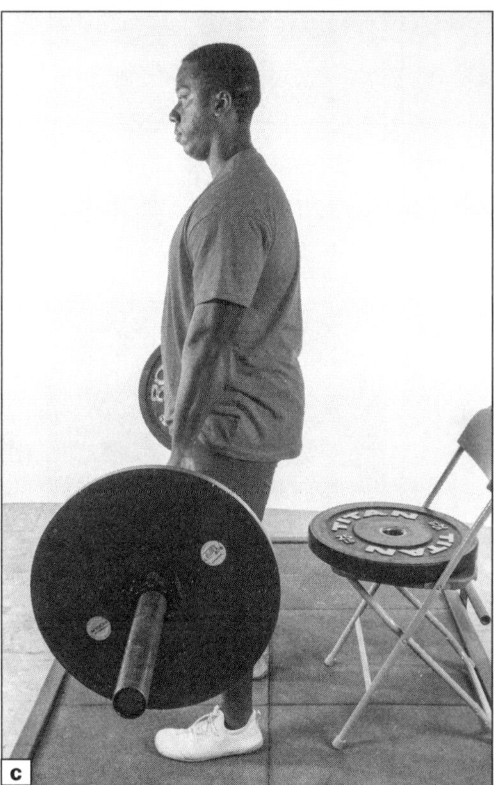

FIGURE 5.37 The full sequence of a chair deadlift. Note how the hips don't immediately rise off the chair to initiate the movement but slide forward to wedge into the bar more.

Deficit Deadlift

The deficit deadlift is not a variation that I used to use very often, but it's become one that I turn to more and more because it is a great solution for insufficient leg drive in the deadlift. The beauty of a deficit deadlift is that you can do it at multiple different heights. The two that I like to use the most are a two-inch deficit and a four-inch deficit.

A two-inch deficit deadlift is a great way to improve starting position and leg drive. It elongates the pull just enough and also helps with grip if that tends to be an issue for you. I have most of my athletes use plates or the two-inch sections of jerk blocks to stand on. The only special instruction from a setup standpoint is if you pull sumo. In that case, use something that will not slide on the floor you are pulling on. The last thing anybody wants is to have plates slide out from under your feet during a pull, driving you into a full split.

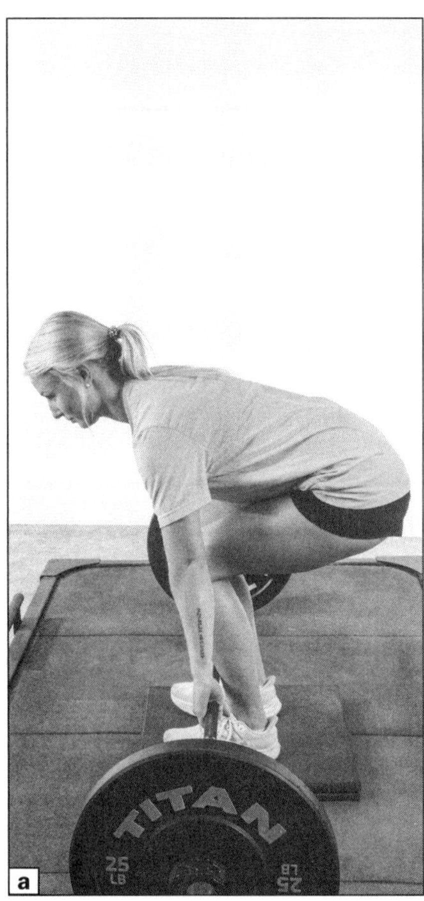

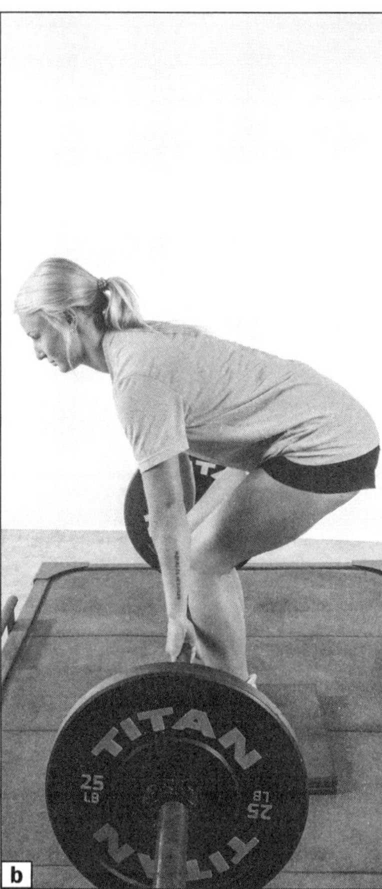

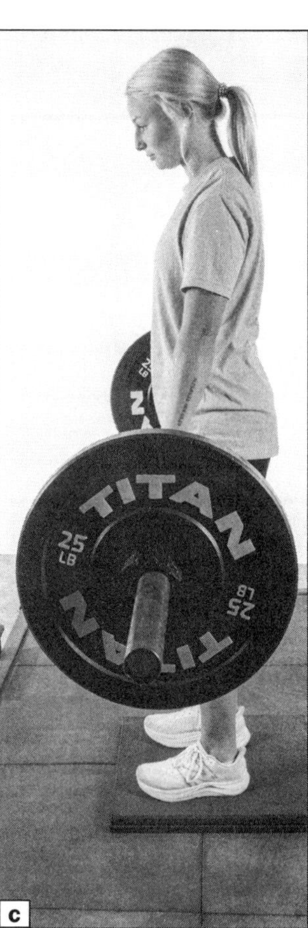

FIGURE 5.38 Full sequence of a deficit deadlift. Note that the knees aren't locked when the bar is at mid-shin, which some lifters may be tempted to do because of the deficit. Maintain the same positions you would in a deadlift from the floor, with only the start position be slightly different.

A four-inch deficit deadlift is a whole other animal. Four inches or greater for a deficit deadlift can be a difficult position to get into, and for many athletes, it will force more knee flexion and possibly some upper- and lower-back flexion. It's a hard position, but that doesn't mean it's not safe. It's important to recognize that the position itself is going to limit the amount of weight you will be able to lift, but that's the point here. With this start position, you can build up those areas and challenge the posterior chain through a greater range of motion. This deep of a deficit isn't for everyone, but if you are a competitive powerlifter with a stagnant pull, this is a variation to try.

To do a deficit deadlift, stack up plates or use a box to create the prescribed height. The plates should be in the same position your feet would be in because you will then stand on them. From here, everything is the same as it would be for your normal conventional or sumo deadlift (see figure 5.38). There is one more thing to keep in mind here: The deficit can make wearing a belt very uncomfortable. I suggest skipping the belt for the first couple of sessions while you figure out the movement.

Block Deadlift or Block Pull

The block deadlift is the same as the deficit deadlift, except here the bar is elevated to make the pull shorter. A two-inch elevation is perfect for people who struggle to get into a good starting position and maintain it. I've seen countless lifters get into a good position and then as soon as they start the pull, it falls apart. The slight elevation of the bar in this block pull gives them just enough room to maintain that position and to build it better. On top of that, I've also found it to be a very good predictor of performance a few weeks out from a maximum test or meet (there will be more on programming in that chapter). Also note that I very specifically use only a two-inch pull. I have seen so many people use block pulls at the knees to try to improve lock-out and, sadly, it just doesn't carry over. When I see a weak lock-out now, I look earlier in the pull for when the bar gets away from the lifter.

To set up for the block pull, do everything you would normally do to set up to the bar. Pull the slack out and be ready. At this point, you shouldn't be in your normal start position (see figure 5.39*a*). Instead, you should be exactly where you would be if you had pulled the bar two inches off the ground. Your shins should be slightly more vertical, your upper body and your hips should be slightly higher (not taller, but higher compared to normal,) and your knees should be slightly less flexed. For any block pull of any height, the start position needs to be where the bar would be during your deadlift if the bar were in that exact position. This is what is going to train that position. Then pull the slack out of the bar, and pull the bar to lock-out (see figure 5.39*b* and *c*).

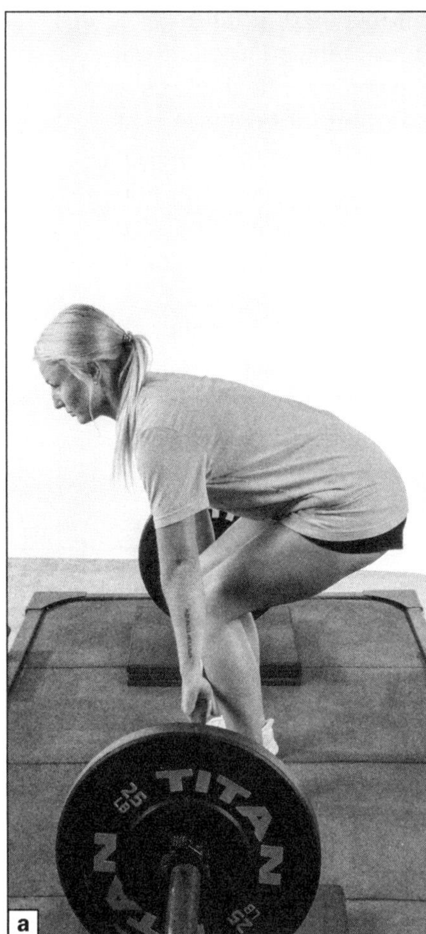

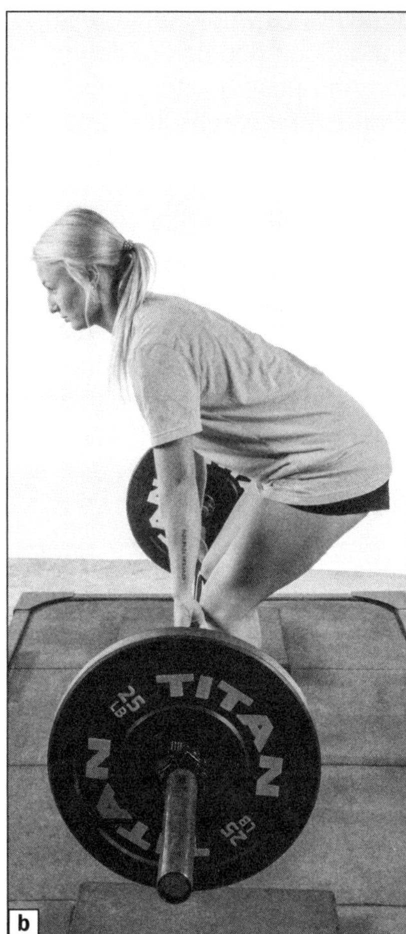

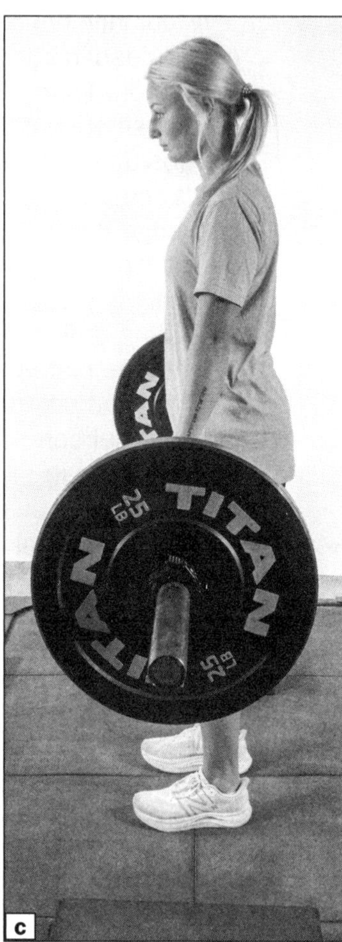

FIGURE 5.39 The full sequence of a two-inch block deadlift. Note that in the start position, the shins are already vertical because this is the position the bar and the lifter would be in at that point in a deadlift from the floor.

Kettlebell or Dumbbell Deadlift

For the complete beginner, there can be some limitations with the barbell deadlift. One of them is weight. Most gyms don't have bumper plates to elevate the bar to the right height, and putting 45-pound (20 kg) plates on each end to get to that height would mean starting at 135 pounds (61 kg). That is quite a lift to start off with. Another limitation is the position of the bar. The way the bar-lifter unit works with the deadlift, the bar isn't completely centered. It's always going to be slightly out in front, making finding the center of gravity a bit harder for beginners. Both of these issues can be resolved by using a different tool: a kettlebell or dumbbell.

I prefer a kettlebell, but an upright dumbbell also works in a pinch. This allows you to straddle the weight so that it's right over the center of gravity. The rest of the lift remains the same with one small layer of difficulty removed. This makes for a great entry point and learning tool for new lifters as well as for people who don't have the base strength to lift the barbell. See figure 5.40 for an example of a kettlebell deadlift.

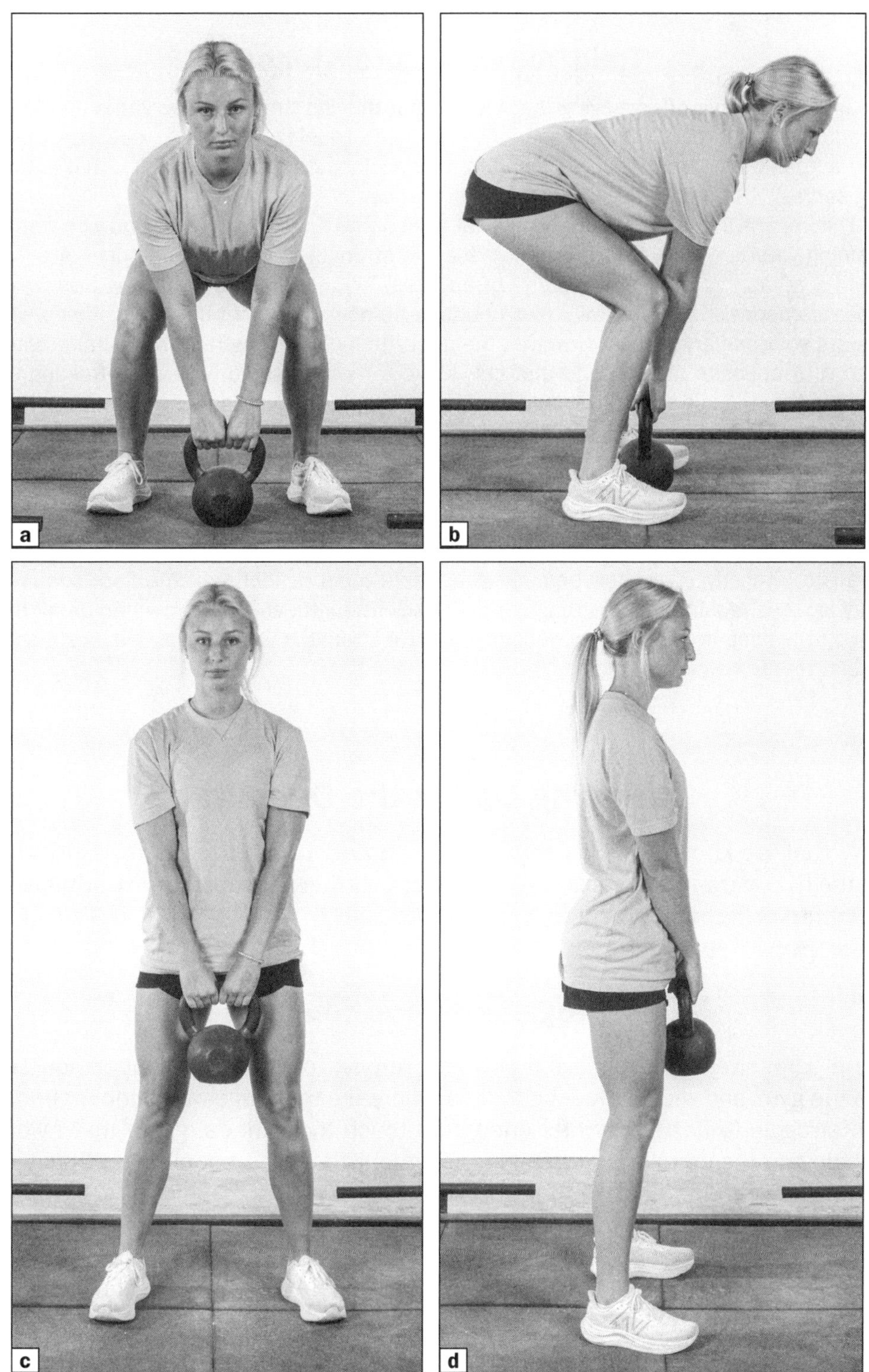

FIGURE 5.40 The kettlebell deadlift. Note that the kettlebell starts between the feet, making the bar-lifter center of gravity much easier to manage.

Train Your Opposite Stance

I want to start this off by saying that I know that this isn't really a true variation of the deadlift. It is, however, a huge gap in most people's training, and it's a weakness that I see across the board in programs and in the development of the deadlift. What is this big secret? It's simple: Train your opposite stance.

This means that if you pull conventional, take some time to pull sumo and vice versa. Training your opposite stance will increase the strength in your main stance, and I've seen it reliably do so with hundreds of athletes. This is now the first thing I do when I see someone's deadlift stall. Your opposite stance will start off weaker; that's why it's not your primary stance. However, the opportunity for strength growth is far greater with your opposite stance, and that can stoke a more positive outlook in training as you progress. Additionally, training your opposite stance can identify weak points that may be holding back progress with your primary stance. For example, some sumo lifters start to miss lifts because of weakness in the lower back and the posterior chain that makes the phase of the lift from the knees to lock-out more difficult. With the conventional deadlift being slightly more focused on these areas, training conventional deadlift as a sumo deadlifter can improve these weaknesses and improve the sumo deadlift. Similarly, some conventional deadlifters miss deadlifts off the floor because they lack the required quad strength, upper-back strength, and positioning to break the bar off the floor. Training sumo deadlifts can build strength there, helping a conventional deadlifter lift more weight.

Warming Up for the Deadlift

Now that we know how to deadlift, how should you get ready to do it? Here are the five warm-up exercises that I cluster together the most for my athletes on deadlift day and what they do.

Progressive Toe-Touch

The progressive toe-touch is the perfect exercise for those days when you step into the gym, and you just feel tight. It can increase the range of motion for people who struggle to flex forward far enough to touch their knees. (Note that I would still elevate the deadlift as the main movement for these people, and then work my way down to the floor as they got better).

To do it, grab a two-by-four-inch board from the hardware store. It just needs to be long enough to get both your feet on it. Bring your feet together, and start with your toes on the board. Flex forward and try to touch your toes (see figure 5.41*a*). There is no need to brace hard here, just breathe normally. Reach as far as you can, pause for two seconds, and then come all the way back up to standing. Repeat this five times. Then step off the board, and do the same thing with your feet flat on the floor for five more reps (see figure 5.41*b*). To wrap up, step back onto the board, this time with your heels on the board and your toes on the ground (see figure 5.41*c*). Do five more reps, and you're all set. It's that simple. Cluster this in with your deadlift warm-ups to feel more comfortable in your approach to the bar.

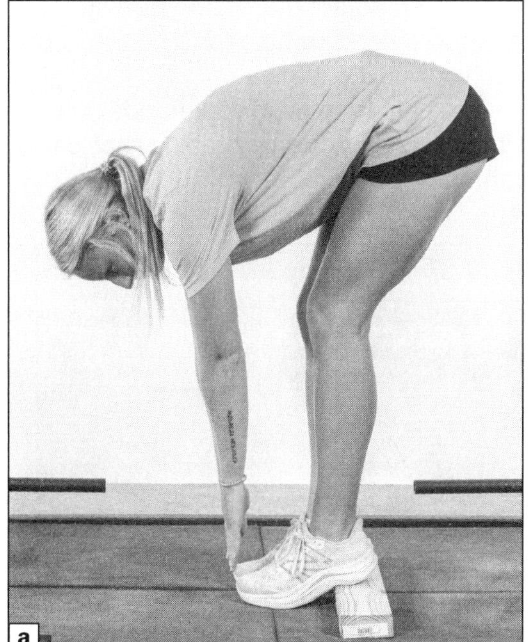
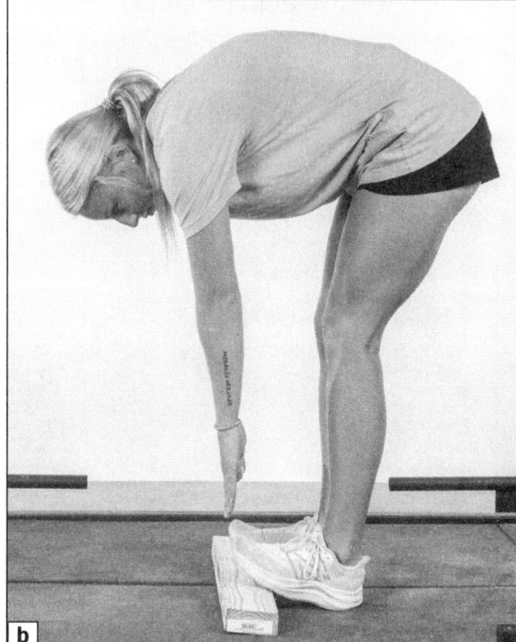
 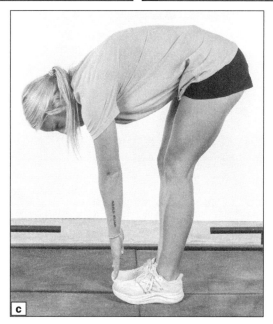

FIGURE 5.41 The progressive toe-touch: *(a)* heels up, *(b)* toes up, and *(c)* feet flat. Remember that there is no need to brace hard here. Allow yourself to go through the range of motion smoothly.

Active Straight-Leg Raise

Next up is an exercise I love to couple with the progressive toe-touch. This works based on a similar idea of increasing tolerance to stretch. Where the toe-touch uses gravity to help move you into these positions, the active straight-leg raise uses active movement to accomplish this.

Start by lying flat on your back with your hands at your sides, your legs stretched straight out, and your feet together (see figure 5.42*a*). Raise one leg up as high as you can while keeping it straight (see figure 5.42*b*). As soon as your knee starts to bend *or* your down foot starts to turn out, stop there and hold for a breath. Do this five times on each side, and move on to your next exercise.

If this is difficult for you, a trick you can use to help is to push your hands down into the floor as hard as you can. This will produce a reflexive bracing that can give you a little more stability for this movement.

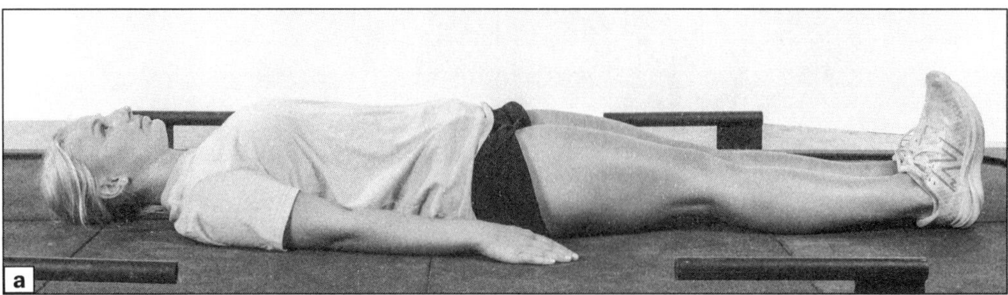

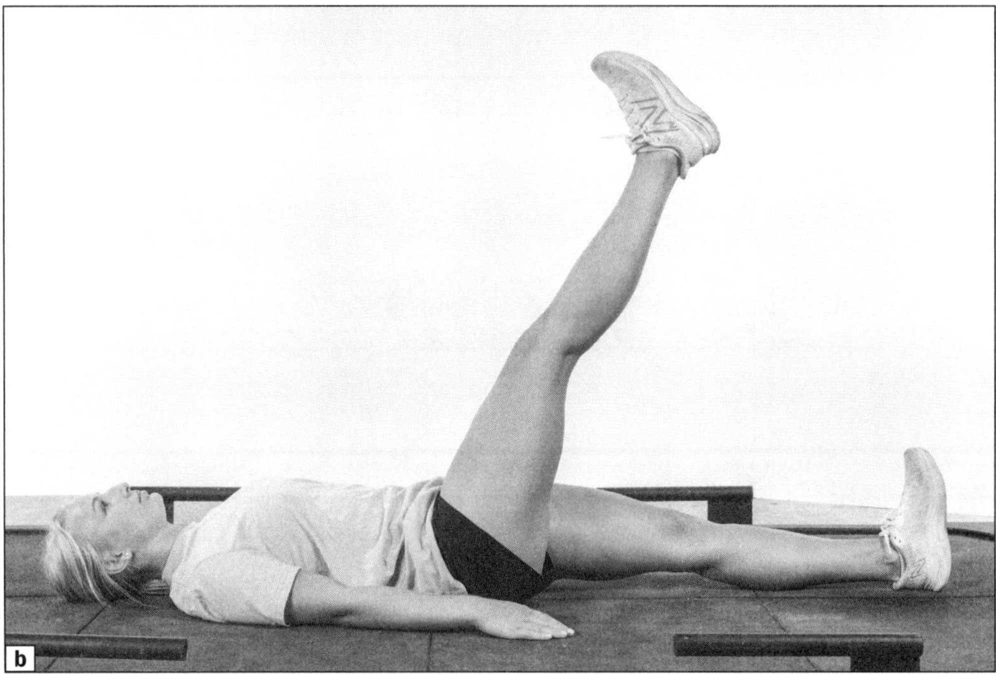

FIGURE 5.42 The active straight-leg raise: *(a)* start position and *(b)* the position with the leg up. Note that both legs stay completely straight.

Lat Pull-Over

"I can't feel the *long arms* cue. I've tried and just can't find it." I hear this a lot when people are starting out. They try to make their arms long and pin them down to their sides, but they can't get the feel of the tension. Many times, this comes from not understanding the feeling they're looking for and, possibly, lacking requisite strength to feel it. This is where a lat pull-over can come in handy. I've not found an exercise that can help re-create this feeling better. Especially after 12 to 15 reps here, there should be enough blood in the lats that they start to feel tighter. If you have a hard time finding the locked-in upper-body feeling, cluster this in with your warm-up sets.

Use a lat pull-down machine or a band that's secured at a high point over your head. Grab the implement with your arms straight all the way overhead (see figure 5.43*a*). Keeping the arms straight, pull down until your hands are by your sides or the lat pull-down bar hits your hips (see figure 5.43*b*). Make sure that when you are here, you keep your arms straight and try to pin your elbows to your sides. From here, bring the weight slowly back to the start position overhead, and allow the weight to create a big stretch at the top. Then initiate the next rep. Choose a weight that you can do for around 15 reps.

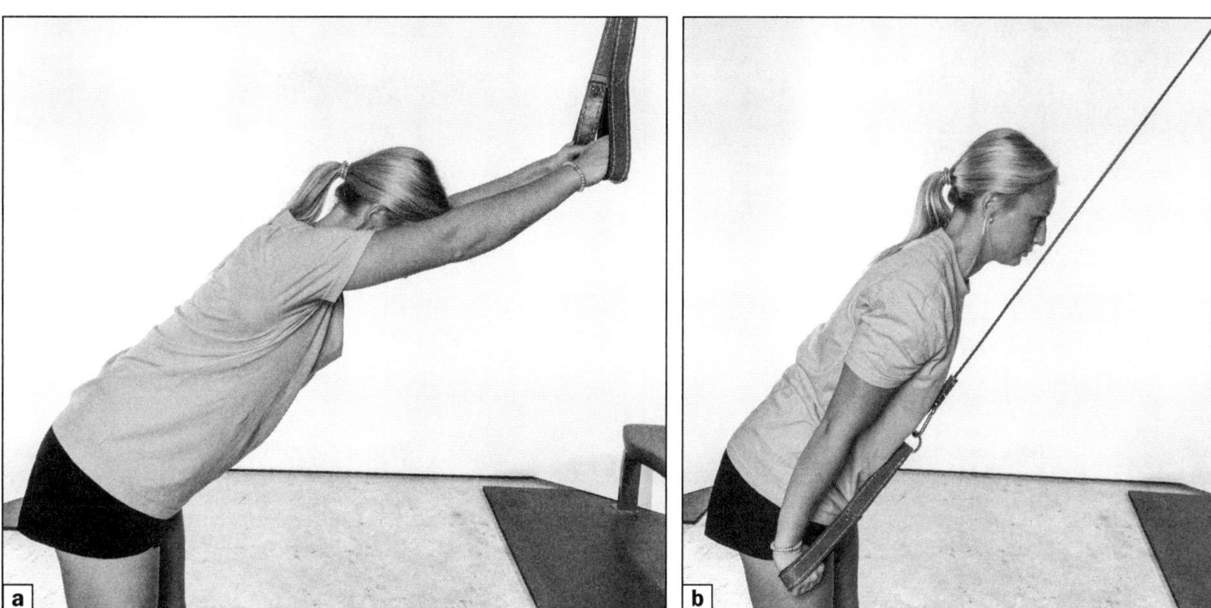

FIGURE 5.43 The *(a)* start and *(b)* end position of a lat pull-over. Keep your arms straight, and look to get a big stretch at the top when you return to the start position.

Thoracic Extension with a Foam Roller

That's right—the foam roller is back! I don't use these in the traditional way, but they can still be a great tool to use for a warm-up. This exercise specifically targets that sticky thoracic extension, or upper-back extension, that so many of us feel. Many people spend most of the day in one position: sitting. So there may be days when you just feel stiff or struggle to get into the upright position that's needed for an efficient pull. If that's the case, grab a foam roller and get to work.

Start with the roller at eye level and pin it against a wall with your wrists. Keep your wrists shoulder width apart, and keep your palms facing each other (see figure 5.44*a*). You don't have to lean hard into it here, just put enough pressure on it to keep it in place. Your arms should be parallel to each other. Breathe normally and then start to roll the foam roller up the wall, letting your chest and your shoulders fall toward the wall. Go as high as you can while keeping your arms parallel to each other (see figure 5.44*b*). It's common—though not required—to feel a pop in your thoracic spine as you go through this. Hold this top position for one long inhale and one long exhale, then return to the start position. The idea here is to feel the thoracic spine extend as the arms go up with the roller and to use the leverage created to move into more extension. This will help to build more tolerance to this position. Do this for five reps, and move on to your next exercise.

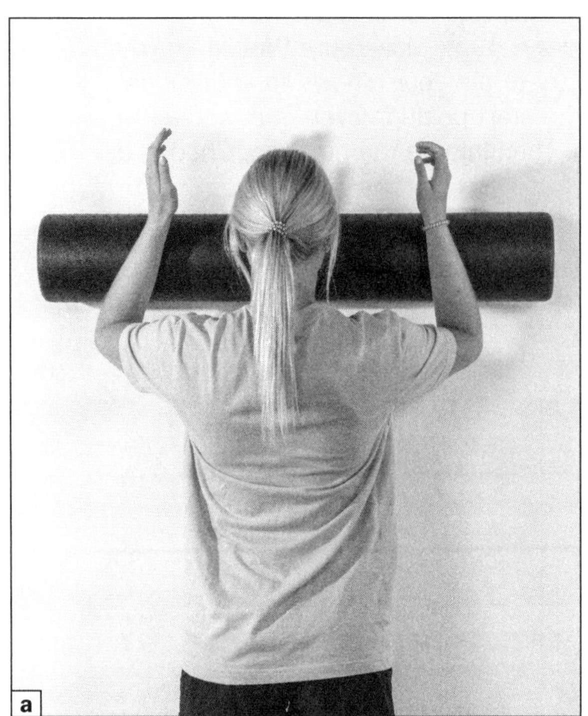

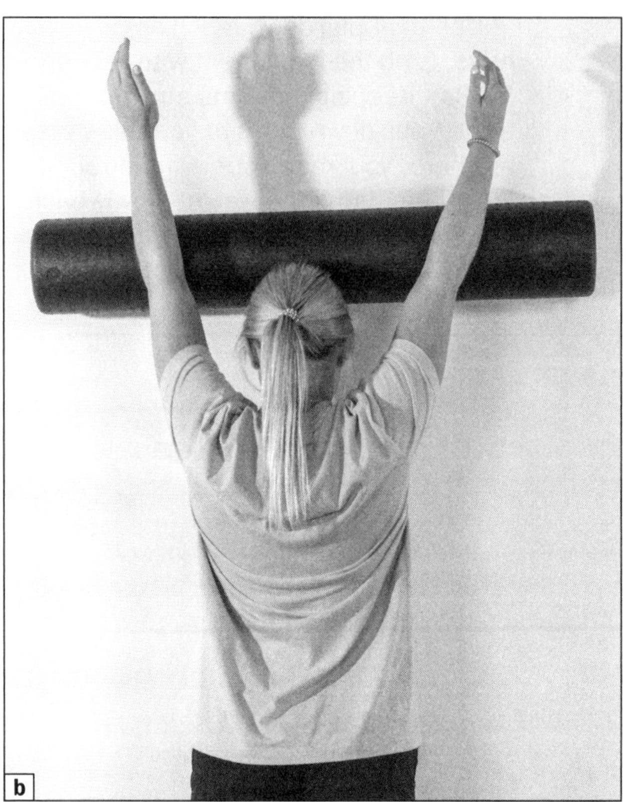

FIGURE 5.44 Start and top position of the thoracic-extension drill with a foam roller. Note that the arms stay parallel to each other and that the athlete isn't forcefully leaning into the roller in the top position.

One-Inch Drop Pull

This is my favorite position-specific drill to warm up with. It is all about the start position and balance. Also, it's literally the first part of the deadlift, so it directly carries over. This exercise will help you build your start position and feel more balanced in your pull, all while warming up the exact muscles you are going to use.

To do this, set up in your normal deadlift position or in the one you are going to use that day (see figure 5.45*a*). Everything stays the same. Initiate your deadlift, and then stop one inch off the floor (see figure 5.45*b*). Pause here for a moment, and then drop the bar. I mean drop it: Open your hands, and let it free-fall. Did you fall backward? You shouldn't, because the start should be a balanced press off the floor, not a pull back (see figure 5.45*c*). You should be able to drop the bar and stay completely motionless (outside of being startled from the noise). I like to use this as the last exercise in the warm-up cluster and roll it right into the deadlifts. All you need is two to three reps, and then start pulling the first warm-up set. Stop after three rounds of the warm-up or if the weight gets above 50 percent of your one-rep maximum.

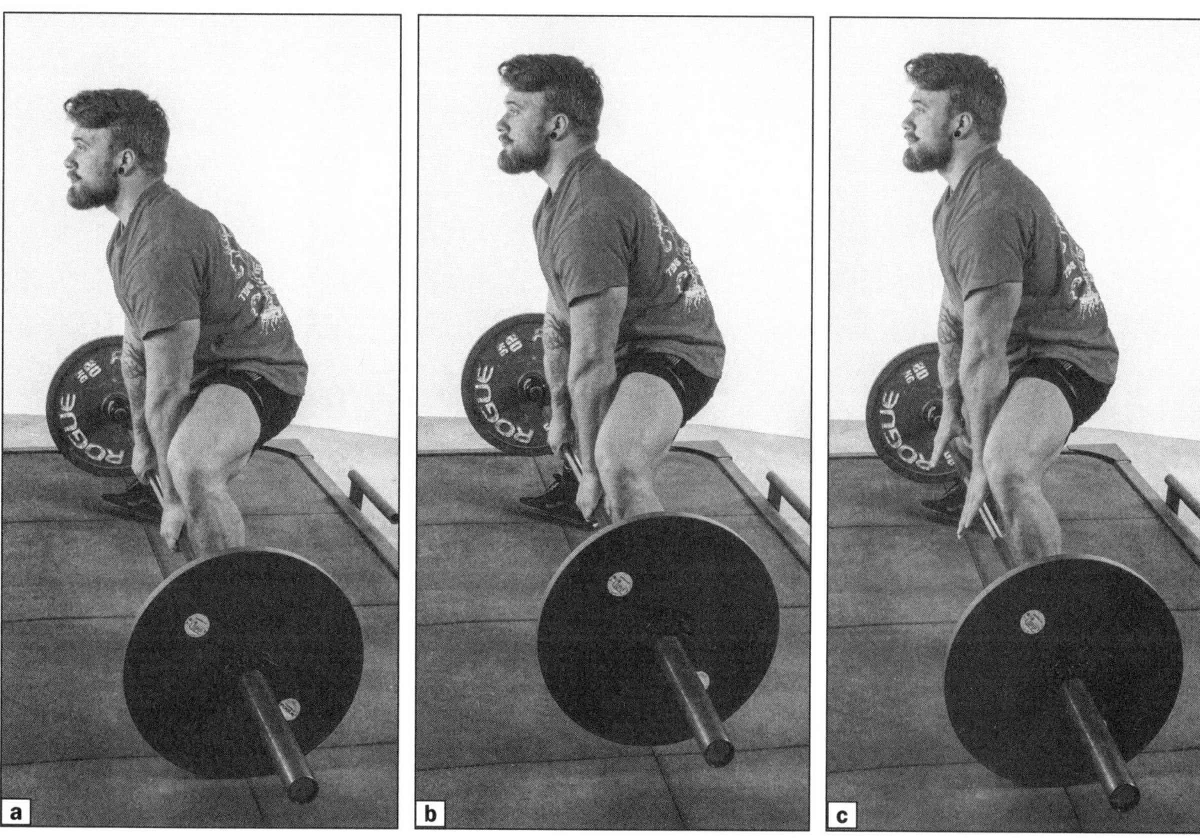

FIGURE 5.45 This is one of my favorite exercises to lock in the start position: *(a)* The start position, *(b)* the pause position, and *(c)* the position of the lifter after the drop. Note that the lifter's position doesn't change from the pause to the drop.

Another one bites the dust. You now know everything you need to know to get started deadlifting effectively and safely. There is one more main movement left: the press. Don't forget to practice what you learned here though. Get to the gym and get in the reps. Find your foot position and the stance you prefer. Practice creating tension in your body before you lift the bar off the floor. Implement the concepts and principles so you can master them. I'll see you in the next chapter.

Chapter 6

The Overhead Press

Everyone calls this lift *the press*, but to be precise you should call it *the overhead press*. This is the last of the foundational movements we will cover, but that doesn't mean it's the least important. Given how often we reach over our heads in daily life, the press is an incredibly functional movement that can also help maintain shoulder health and range of motion. Shoulder health is neglected by so many people. When I was working in a clinic, shoulders were the second most common body part treated, with the lower back coming in second. Most people just don't do much at all with their shoulders from an activity standpoint.

Believe it or not, I considered omitting the overhead press from this book. Why? The overhead press can help with shoulder health and range of motion, but it's not super accessible because like the bench press, the overhead press has a lower strength ceiling than other lifts. A 45-pound bar (20 kg) may simply be too heavy for some, and lighter-weight Bella bars or old barbells with no sleeves are hard to find. Plus, so many people of all ages have range-of-motion limitations in their shoulders, and that may need to be addressed before attempting the overhead press. While neither of these issues will necessarily lead to injury, they can slow down progress and create frustration—the exact opposite of what I'm trying to achieve with this book. However, I decided that the importance of being able to lift weight overhead in terms of quality of life, longevity, and strength outweighed any reason to leave it out. So this chapter will cover the reasons why you should press, the elements that make up a good press, and the phases of the press. Let's get started.

Reasons Why You Should Overhead Press

The relationship between the overhead press and the bench press is actually a pretty close one. Just like you would imagine that the squat and the deadlift would build each other, the bench press and the overhead press complement each other as the core of a strength-and-conditioning program. I've found that the overhead press helps build the bench press more directly than the other way around. It's a great builder for triceps strength and shoulder strength, which tend to be limiting factors when it comes to the bench press, even late in people's strength careers.

Additionally, the overhead press is a great exercise for general shoulder health. There is a misconception that lifting overhead is actually dangerous for the shoulders. In reality, it's important to get into different positions and to load those ranges of motion so that tissues can build tolerance to those positions. The overhead press allows you to go into these positions and to build that tissue tolerance and strength through ranges of motion that the shoulder isn't typically taken through. Too often, individuals discover that they have limited range of motion and limited functionality when it comes to overhead work or the use of their arms overhead. Including the overhead press as a fundamental lift within your program can help prevent this and also keep your shoulders healthy around the other lifts. The truth is, no one lift is any more dangerous than another. Since the shoulder is not often used overhead, the press is a great way to train for increased capacity and decreased risk of injury.

Lastly, the athletic development of the overhead press, which is similar to that of the bench press, helps develop power overhead that can be beneficial in sports like football, swimming, and even baseball. One of the critiques of the bench press, specifically with regard to football, is that players don't lie flat on their back and push somebody away from them, and an offensive lineman doesn't block with their arms just straight out in front of them. However, they do typically block with an inclined angle, and sometimes they lift the defensive lineman up off the ground to the point where their arms are over their head as they press up on this other player. This is known as *pancaking* (so named because the offensive blocker "pancakes" the defensive lineman to the ground), and it's pretty impressive. The overhead press is the lift that can develop that kind of power, which can help you in all of your athletic pursuits.

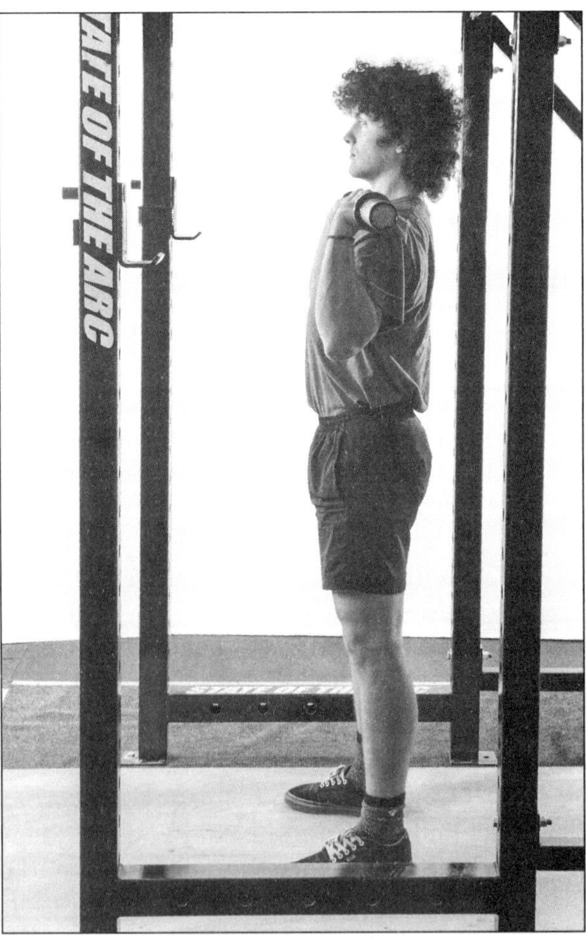

FIGURE 6.1 The press affects the vertical axis of the bar-lifter unit, making stability under the bar paramount. Every degree of horizontal movement of the bar compounds the effect on the bar-lifter unit and makes the lift more difficult.

Elements of the Overhead Press

Here we are going to cover the basic elements that make up the press—the bar-lifter unit, bar path, and bar speed. These elements will help you understand what the lift should look like and help you analyze your lift to make sure you are headed in the right direction.

Bar-Lifter Unit

In the start position of the press, the barbell sits just over your collarbones (see figure 6.1). This puts the bar directly over the midfoot, making the bar-lifter unit fairly balanced over your normal center of gravity. The difference with the press is that the bar travels overhead and creates a long lever arm that affects the bar-lifter unit. Up to this point, we haven't had to talk about the center of gravity and the bar-lifter unit being affected vertically. With the bench, you're supported by a stable object underneath you, and with the squat and the deadlift, the effect of the lever arm on the center of gravity is not as extreme.

What happens in the press is that as the bar travels vertically, moving away from the center of gravity, the bar-lifter unit also moves vertically (not forward and backward like with other lifts). This creates the need for a large amount of stability under the bar to prevent it from moving forward or backward. Any forward or backward movement of the bar makes it exponentially more difficult to keep the bar over the center of gravity.

Bar Path

This effect of the bar moving vertically is precisely why the bar path has to be a completely straight line from the start position to lock-out. There is no debate on this like there is with the bench press. In the overhead press, the bar needs to move perfectly vertically. This does create a small issue with your head being in the way of the movement of the bar, but in this case, we will move the body around the bar as opposed to the bar around the body. This will be covered in the execution sections of the chapter, but I want to make it clear here that if you move the bar forward to get it around your face, you make the lift much harder. A straight vertical line is the bar path you need.

Bar Speed

Just like with other lifts, the bar speed changes throughout the press. The first peak velocity happens right off the chest. As the bar approaches your chin, it slows down as you move your head out of the way and is at its slowest around your forehead. Once the bar gets past your forehead and you start to move your head back under the bar, there's a second peak velocity. It slows again just before lock-out as with the other lifts.

The transition point around the face and forehead is a common sticking point for many people not only because the bar slows down but because it can drift forward slightly, and then it's hard to bring it back to over the center of gravity. For this reason, it's one of my favorite spots to incorporate pause work to solidify this position.

The Phases of the Overhead Press

It's time to learn how to overhead press. If you've skipped ahead to this part because you want to unlock the secrets of a strong overhead press, please go back and start from the beginning at the squat. No skipping the line! For the rest of you, let's start with the phases of the press and how to execute the lift overall. Something to keep in mind is that the range of motion for the overhead press is very short and that the lift starts with the concentric phase. As with the deadlift, the errors on the press tend to occur more often on the way up than on the way down, so I will address common errors all in one section rather than throughout the phases of the lift itself. Let's get into it.

Start Position

A solid start position for the press is a requirement, just like with the other lifts. It's especially important with the press because the shorter range of motion leaves less room for error than there is with something like the squat. If the bar is a little out in front in the start position, it makes the whole lift so much harder. Here is how to get set up for success with the press.

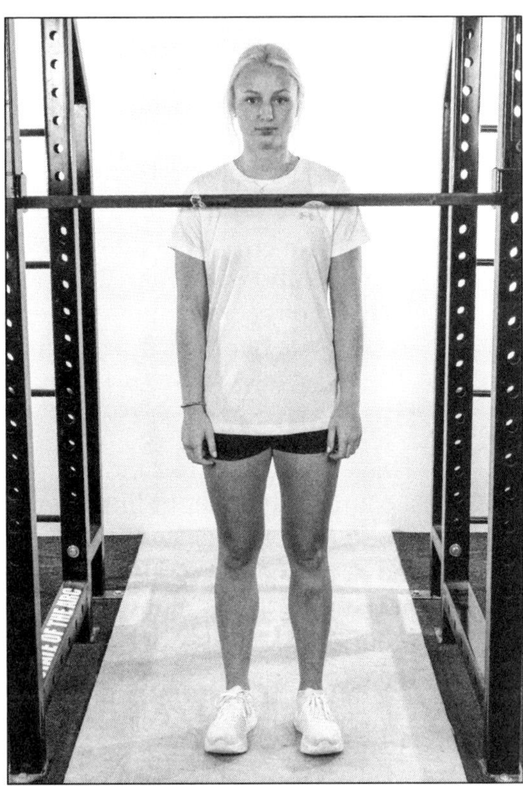

FIGURE 6.2 An example of the proper bar height in the rack to begin the setup of the press.

Set Up the Bar

The bar should be set in the rack at roughly the same height as it would be for your squat—with the same caveat that a little too low is better than a little too high. Set the bar in the J-hooks at a level just below your collarbone so that the bar is right at the top of your chest (see figure 6.2). This will let you unrack the bar safely and have enough space to clear the J-hooks without having to do a quarter squat in an awkward front-rack position.

Position the Hands

Next, you need to position your hands. Start with the same standard grip for the overhead press as for the bench press. In this case, your hands should be just outside shoulder width. The easiest way to set this up is to bring your hands up to your shoulders, slide them out to where they're just outside shoulder width, and then grasp the barbell. Then take the measurement by looking at where your hands are in relation to the power ring, or that first ring inside the barbell. This will give you a consistent reference point for where to grip the barbell so that you can go through this process quicker from set to set. Use a full-hand grip (see figure 6.3); don't unloop the thumb or use a suicide grip like we talked about in bench press. Use a full-hand grip and squeeze tight—like you're choking the bar while also pulling it apart.

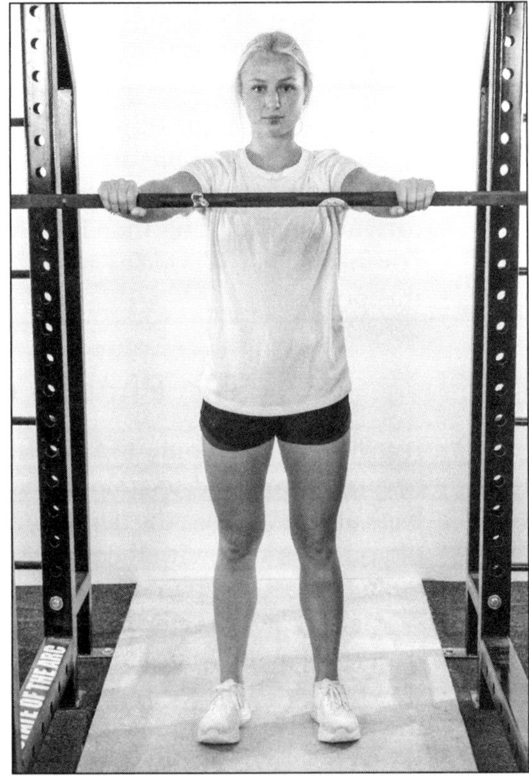

FIGURE 6.3 For the standard grip, make sure to grasp the bar with your thumb looped around it.

Get Under the Bar

Once your grip is set, you can start to work yourself underneath the bar. Think about pulling yourself into that position. Set your feet directly underneath the barbell at just outside shoulder width, just as you would for a squat. While still grasping the barbell, pull your upper body underneath the bar, and rest the bar directly across the front of your shoulders. Your elbows should be stacked directly underneath your wrists, making your forearm vertical. Your chest should stay nice and tall in this position (see figure 6.4). A cue that we have used a lot through the book is putting your shoulder blades in your back pockets, and it still applies here.

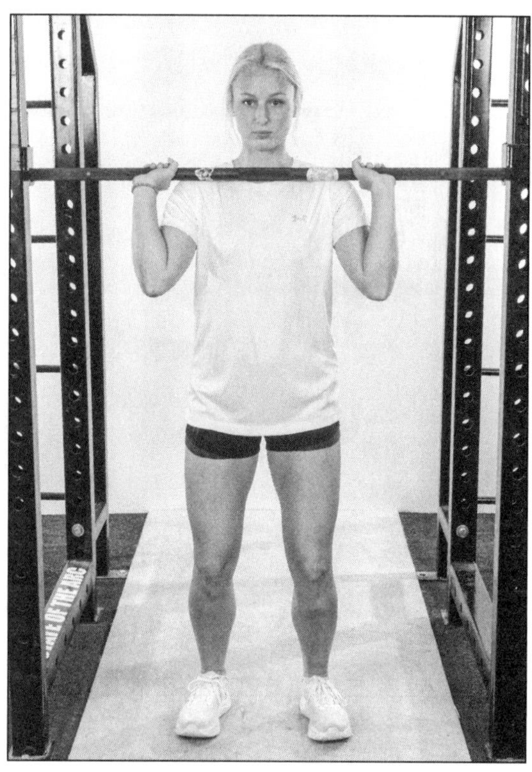

FIGURE 6.4 The proper position of the barbell for the press. The elbows should point down and the bar should be as close to the collarbones as possible.

As you tuck those shoulder blades into your back pockets, you should feel your chest drive into the bar more. The key to a strong overhead press is the foundation, or stability, you create underneath it. As with the squat, you want as much contact with the barbell as possible when you're in the start position. By tucking the shoulder blades into the back pockets and driving your chest up toward the bar, you create more contact with the barbell and build a more stable foundation to press from.

At this point, your hands should be fully grasped around the barbell, the barbell should be across the front of your shoulders, your chest should be nice and tall, your knees should be slightly bent, and your feet should be directly underneath the bar just outside shoulder width. Now you're ready to unrack the barbell and walk out to the start position. This part is going to sound really, really familiar.

Unrack the Bar

The way to unrack the bar and get set is the exact same way you would walk out a squat. Extend your knees and stand straight up underneath the barbell, creating enough height for the bar to clear the J-hooks. From here, take that same three-step approach to step away from the J-hooks, and remove the bar from the rack. If you need a refresher: It's one step straight back, another step straight back, and a third step to set your stance, which should be just outside shoulder width apart (see figure 6.5).

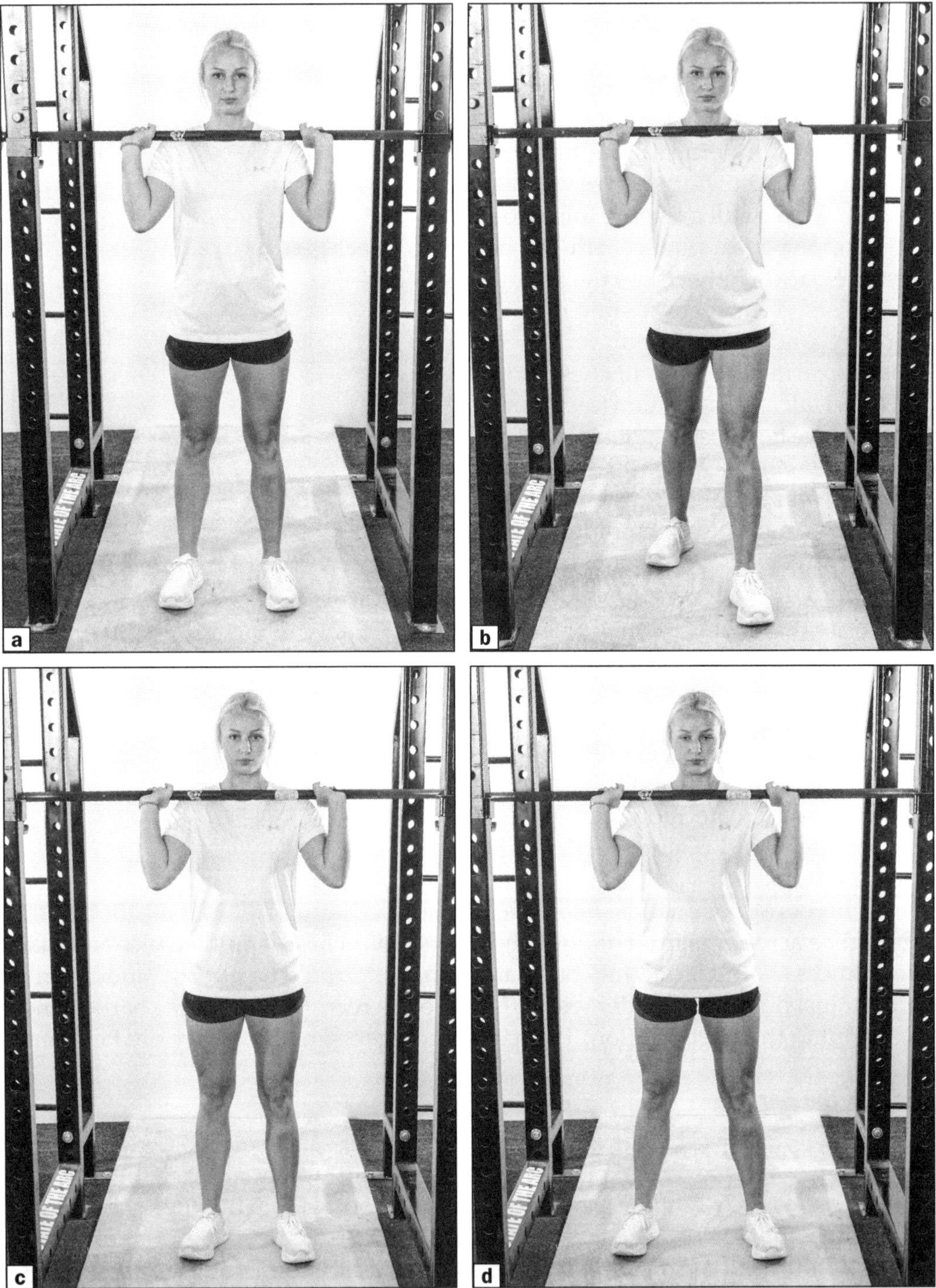

FIGURE 6.5 A look at the proper positions to unrack the barbell in the overhead press: *(a)* the unrack, *(b)* the first step straight back, *(c)* the second step back, and *(d)* the third step to set the width of the stance.

Once you've walked the bar out, your upper body should still be set in place and ready to press. The position you're in shouldn't be drastically different from the position you just used to unrack the barbell. Maintain tension by keeping those shoulder blades pinned into your back pockets, and keep a firm grasp on

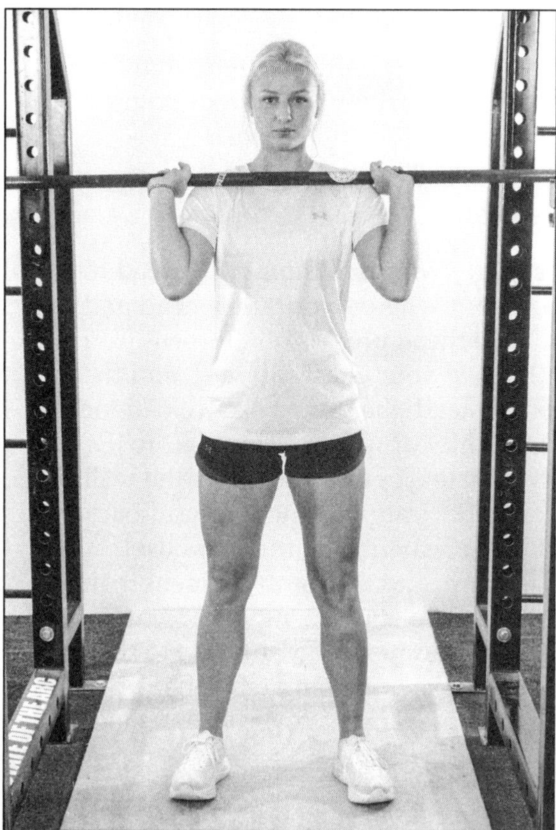

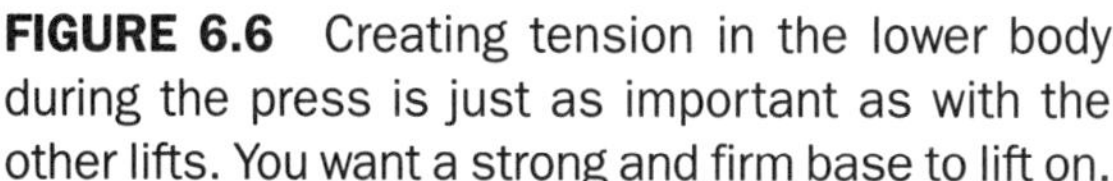

FIGURE 6.6 Creating tension in the lower body during the press is just as important as with the other lifts. You want a strong and firm base to lift on.

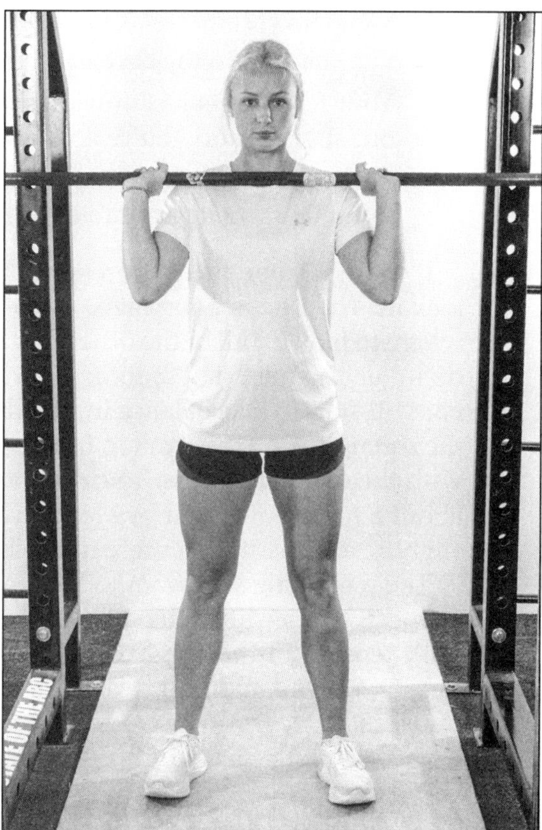

FIGURE 6.7 Starting position for the overhead press with the lifter ready to begin the ascent.

the barbell by trying to pull the bar apart. Next, you need to create tension in your lower body. A very common mistake with new lifters is trying to execute the overhead press without creating a lot of tension through the lower body to help stabilize the lift. This results in the bar getting about halfway up, the foundation underneath wobbling, and the lift being more difficult (if not an outright failure). Create tension in your lower body the same way you do with the deadlift or the squat: Set your stance at just outside shoulder width with your toes pointed out so that you can spread the floor apart (see figure 6.6).

Squeeze your glutes as tight as possible to lock in that position. Think of the setup for the overhead press as being similar to what it is for the vertical bench press. There should be no forward or backward hip movement and no movement in the feet, because if either of those two things happen, the bar-lifter unit becomes unbalanced and the center of gravity becomes inconsistent.

Before we move on to the ascent, let's take a minute to recap the start position, as shown in figure 6.7, and check where we are at this point:

- Your hands are grasped tightly around the barbell just outside shoulder width.
- Your elbows are stacked directly underneath your wrists, creating a vertical forearm.

- Your chest is tall, and your shoulder blades are "in the back pockets," pulling your chest into the barbell to create more tension.
- Your feet are set just outside shoulder-width apart with your toes pointed out slightly, and you're actively trying to spread the floor apart.
- Your legs are locked, your glutes are squeezed, and your lower body is tight, limiting its availability for movement.

It's almost time to start pressing, but there are two more things you need to lock in. The first is your gaze. We've talked about where to put your head and where to look for all of the other lifts, and the overhead press is no different. You definitely do not want to look down. That'll drive your chest forward, and the bar will start to lose balance in that direction. Instead, the same gaze we had for the squat—10 to 15 feet out in front of you or slightly upward—is the gaze to use with the overhead press. To drill it with my athletes, I put a sticker on the wall about a foot above their eye level. This allows the lifter to bring the head back slightly, making it easier to get the chin out of the way during the press itself.

The next thing you want to lock in is your brace, and this is no different than any of the other lifts either. Once you're in that solid start position and you've built tension in the upper and lower body, breathe in deeply, filling that 360 degrees of your abdominals and creating all of that pressure and tension in your midsection. Now you've created the foundation to press the bar overhead without letting anything else move.

The Ascent

The goal of the press is to move the bar in as straight a line as possible until it is directly overhead. To accomplish this, keep your wrists stacked vertically over your elbows, just like you do in the bench press. Unlike the bench press, however, the overhead press doesn't start with a lowering phase. You have to create that power out of the starting position like you do with the deadlift. To initiate the press, I tell my athletes to think about punching the sky. Keep your knuckles up and your wrists stacked, and then drive your hands and arms straight up, pressing the barbell in a straight line off your shoulders (see figure 6.8).

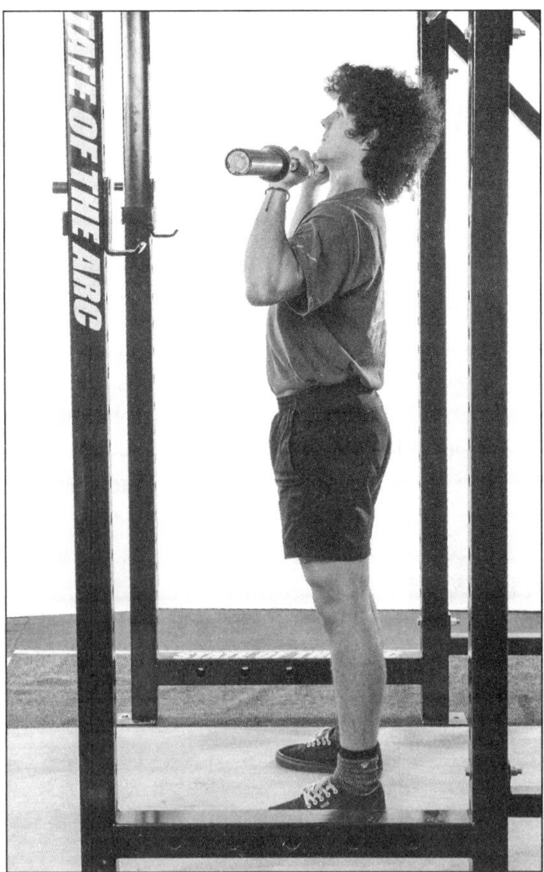

FIGURE 6.8 The first portion of the press should be a straight line off the shoulders to just under chin height.

During the early portion of the press, your elbows should stay directly under your wrists and remain pointed relatively straight forward. As the bar elevates and approaches, your elbows will need to flare out in order to keep the bar

What Do I Do With My *Face!?*

Every single person who has pressed has smashed the bar into their chin at some point. Every. Single. Person. Hopefully, reading this book will help prevent it from happening repeatedly. As the bar starts to move vertically, you have to get your head out of the way in order to keep the bar path in that straight line. If the bar is pushed around the head, as opposed to the head moving away from the bar, it's more likely to get stuck at right about forehead level and not move from there.

There are two things to do here, and one of them is already done: Your gaze is already set slightly upward. That gives you some room, but it may not be enough. To make more room, slide your head and chin back as the bar starts to rise (see figure 6.9).

For many, this will be enough room to clear their face from the bar and allow it to pass freely. Others may still need more room. In this case, a slight lean backward can give you the last little bit of room you need. By "lean backward" I mean about an inch of torso drift back (see figure 6.10).

It's not that a larger amount of lean backward is going to cause injury, but in terms of strength and execution, it's less sustainable for a beginner. It also creates more room for error. I want you to master the press before trying to utilize an advanced competition technique.

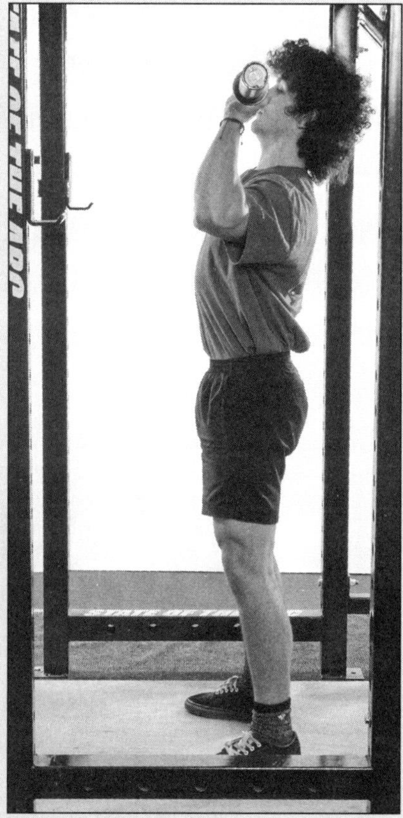

FIGURE 6.9 The head and chin should move as one unit to get out of the way of the bar. This will keep the straight-line bar path.

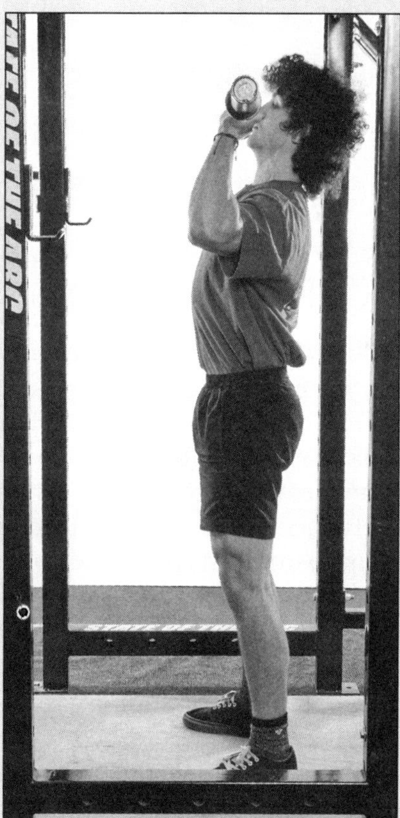

FIGURE 6.10 The lean backward doesn't have to be extreme. This example shows enough backward lean to get out of the way of the bar without losing balance.

traveling in a straight line (see figure 6.11). Allow this to happen naturally, and keep pressing. I've seen many athletes try to keep their elbows straight forward through the press, and it only leads to the bar being pushed forward.

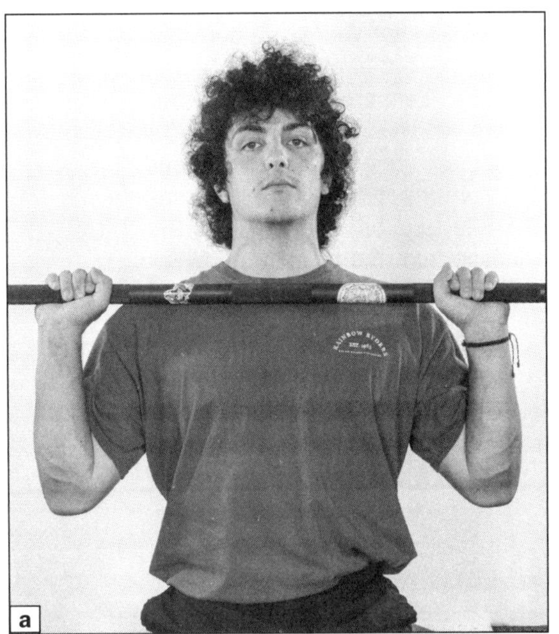

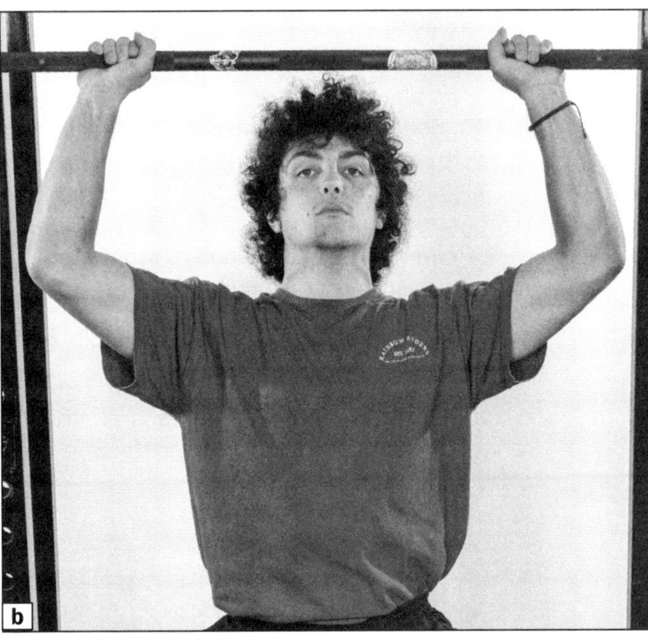

FIGURE 6.11 The elbows will naturally flare out during this portion of the press. Don't fight this from happening.

As the bar passes your forehead, keep pressing it straight up all the way until your elbows lock out. As your elbows begin to lock out, shrug your shoulders up toward your ears—as if you were shrugging "I don't know" but with your hands over your head (see figure 6.12). This will finish the press in a completely straight line, safely lock in the bar overhead, and set you up to bring the bar back down in a safe manner.

Note that I did not mention the lower body at any point in the movement. It should be completely stationary through the entire lift. There should be no dip or knee bend used to initiate the press. There should be no thrust of the hips forward through the sticky points. The lower body needs to be locked in through the whole press. Get tight and stay tight.

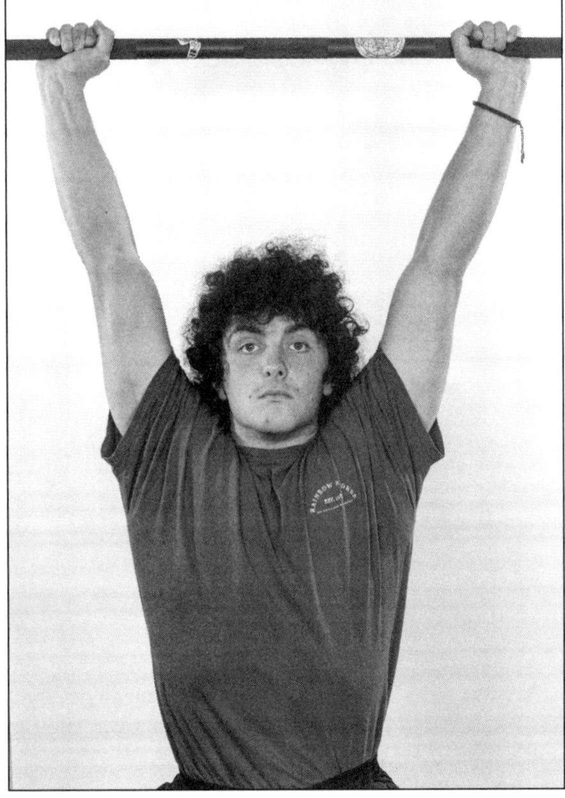

FIGURE 6.12 A cue of "shrug at the top" can help you to remember to keep pressing until you're fully locked out.

The Lock-Out

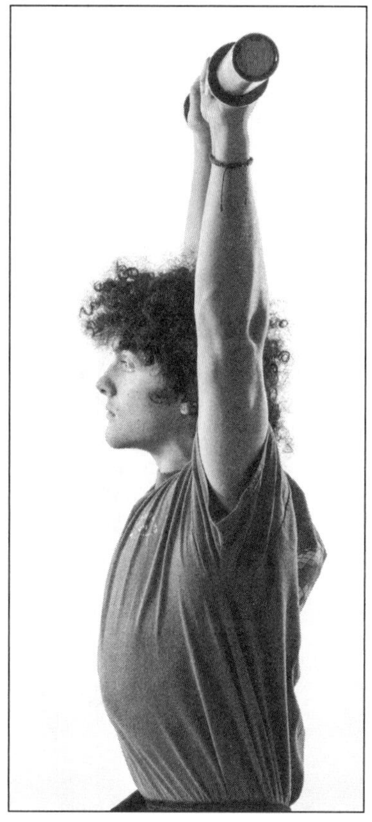

FIGURE 6.13 A full and stable lock-out position for the press. The lifter and the bar should be completely motionless in this position.

The lock-out of the press needs to be locked in before we start the descent. Unlike the bench press, where you have a large stable object supporting you, all you have to support you in the press is yourself and the tension you've created. I've seen many an athlete lose balance, lose tension, or not get to a completely motionless state before starting the descent in the press. This can lead to an inconsistent bar position on the way down, making consecutive reps harder.

This is where you need to exercise patience. In the lock-out position, your elbows should be completely extended with your shoulders shrugged up toward your ears, and your head should be aligned with your shoulders. Your hips and legs should be squeezed tightly under you, and your knees should be completely locked out (see figure 6.13). You and the bar should be completely motionless. This is the lock-out position that will create consistency.

One common mistake I see executed and taught in the press lock-out is an over extension of the head forward past the bar. I understand why this is taught to help standardize the position for people, but it's ultimately not necessary, and it doesn't create more stability or tension in the lift. The key to creating that is the shrugging up of the shoulders, so don't worry about trying to shove your head maximally forward. Get your head back in-line with the rest of your body, and lock the bar in with the shrug.

The Descent

"It's time to bring the elevator down!" This is the cue that I like to use when teaching the descent of the press. Think of a descending elevator that is full of passengers. It shouldn't crash down and make everyone fall over, but it also shouldn't move so slowly that the passengers become impatient.

When you are ready to bring the bar back down, unlock the elbows and the shoulder shrug holding the bar overhead. Now reverse everything you did during the ascent of the press. The key is to keep enough pressure on the bar that it doesn't free-fall. You should maintain control while bringing the bar back down to your shoulders, quickly moving your head and face out of the way. As the bar passes your chin, bend your knees to create cushioning for when the bar returns to your shoulders (see figure 6.14) Essentially, you use your lower body as a spring to catch the weight. If you have another rep to do, extend your knees, lock in your lower body again, and press.

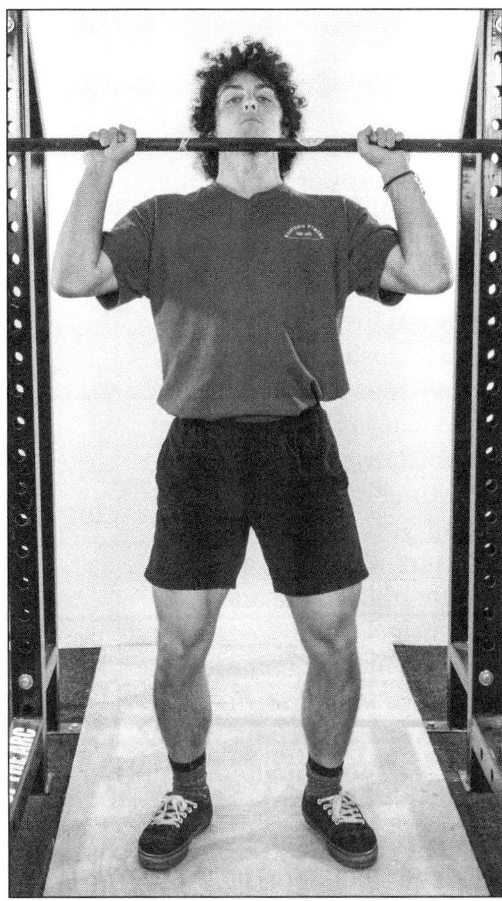

FIGURE 6.14 For the descent, start by unlocking the elbows and controlling the bar down as you bring your head back. Then bend your knees to help you "catch" the bar and soften the impact when it reaches your shoulders.

Common Errors in the Press

There are three errors I see most often in the overhead press: the wrists not remaining stacked, the elbows flaring out early, and too much lower-body movement. In truth, the number one reason why all three of these things happen is the same: too much weight on the bar. Of the four lifts, the overhead press is the lightest by far in terms of how much total weight you can lift, which means that adding weight will have more of an impact. I've run into far too many accounts of "it was only five more pounds than last set." On a percentage basis, a 5- to 10-pound (2 to 5 kg) increase is much greater with the overhead press than it is with the squat or deadlift, where your absolute weight is likely much higher.

If you can't stack your wrists vertically through the movement, focus on turning your knuckles up —like you do with the bench—and find a weight that lets you maintain that position. Get reps there until you can maintain that position better. If your elbows flare early, the bar is simply too heavy or you're performing too many reps in the set. There is a caveat here regarding lower-body movement. The bar being too heavy is certainly an issue because it requires more stability under it to press well. The other factor, however, is how well you can create tension in that position. Here's a check list for when you're in the start position:

Are your feet firmly planted and spreading the floor?
Are your knees locked?
Is your butt tight?
Are your shoulder blades "in the back pocket"?
Is your gaze slightly upward?
Do you have a tight grip?
Have you taken a big breath?

Running through this list should only take a few seconds. Missing one of the things on the list, however, is often what causes the lift to fail.

Overhead-Press Variations

You can just press to build the press. As with other lifts though, there are close variations to the regular overhead press that you can use to spice up your training a bit or to shore up weaknesses. Here are the top four that I use with my athletes.

Pause Press

Just like with the pause deadlift, in the pause press you pause where you experience the first overcoming force in the movement. This tends to be around eye to forehead level for most athletes. Pausing is also a great way to challenge and get a feel for your positioning. If you're not set up well in the start position (see figure 6.15*a*), you'll immediately feel it at the pause.

The goal here is to spend some time around that sticky spot by fully stopping the bar there and then holding it there for at least a one-second count (see figure 6.15*b*). This will help build the position and help prevent the common error of the bar being too far forward, which makes the press more difficult to finish. By pausing here, you can reestablish the proper press position with the bar staying over the center of gravity, and then create acceleration from that spot. To get the bar going again, think about punching the sky. Then the rest of the press is exactly the same (see figure 6.15*c*).

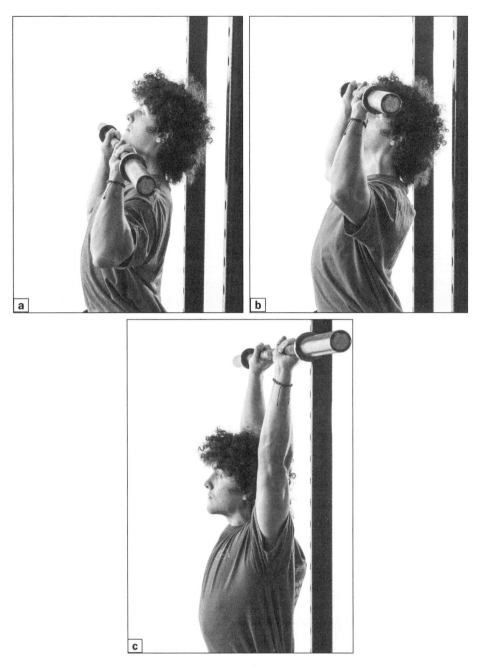

FIGURE 6.15 The three different positions of the paused press: *(a)* the start position, *(b)* the pause position at the sticking point, and *(c)* the lock-out.

The Push Press

Overload is the key ingredient when it comes to getting stronger. It can be tough with the press though, because of its weight ceiling. Adding a single pound (0.5 kg) to a set can be the difference between a make and a miss. Enter the push press.

In the regular press we discussed keeping the legs tight throughout the lift as to not use them to create momentum to drive into the bar. In the push press, this is exactly what you are trying to do. We are trying to create momentum into the bar and make the lift easier. Many people might consider the push press to be cheating, but it's not. It's a very valuable variation of the regular "strict" press.

The big difference with the push press is the drive of the legs to initiate the movement. This should be a sharp and quick dip in the lower body. To do this, set up as you do for the press and get your legs tight. Make sure to still build the same tension you would in the main lift. Once you are in a solid start position and ready to go, bend your knees and push your hips back slightly. This isn't a deep squat—it's a quarter squat at most—and your upper body should remain vertical and not change position at all aside from getting lower to the ground (see figure 6.16). I like to have my athletes think of jumping. In preparation for the jump, you naturally bend your knees and dip the lower body a bit. It's a similar movement here.

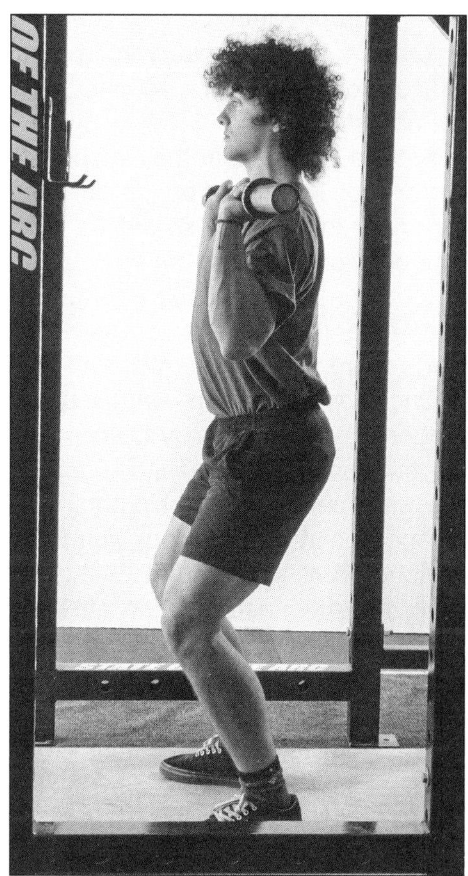

FIGURE 6.16 The dip for a push press doesn't involve a lot of knee bend. It should be quick and aggressive while keeping the bar in contact with the lifter.

One small but important note here: Don't dip so fast that the bar is left hanging in the air. You want that bar to stay on your shoulders and locked in the start position so that when you reverse the dip and drive with your legs, all that force goes into the bar. Otherwise, the bar will be on its way down while you are on the way up, and you will have to overcome the crashing of the bar into you.

Once you are at the bottom of your short dip, drive your legs vertically as hard as you can to start the upward trajectory of the bar. As you start to get to extension, aggressively press the bar overhead to lock-out. If you use enough leg drive, there will be a moment when the barbell will feel weightless. Don't let that fool you into thinking that you don't have to press as hard. The drive of the legs will typically get the bar past the first sticky part of the lift and elevate it to or above eye level. It's still on you to lock it out overhead though, so keep pressing and use that momentum to overload this lift more. Once you have locked out the bar, bring it down to your shoulders the same way you would in a regular press. Bend your elbows, bring the bar down toward your shoulders, and bend your knees to help cushion the bar back into the start position. Now you're ready for another rep. This is a great variation to overload the top portion of the press if you struggle with lock-out, but it is also excellent for creating overall upper-body power.

Pin Press

The pin press is a great variation to specifically work weak points in the overhead press. I use it the same way I use the pin press for the bench, with the main goal being the development of strength and power in the desired position.

The setup requires a rack that you can stand in with enough room to be able to press fully overhead without running into the cross members. This can be difficult for taller lifters, so another option is a rack with long spotter arms that are adjustable.

Set the pins so that they support the barbell at the most difficult portion of the lift for you. This could be just off the shoulders, at eye to forehead level, or even very near lock-out. Next, set up underneath the barbell as you normally would. Your body should be in the same position that it would normally be in at that stage of the press. Pay special attention to where your feet are under the bar; many people set up for the pin press with their feet not directly under the bar, and this leads them to push it forward off the pins.

Once you are set up—with your feet under the bar, your hands grasped tightly around it, and your body braced tightly—you need to create tension similar to the tension you create with a deadlift. You will not pull the slack out of the bar like with the deadlift, but putting pressure into the bar will allow you to find the balance point and will lock you into a better position (see figure 6.17*a*). Then explode. Punch the bar into the air as hard and as fast as possible. You should have maximum acceleration off the pins. Drive the bar up, and push your head through all the way to lock-out (see figure 6.17*b*). To bring the bar back down, reverse the movement the same way you would with a normal press. One thing to note here is that it will be loud when the bar makes contact with the rack, so be ready for that. Reset yourself for the next rep, and repeat.

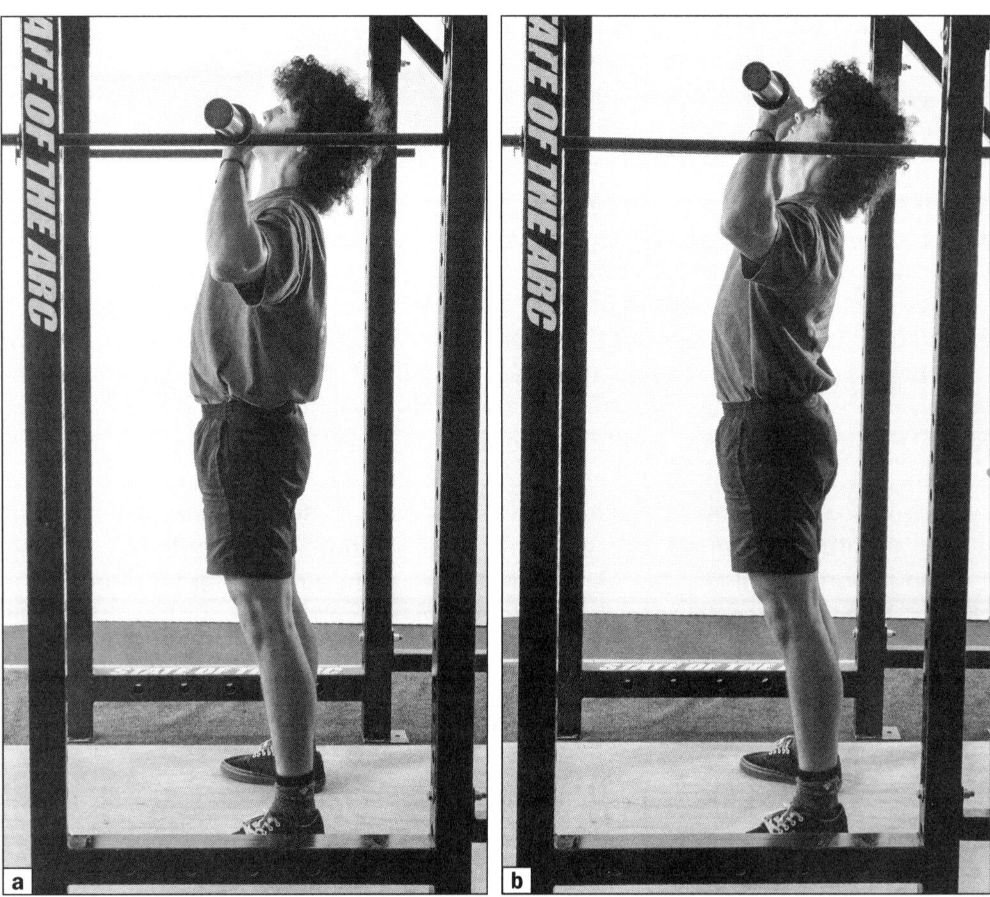

FIGURE 6.17 The pin press: *(a)* the start position *(b)* and the drive off the pins.

Behind-the-Neck Press

This is a controversial one. "You encourage a behind-the-neck press!? What about shoulder health?!" We have covered this concept extensively already, but I want to make it clear: There are no inherently dangerous movements, only inappropriate exercise selections for individuals. I have used the behind-the-neck press successfully for years with weightlifters, powerlifters, Strongman athletes, and the general population. That doesn't mean I use it with everybody. The individual needs to be able to comfortably get into the start position and have the required shoulder range of motion to get there. I test for this by doing a supine shoulder external rotation test.

Lie flat on your back with your knees bent. Bend your elbows and bring both arms up to 90 degrees of abduction so that your elbows are even with your shoulders. Keep your upper arms in contact with the ground. From here, let your hands fall back to the ground in a relaxed manner. If you can get your hands in contact with the ground, move to my next test, which is to give you a dowel rod or a PVC pipe and have you get in the behind-the-neck press start position (described next). If you can do this without pain or discomfort, then we are ready to roll.

What does that start position look like? It looks very similar to your back-squat position. The bar should be across your upper traps and below the C7 vertebra. Your hands should be set on the bar just outside shoulder width, and you should be grasping the bar with your entire hand and with your thumb wrapped around it. Your elbows should be pointed down with your shoulder blades pulling down into your back pockets. Your chest should be tall, your lower body should be tight and spreading the floor, and your brace should be locked in (see figure 6.18*a*).

From here, the execution is the same except you don't need to get your face out of the way of the bar. The bar path should be a straight line up to lock-out. When you bring the bar back to your shoulders, bend your knees slightly to cushion that position (see figure 6.18*b*). The bar should end up directly over your ears, just like in the regular press (see figure 6.18*c*).

So what's the purpose of this variation? With the weight supported on the shoulders in this fashion, the bar is more secure than it is when it's in the front-rack position. This means you may be able to press more weight from this position than from the normal start position of the overhead press. You also may be able to create more of a straight-line press with the bar already being behind your head. Overload is a large portion of progress, so if I see the overhead press stalling with my athletes, I use this variation to drive more overload and stoke progress.

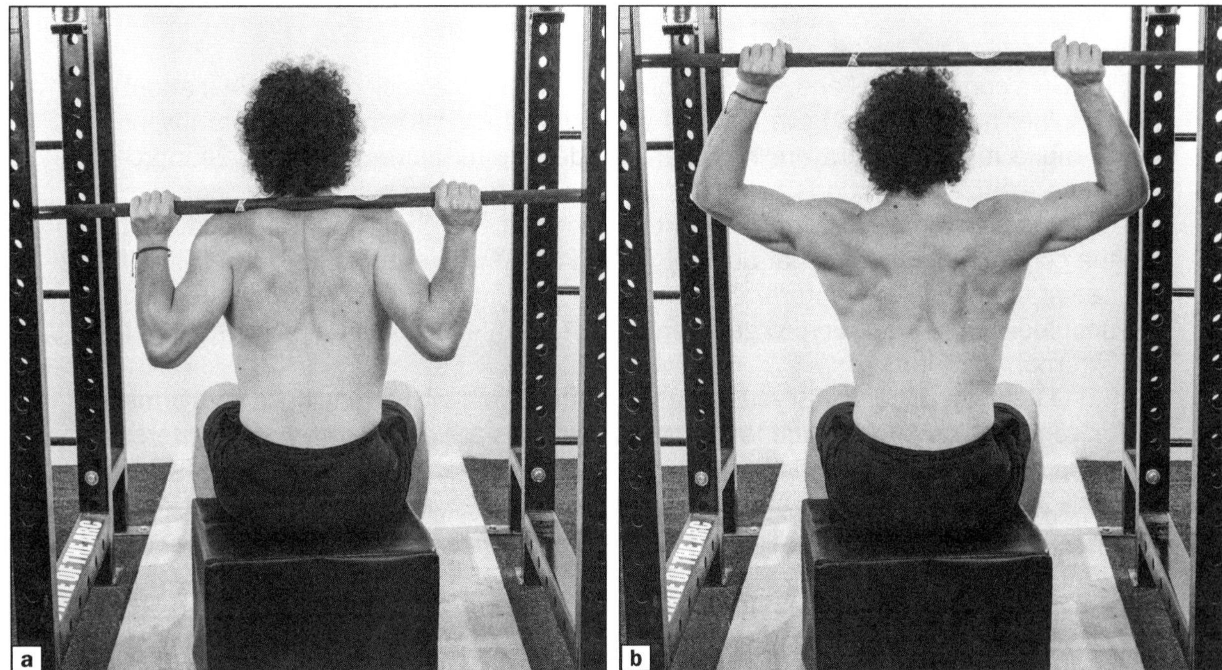

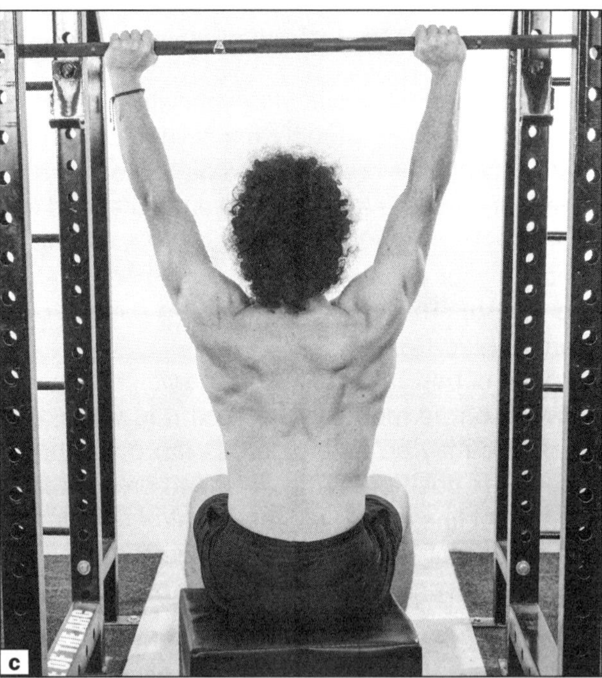

FIGURE 6.18 The behind-the-neck press: *(a)* start position, *(b)* the bar passing the head, and *(c)* the lock-out.

Warming Up for the Overhead Press

This section is going to feel like a review. I think there is elegance in simplicity, so many of the warm-up exercises that I use for the press are the same ones that I use for the bench and the squat. They have proven time and again to be the most effective exercises to cluster in a warm-up. I could put new ones in here just for the sake of newness, but the honest truth is that when I've tried them, they just haven't been as effective. The big lesson to learn here is that effective training doesn't require a huge encyclopedia of different exercises. Effective training is doing the same, simple things, over and over, until you become an expert in them. So let's look at the exercises I use to warm up athletes for the press.

Half-Kneeling Arm Circles

Again, if you've read through previous chapters, this exercise will be familiar! Tightness in the anterior shoulder, or pec, is a common complaint from people when they first start pressing overhead. Stand next to an empty wall—I suggest dry wall or something smooth because you will be dragging your arm on the surface. Go down on your knee that is closest to the wall (see figure 6.19*a*). Both your bottom knee and your top knee should be bent at 90 degrees. There is no need to lean forward. You should be close enough to the wall that your shoulder is just touching it. If being this close to the wall is too hard or if you aren't able to get your arm all the way around in the circle, slide away from the wall until you can. Extend the arm closest to the wall straight out in front of you with your palm facing away from the wall (see figure 6.19*b*). Squeeze your glutes tight. You should feel a decent stretch in the front of your hips. From here, bring your arm overhead as you work it around in a circle on the wall (see figure 6.19*c*). As your arm gets behind you, allow your hand to naturally turn over so that your palm is facing the wall (see figure 6.19*d*). Keep working that arm around and as it approaches your hips, you can turn your hand back over (see figure 6.19*e*). Do this for five to eight reps on each side, and then move on to the next part of your sequence.

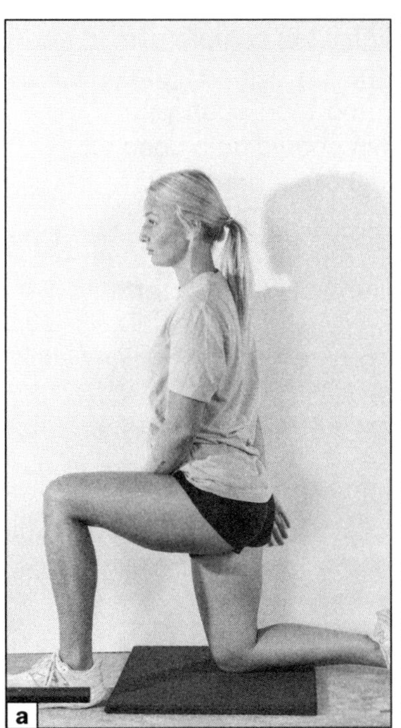

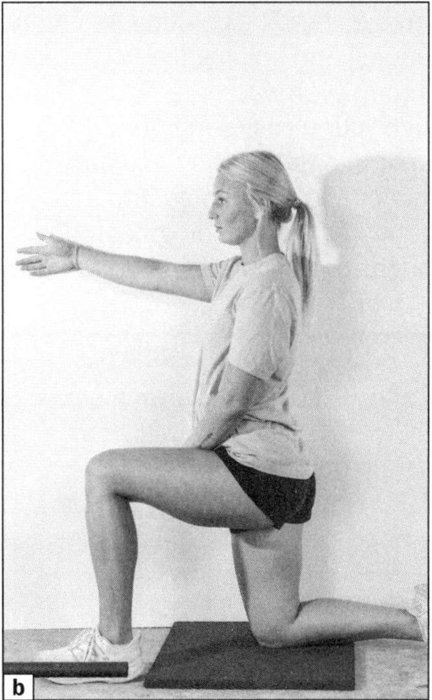

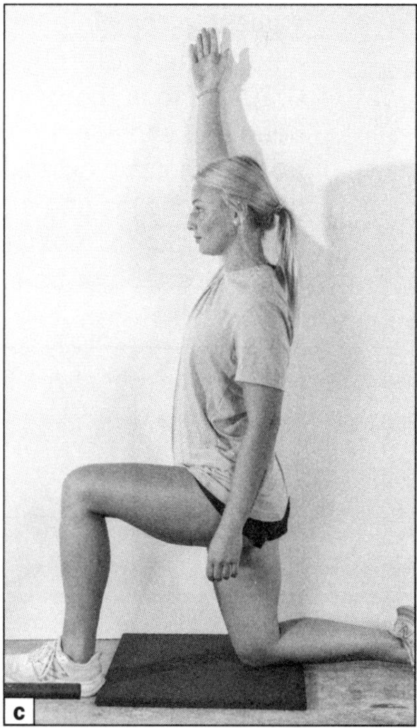

FIGURE 6.19 Half-kneeling arm circle.

(continued)

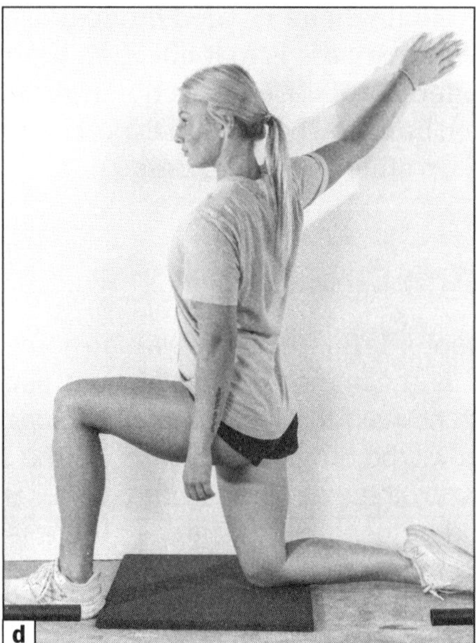

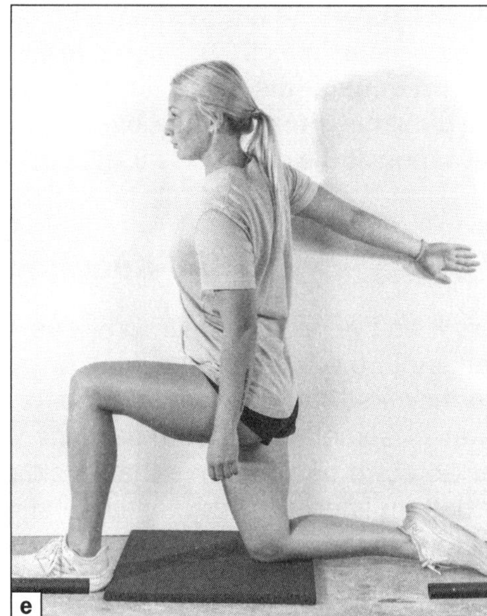

FIGURE 6.19 *(continued)*

Kettlebell Sots Press

This can be done from a deep squat or from a standing position, and it's best used on those days when you just don't feel like you can extend through the upper-back area. Grab a kettlebell (or dumbbell) and hold it at your chest. I suggest using one that you think is going to be far too light. Trust me—this is a tough one. It's easiest to complete this from a standing position and more difficult to complete in a deep squat. Start by standing and holding the kettlebell by the horns (see figure 6.20*a*). Press the bell directly overhead (see figure 6.20*b*), and then push your head and shoulders through your arms (see figure 6.20*c*). This should help open up that thoracic extension. If this is too easy, you can move right to a deep-squat position or even use a chair or a low box to go into a seated position. This will be much harder for most, so master the standing position before moving on. Five to eight reps tend to be enough. Then you can move on to the next in your cluster.

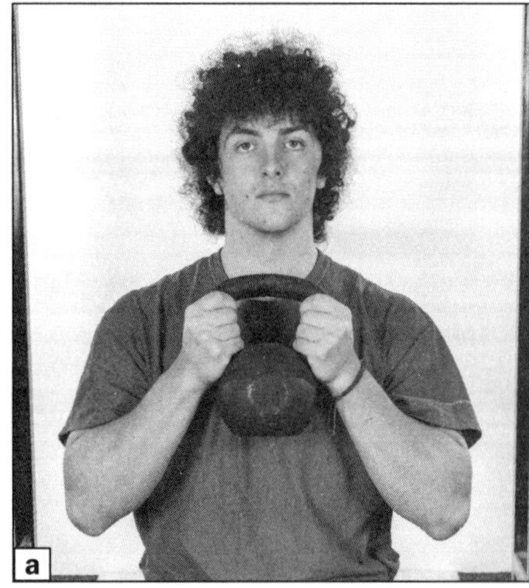

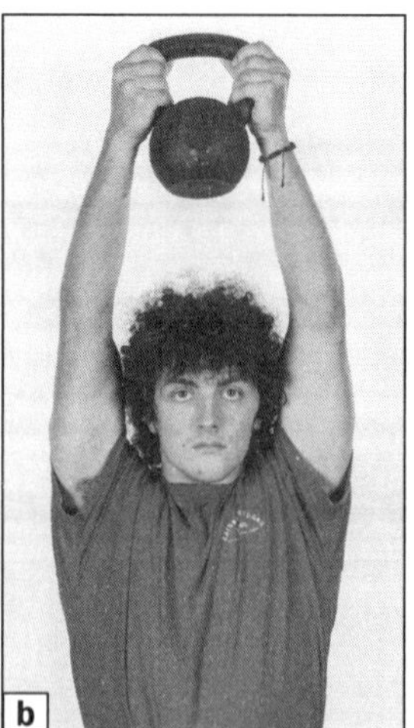

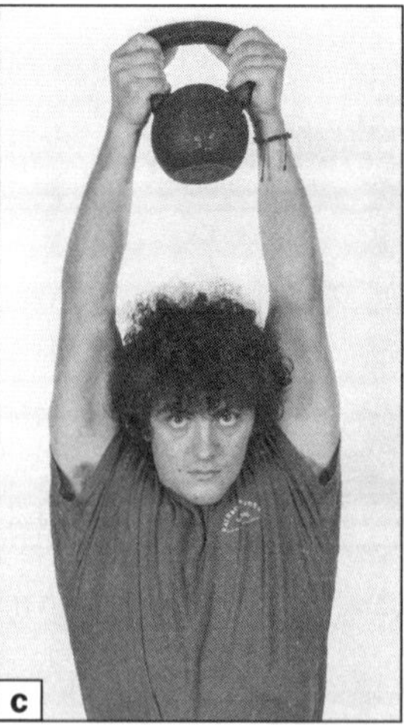

FIGURE 6.20 Kettlebell sots press.

Half-Kneeling Kettlebell Press

The initial setup will be the same half-kneeling position as with the arm circles (minus being right next to a wall). Grab a kettlebell (or dumbbell) and hold it in the hand on the same side as the downed knee (see figure 6.21*a*). Brace tightly, like you would before you bench or squat, then pull the shoulders down into the back pockets and press the bell overhead (see figure 6.21*b*). The key here is to get your biceps to your ear while not leaning back or letting your chest open up to the ceiling. Sets of eight work well here, using a weight that is relatively light.

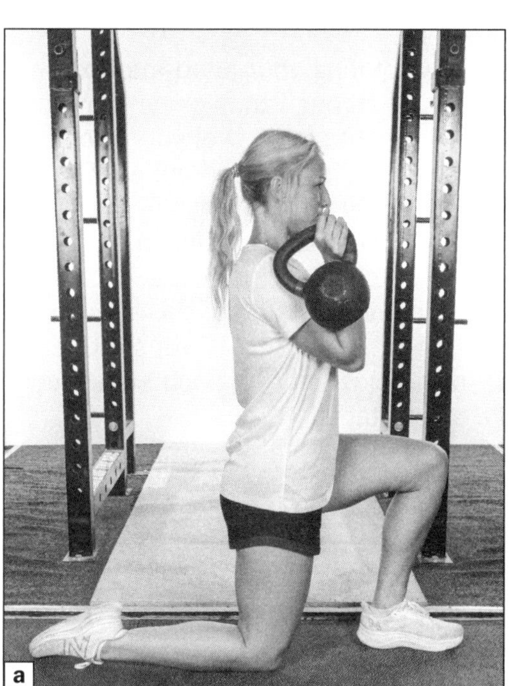

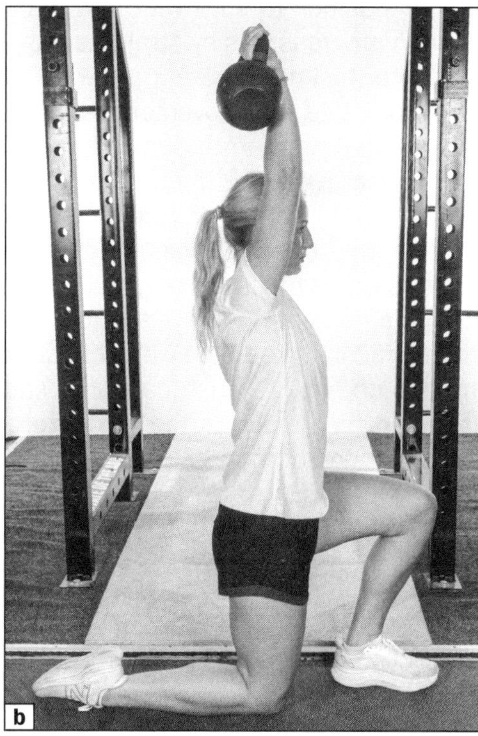

FIGURE 6.21 Half-kneeling kettlebell press: *(a)* The start position and *(b)* the lock-out position. Note that the athlete isn't leaning back at the lock-out position but instead is sitting tall.

Kettlebell Arm Bar

This is the only new exercise in this section, and it will be the last one. I love this exercise. I almost put it into the bench section earlier, but there were already enough exercises there. This exercise is incredibly scalable, and it's excellent for working the shoulder through internal and external rotation in a controlled manner.

Start by getting a light kettlebell (or a dumbbell) and lie on your side. Using the arm that is closer to the ceiling, press the weight up so that your arm is straight up in the air (see figure 6.22*a*). Your bottom arm can be tucked under your head or reaching out in front of you, whichever is more comfortable. The easiest lower-body position to start with is with both your knees bent, known as *hook lying.* You can progress this by straightening your bottom leg while keeping your top leg bent with the knee tucked up toward your chest.

To complete the movement, start by simply rotating your hand into external and internal rotation and letting the shoulder go through that range of motion with it (see figure 6.23*b* and 6.23*c*). Keep the weight stable over your shoulder; it may start to wobble around a bit as you move. This is normal. With each rep of rotation, try to turn the hand a little more.

If this is easy, the next step is to start to turn your chest to the floor as you keep your arm straight up in the air. You will feel a stretch in your chest, and it will be more difficult to keep the weight in position. Remember that this is a warm-up, so there is no need to push past your capabilities here. Do 8 to 10 reps with each arm, and then move to the next exercise in the cluster. With each subsequent set, the range of motion will become more comfortable.

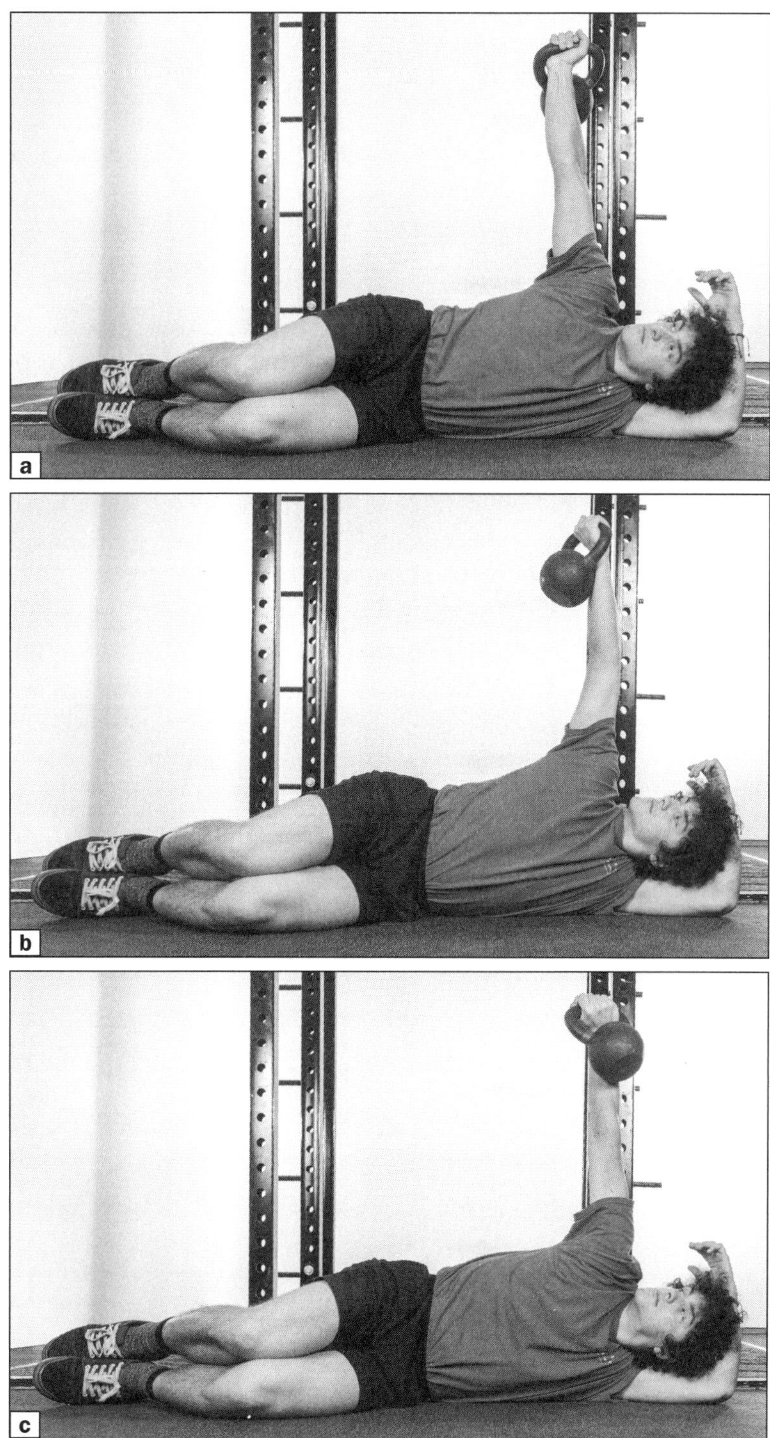

FIGURE 6.22 The kettlebell arm bar.

That's it. You have completed the four foundational barbell movements and are ready to start training to new levels. The journey isn't over yet though. What else is there to do in the gym? How do we create a program and what else do we fill it with? Let's find that out now.

Chapter 7

The Accessory Lifts

The first half of this book is all about the main movements—the big four, so to speak—and about unlocking the power of the bar. For a complete program that will help you achieve your goals however, you need something else as well: accessory, or supplemental, exercises. As you were reading the first part of this book, perhaps you found yourself thinking "What about the other exercises I see people doing?" Most of those exercises fall into this broader category. In this chapter, we will break these down based on specific movement patterns, but in general, anything that isn't a squat, a bench, a deadlift, or a press is an accessory exercise that can help build the performance of those four lifts.

Why do they need to be part of the overall program? There are two big reasons to incorporate accessory lifts into your program. The first one is novelty. I've done and seen programs that focus on just the big four. Repeating those lifts over and over, day after day, can lead to burnout, boredom, and a stagnation in progress. Programs like this can definitely be effective, but they run the risk of becoming tedious and difficult to complete from a compliance standpoint. By adding accessory exercises, you can incorporate novelty into the program on a more regular basis and stay more engaged with the exercise and program as a whole. This novelty also leads to motor-pattern learning and to increased strength in the main movements.

The second big reason to incorporate accessory movements is hypertrophy. The old adage goes that a bigger muscle is a stronger muscle. You can get bigger using just the big four, but I wouldn't say it's the best route to take. Accessory exercises can help you to isolate weak points in a lift and then target and strengthen those muscles more directly. This creates more growth, leading to better progress over the long term. Plus, most of us lift so that we can look like we lift. Accessory exercises help with that.

There are endless ways to categorize exercises and overcomplicate this aspect of training. So to create and outline categories of accessory exercises for my athletes, I use a tried-and-true formula from the *great* strength coach, Dan John. I have tried others, but I keep coming back to this. It's simple. It's effective. It's damn near perfect. As a matter of fact, I've only added one category to it over the years. Without further ado, the following are the six categories of accessory exercise that we will cover.

- *Push.* An exercise that requires you to move the weight away from your body with your upper body.

- *Pull.* An exercise that requires you to bring the weight closer to your body, especially with your upper body.
- *Squat.* An exercise that involves knee and hip flexion (i.e., bending) with one or two legs. A favorite exercise of mine—from a squat-accessory standpoint—is the lunge.
- *Hinge.* An exercise where your hips push back and you go into hip flexion without much knee flexion. Think about sticking your rear end out to close a car door.
- *Carry.* Exercises in which the athlete walks with weight on their back or in one or both of their hands. Carries are grossly underutilized in most training programs. While they may not have direct carryover to the big four, they do help build core strength and conditioning to improve recovery. Carries make the entire program more well-rounded, especially for athletes who want to focus on strength while still maintaining some cardiovascular endurance. Due to the decreased impact, carries allow you to get the required heart-rate increase from walking with less recovery cost than running.
- *Core.* Core exercises are defined as exercises that help improve the stability and strength of the trunk itself. You will often hear that if you squat, bench, deadlift, and press then you don't need extra core exercises, but I disagree with this. I don't think you need to do super-complex core exercises, but it is effective to train the core on its own in order to build as much strength as possible there. It's very frustrating if your core is the weakest link in the lift. You can prevent that from happening with a few simple exercises.

The accessory exercises provided here are not intended to constitute an exhaustive list of all the possible exercises you could ever do. There are thousands of exercises to experience during your lifting journey. You will also notice that some of these are compound movements that hit multiple muscle groups, while others are isolation movements that are more specific to common weak points in the lifts. Think of this list as the greatest hits of basic exercises that can fill out your program for years to come.

Push Accessory Lifts

Let's start with the push accessory lifts. These are often coupled with the bench press or the overhead press in a program so that pressing and push movements occur on the same days. They help support the growth of upper-body muscles like the triceps, pecs, anterior delts, and other pressing-related muscles. It's important to include them in your program so that you aren't relying only on the bench press and the overhead press to build the required muscle to get stronger. These accessory lifts provide the added benefit of allowing you to press from different angles and with different ranges of motion, helping you to stay healthier in the long run and keeping training more interesting.

How Hard Do I Train Accessories?

The absolute basics of programming will be covered later in the book, but one question to answer early is how intensely to train the accessory movements. There is a lot of debate about whether these should be trained to absolute failure when the muscle can't effectively contract anymore, to technical failure where form breaks down and the set stops, or if you should stop the training when there are still a few reps left in the tank. Going to muscular failure is great for hypertrophy. In my opinion, however, the recovery cost is far too high to do this on a regular basis. That leaves us with two options: training to technical failure or leaving reps in the tank (stopping at a certain rate of perceived exhaustion, or RPE). These two methods have two specific timelines in programming for me.

I save going to technical failure for the off-season when there is no plan to test a maximum weight in the near future. You take each set of each exercise to the point where your technique begins to break down. That can mean having a little too much elbow flare, or letting the chest fall, or not being able to maintain position because of fatigue. Whatever it is for you, that's when you cut it off. While RPE has a component of technical failure, it normally occurs at RPE 9 and RPE 10. Also, being able to accurately gauge RPE is a skill, so I find it best to start by separating these two.

The next option is to leave a few reps in the tank, or to stop at a specific RPE target. For many, RPE 6 to RPE 8 is when they are two to four reps away from technical failure. This option gives you enough stimulus to maintain progress without taking recovery away from the big lifts. I prefer to use this method during the competitive season as early as six weeks before a competition or a testing day for new one-rep maximums. It gives you enough room to push the big lifts hard and to nail down technique at heavier loads. Each method has its time and purpose; use both of them wisely as you progress.

Arnold Press

Named after the legend himself, Arnold Schwarzenegger, the *Arnold press* is one of my favorite overhead presses. This press is unique in that it adds a rotational aspect to the overhead press. I've found that this helps my athletes stay healthier while pushing themselves on the overhead press, probably because of the greater range of motion and the more natural rotation that this exercise allows the shoulder to go through.

The Arnold press is typically performed using dumbbells, but it can also be done using kettlebells. You can do it standing or seated on a bench. If you're standing, take the same stance that you would for an overhead press. If you're seated, the stance should be slightly wider than shoulder width and you should create tension in the lower body like you do for the bench press.

The easiest way to get the dumbbells to your shoulders is to have someone assist you, one dumbbell at a time. Make sure the person assisting you uses both hands with each dumbbell. They shouldn't grasp the handle of the dumbbell; in addition to being awkward for the lifter, it's also not a secure grip on the weight. Instead, they should grab both ends of the dumbbell and then help you bring it up to shoulder level. If you can't get help, the next best thing is to kick them up. The heavier the dumbbells get, the harder it becomes to kick them both up at the same time, so I suggest you do this one side at a time. Rest the dumbbell vertically on your knee. In one continuous movement, lift up your knee and lift the dumbbell up with your arm to shoulder height. I like to do this on my nondominant side first, so if you are right-handed, kick up the left side first. Then kick up the other dumbbell, and we are ready to press.

The Arnold press has one small detail to it that sets it apart from other press variations. With most, you start in a neutral position with your hands just outside your ears and your palms facing in (see figure 7.1*a*). For the Arnold press, on the other hand, you start with your hands in front of your face and your palms facing toward you. To perform the movement, start to press the dumbbells up and as you press, allow your shoulders to naturally internally rotate into the finish position (see figure 7.1*b*). At the top, your palms should be facing away from you and straight forward (see figure 7.1*c*). Then pull the dumbbells back down into the starting position, externally rotating and turning your hands back toward your face (see figure 7.1*d*).

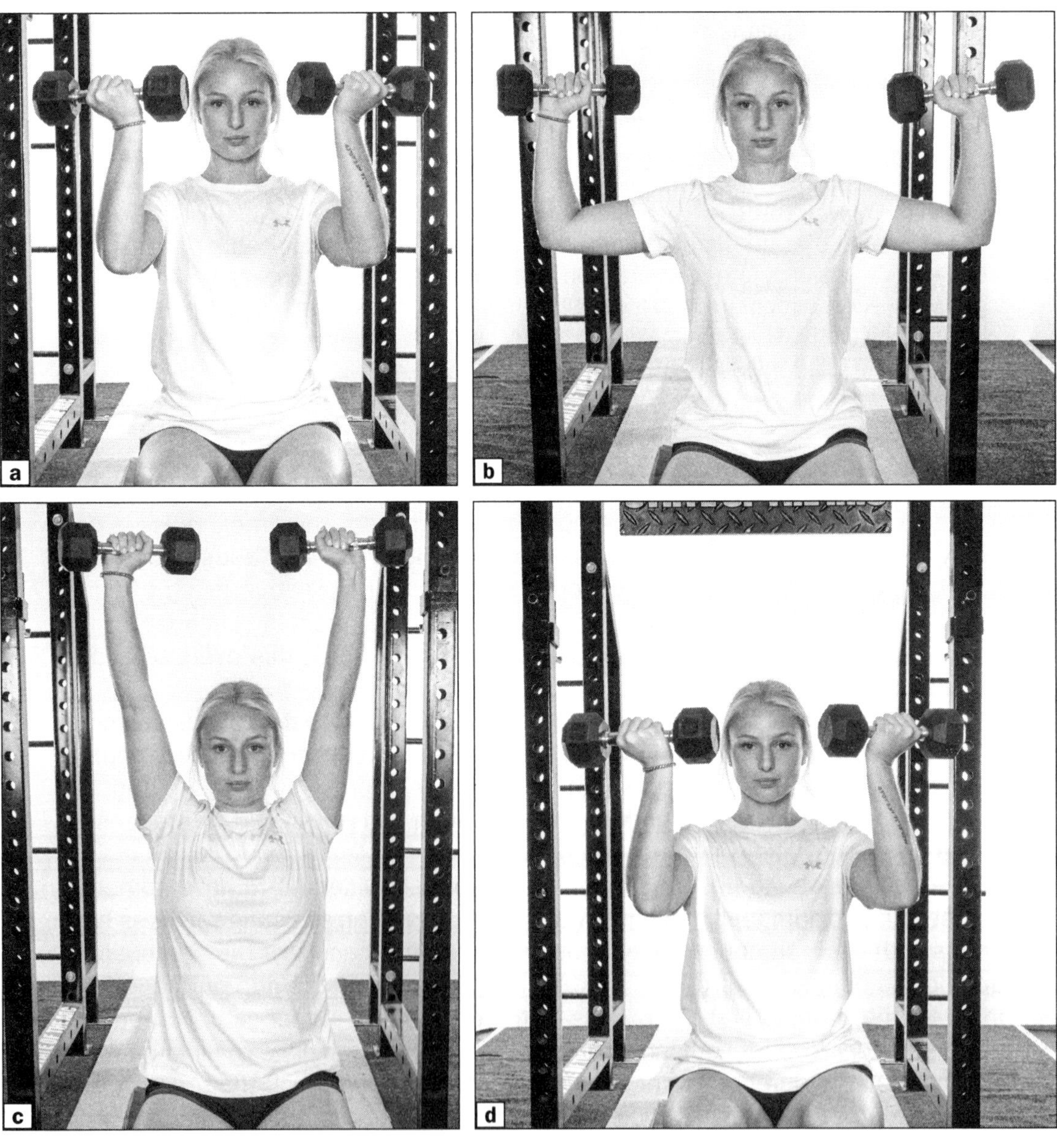

FIGURE 7.1 Full sequence of the Arnold press: *(a)* The start position, (b) the external rotation of the shoulder at the midway point, (c) the lock-out, and *(d)* back to the start position.

Triceps Extension

For pressing, the chest, shoulders, and triceps are universally understood as the prime movers of the lifts. However, if there is one muscle group I consistently see lag behind in performance, it is the triceps. As I tell my athletes, "You can always use more triceps." This basic triceps-extension exercise is super simple and incredibly effective.

This can be done using a cable machine with the rope attachment, a triceps handle, or a regular single-arm handle. It can also be done using bands that are securely attached to a rack. Stand tall with your arms at your sides, then bend your elbows fully to grasp whatever implement that you're using (see figure 7.2*a*). Keeping your arms tight to your sides, extend your arms all the way until your elbows are fully extended. This is the lock-out of this movement. Some people may add a twist to this by spreading the rope attachment or the bands apart at the very bottom. The main thing is to go from full elbow flexion to full elbow extension in one clean movement (see figure 7.2*b*). Once you're to lock-out, unlock your elbows and return them all the way to a fully flexed position *without* letting your torso move forward or backward. Since the triceps are a smaller muscle group, I have my athletes do much higher reps with these. Often, it's sets of 15 to 20 reps with some workouts including 100 total reps. The smaller muscle groups recover faster, allowing you to train this at a higher volume more frequently and more often in the program.

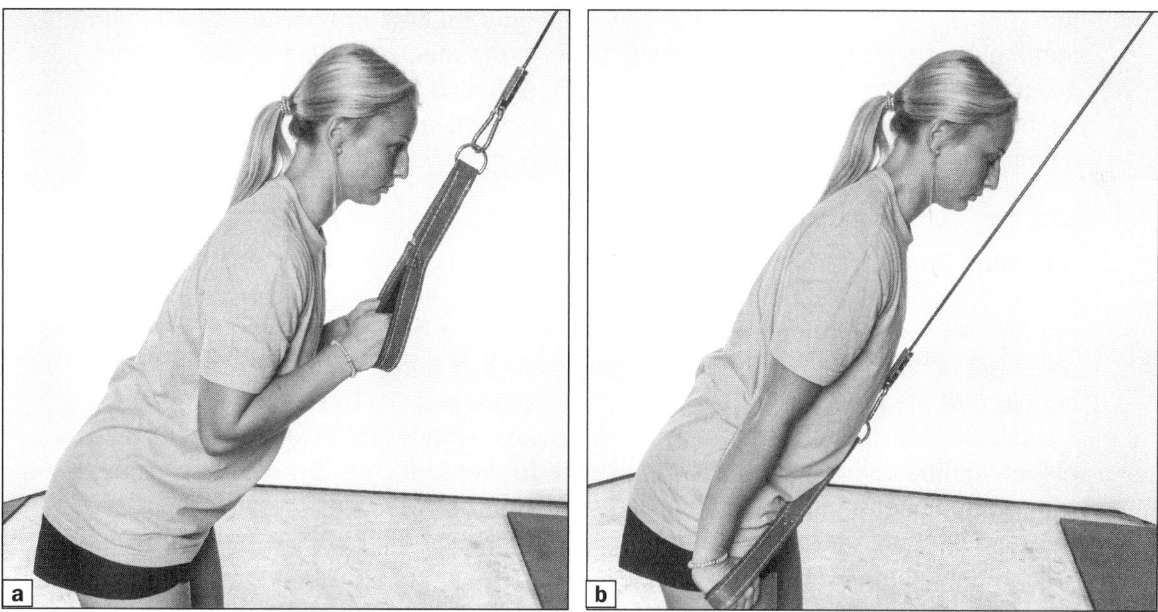

FIGURE 7.2 Start the triceps extension by standing tall with your elbows in as much flexion as possible. At the lock-out, your elbows should be fully extended, and you should be flexing your triceps as hard as possible.

Arm Raise

The arm raise focuses on the three heads of the deltoids (anterior, medial, and posterior), which are the muscles of the shoulder that are commonly understood to create the rounded-shoulder look that is typically found with very strong pressers. Arm raises are a great way to isolate these muscles and build them without increasing pressing volume.

There are three variations of the arm-raise exercise—the lateral, the front, and the reverse. They are similarly executed, typically using dumbbells. We'll start with the lateral arm raise, since it's the one that most people are familiar with, and then carry those instructions over for the other two. The lateral arm raise is one of my biggest go-to accessory movements for shoulders. Start in a standing position (you can also do these seated) with the dumbbells straight down at your sides and your palms facing your body (see figure 7.3*a*). The key through this movement is to not use momentum and to keep the arms straight as you raise your hands up to shoulder level. To do this, brace as we've discussed previously and then—without rocking your torso back and forth and while continuing to stand tall—lift your arms out to the sides until your shoulders are at a 90-degree angle and your arms are parallel to the floor (see figure 7.3*b*). I like to hold this position for one to two seconds, and then slowly lower the weight back down to the start position. You should feel the muscles working in the front of the shoulders.

The front raise is executed in the exact same manner as the lateral arm raise, but you bring your hands straight out in front of you to shoulder height. Throughout this movement, remain tall and keep your palms facing the floor so they remain in full pronation. Stop the motion when your arms reach the height at which they are parallel to the floor (see figure 7.4*a*). Again, hold this position for one to two seconds, and then slowly lower the weight back down to the start position (see figure 7.4*b*) You should feel the muscles working around the entire shoulder.

The one difference with a reverse arm raise (also known as a *reverse fly*) is that you do it in a bent-over position. Everything else remains the same. Hang your arms straight down toward the floor with your palms facing each other so you're in a neutral grip position (see figure 7.5*a*). Then raise your arms until they are parallel to the floor (see figure 7.5*b*). Again, hold this position for one to two seconds, and then slowly lower the weight back down to the start position. You should feel the muscles working more toward the back of the shoulder.

Just like the triceps extensions, these work smaller muscles that can take higher volume during sets. I program these for sets of 15 to 20 reps, especially with my beginner athletes. Once acclimated, they can add some weight and lower the reps. Setting up specific sets, reps, and frequency through a training block will be covered more in the programming section.

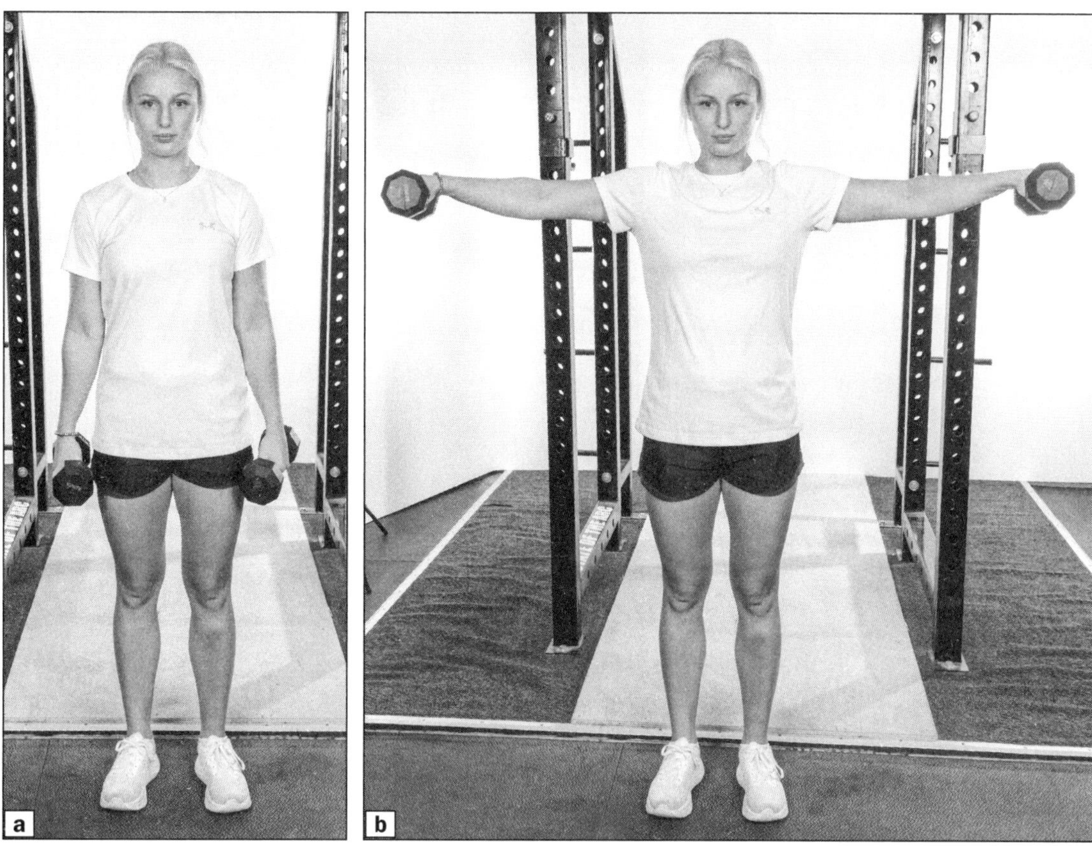

FIGURE 7.3 The *(a)* start position and the *(b)* finish position of the lateral arm raise. Note that the arms do not go so high as to be overhead and that the athlete isn't leaning back.

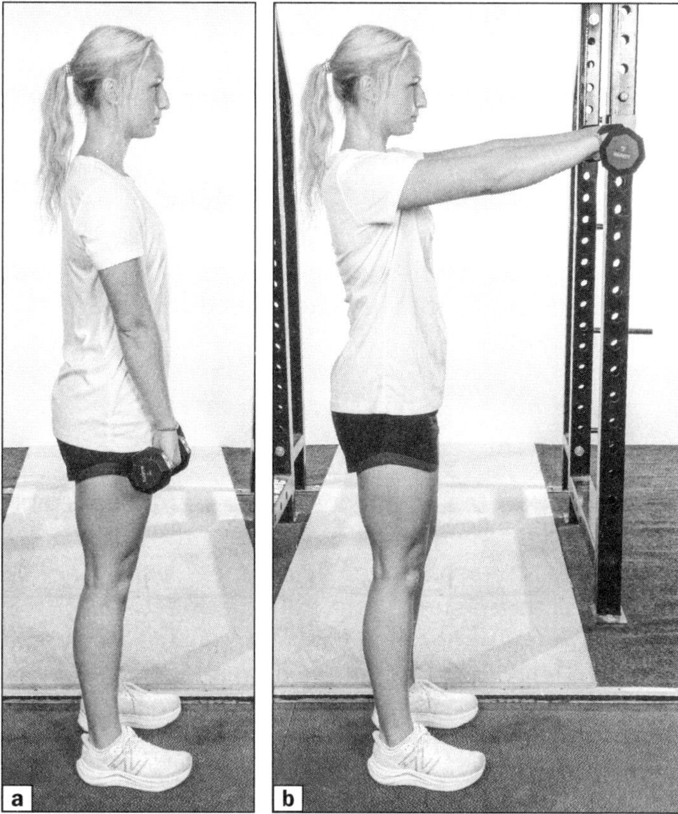

FIGURE 7.4 As with the lateral arm raise, the front raise shouldn't be elevated to an overhead position. Instead, stopping with the arms parallel to the floor is optimal.

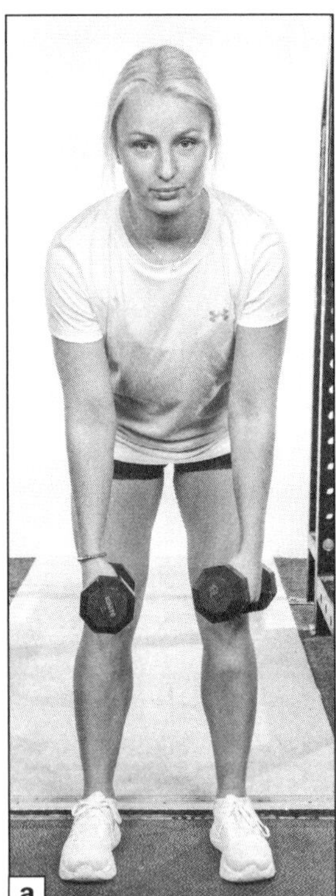

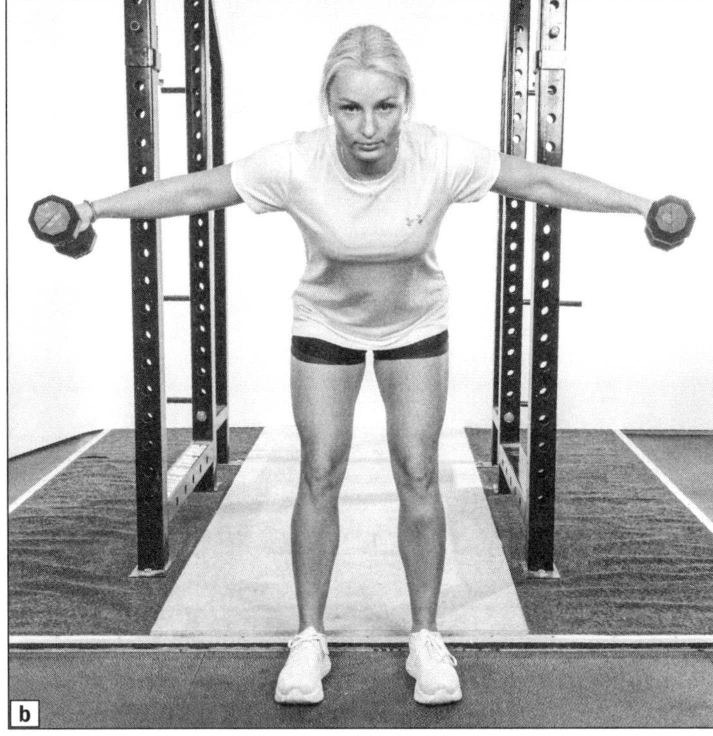

FIGURE 7.5 Unlike the lateral and front arm raises, the reverse arm raise, or reverse fly, uses a neutral grip and is performed bent over.

Pull Accessory Lifts

On to the pull accessories. These exercises are typically used in a program across many days: on bench-press and overhead-press days, but also on deadlift days. They help to build the upper-body pulling muscles like the biceps, the lats, all three segments of the traps, and others. This pulling musculature is incredibly important. Even though these muscles aren't the primary movers in the big-four lifts, they contribute massively to positioning. A great example is the deadlift, where the bar is slightly in front of the lifter. Here, strength in the upper back and in the lats helps to keep the bar close and to maintain the thoracic spine position that allows a vertical bar path. Deadlifting alone isn't enough to build all the muscles needed, so adding in pull accessory exercises throughout your program is necessary. Here are my go-tos.

Lat Pull-Down

The largest muscle in the upper body is the latissimus dorsi. It is an incredibly powerful muscle, and it's responsible for many, many functions of the upper body. When lifting big weights, the lats are a core component in creating stability, power, and an efficient brace. You can get huge, strong lats from just deadlifting. The problem is that you can't deadlift three to four times a week to get the stimulus required to grow the lats this way. Deadlifting that often is too difficult to recover from, so it's essential for us to find other ways to build the lats. My initial starting point for most athletes is lat pull-downs. It's the best entry point because some people can't complete a full pull-up (we'll cover that next), and the lat pull-down is a great building block to get there.

The lat pull-down machine can be a little funky the first time you operate it. There's a leg pad that's supposed to help lock you in, and the bar seems far too far away when you're sitting down all the way. Let's outline how to actually use this piece of equipment and get the most out of lat pull-downs. The first thing to adjust is the leg pad. In a seated position, pull the pin and bring the leg pad down so that it is just in contact with the top of your thighs. This pad keeps you from being lifted into the air when you pull the handles down to execute the movement. The next step is to stand up and grab the bar with your hands placed just outside shoulder width apart and your palms facing away from you. There are a variety of ways to grip for a lat pull-down. Let's start with a double overhand grip that's slightly outside shoulder width. Now start to sit down, allowing your arms to extend until tension is put through the bar. Continue to sit down until you are in the fully seated position, and you have started to pull the weights up (see figure 7.6*a*). This is the start position of a lat pull-down.

From here you will start to hear some very familiar cues. To initiate the movement, take your shoulder blades and put them into your back pockets. Once that is locked in, pull down with your arms and try to squeeze your elbows into those back pockets as well (similar to the way that you set up underneath the barbell to squat). You can lean your torso back slightly to allow enough room for you to pull the bar all the way to the top of your chest (see figure 7.6*b*). Once the bar is touching your chest, hold the position for one to two seconds, and then slowly allow the bar to return to the start position, relaxing the shoulders out of that back-pockets position and allowing the weight to stretch your lats all the way out. Reset the shoulder blades into the back pockets to initiate the next rep, and you're ready to rock and roll. The stretch at the top of the lat pull-down is very important to maintain full range of motion through this lift. One error that I frequently see with this lift and with pull-ups is not allowing that stretched position at the top. Allow the weight to stretch you out to get to full range of motion.

When it comes to sets and reps for lat pull-downs, it's very athlete dependent. With the ability to adjust the weight, lat pull-downs are very scalable so I tend to program anything between 8 and 20 reps.

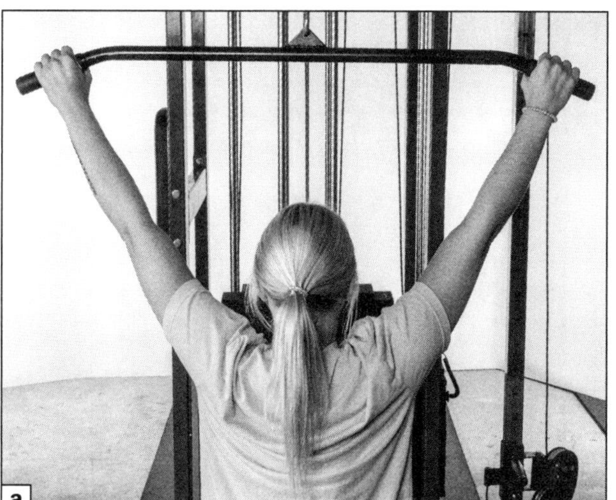

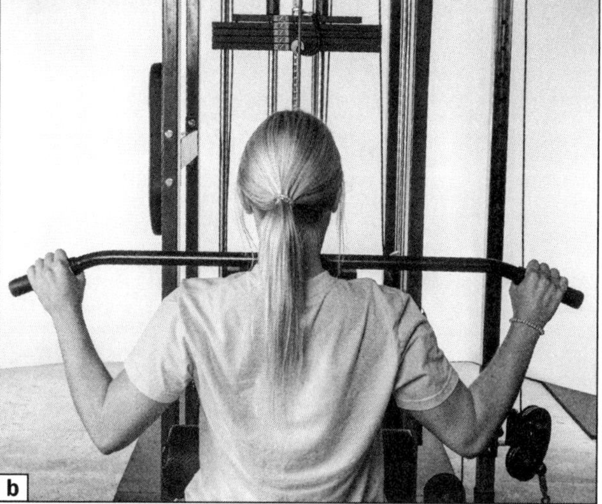

FIGURE 7.6 *(a)* Start the lat pull-down in a fully stretched position, *(b)* pull the bar all the way down to the top of the chest, and then slowly return it to that fully stretched position. Don't miss out on the stretch here.

Pull-Up

Pull-ups are the next progression after lat pull-downs. It is possible to suspend bands from the pull-up bar to add some assistance, but I haven't found that this builds people into pull-ups as quickly as lat pull-downs do, especially because the band changes the pattern slightly. The start position for a pull-up is very similar to that of a lat pull-down. However, you don't have any assistance from a machine. To get into position, you can either jump up to a pull-up bar or use a stool or a box to step up to a pull-up bar (see figure 7.7*a*). Use the same grip you use for the lat pull-down: the double overhand with your hands just outside shoulder width apart. Initiate the movement in the same way you do with lat pull-downs by pulling the shoulder blades into the back pockets. Then pull yourself up until your chest touches the pull-up bar (see figure 7.7*b*). Hold there at the top for one to two seconds, and then slowly lower yourself back down to the start position, going into that stretch at the very bottom again.

As with lat pull-downs, sets and reps for pull-ups are athlete dependent. Once an athlete is able to do three unbroken reps of pull-ups, I start to incorporate them within their program and build them up to being able to do sets of 10. If you can't do three unbroken pull-ups, a great variation is an eccentric-only pull-up where you jump from a box to the top of the pull-up position, and then very slowly lower yourself down to the start position. If you find yourself getting frustrated by doing a lot of lat pull-downs and not seeing the pull-ups increase, add this little wrinkle in and it'll help you get there.

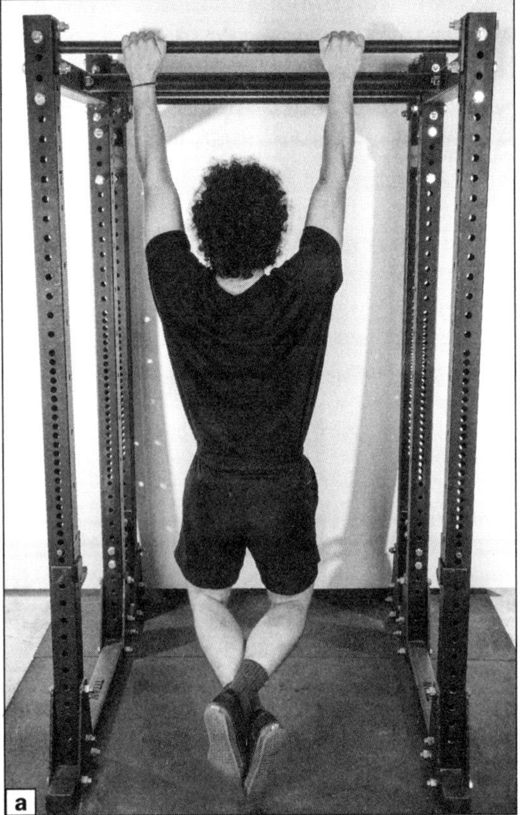

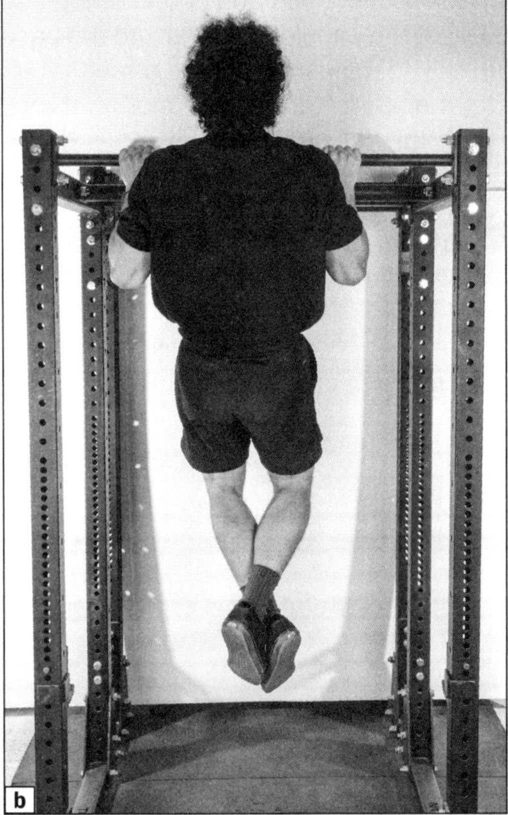

FIGURE 7.7 Just like with the lat pull-down, *(a)* start in a fully stretched position with pull-ups. *(b)* Pull yourself up to the bar, getting your chin over the bar and raising yourself to top of chest height, then slowly return down to the full stretch position.

Pendlay Row

The Pendlay row is by far my favorite row variation. Named after the late great weightlifting coach Glenn Pendlay, this is a bent-over barbell row where each rep starts on the floor. A common error in a normal barbell row is allowing the torso to get more and more vertical throughout the position and throughout the reps. The Pendlay row prevents this by starting each rep on the floor. This added constraint keeps you consistently in the position so that you get the most out of the movement.

I have slightly modified this movement for our purposes because it was originally designed for competitive weightlifters to help them build immense pulling power. To set up for the Pendlay row, get the bar to the proper height, or the height it would be if it were on the floor with 45-pound (20 kg) plates on each end. For most lifters, that puts the bar at about mid-shin height. However, you may not be able to row that much weight to start, so you may need to use 25-pound (11 kg) plates or even an empty bar. When an empty bar is resting on the floor, it's too far away from you, and you'll need to elevate it up to mid-shin to execute this row correctly.

If you have access to bumper plates, then you're in luck because you can put 5- or even 10-pound (2 kg or 5 kg) bumper plates on a barbell and get it to the height that you need for this exercise. If those aren't an option, you can elevate the bar on a box or a similar platform to get it roughly the height that it would be if it had 45-pound (20 kg) plates on it, or around mid-shin (see figure 7.8*a*).

Once the barbell is in position, set up with your stance just inside shoulder width like you do for the deadlift. To approach the bar, hinge your hips while keeping your back nice and flat, bend your knees slightly, and grasp the bar using a double overhand grip with your hands just outside shoulder width. At this point your torso should be parallel with the ground. The difference here from the deadlift is that the barbell should be farther away from you with the barbell directly under your shoulders. To get the bar moving, grasp it tightly, pull the shoulder blades into your back pockets, and then pull the bar all the way to your sternum (see figure 7.8*b*). Hold for one to two seconds at the top, and then lower the barbell all the way back down to the ground. The elbow position through this lift can vary. For the original Pendlay row, the elbows stay high, perpendicular to the shoulders. For my modification, I instruct my athletes to keep the elbows at about 45 degrees or cue them to think about their armpit and elbow making a slice of pizza. Either way, the barbell should touch anywhere between your nipple line and the bottom of your sternum when you're at the very top of the lift. With this being a slightly more explosive movement and involving larger musculature, I like to program this for 8 to 12 reps per set.

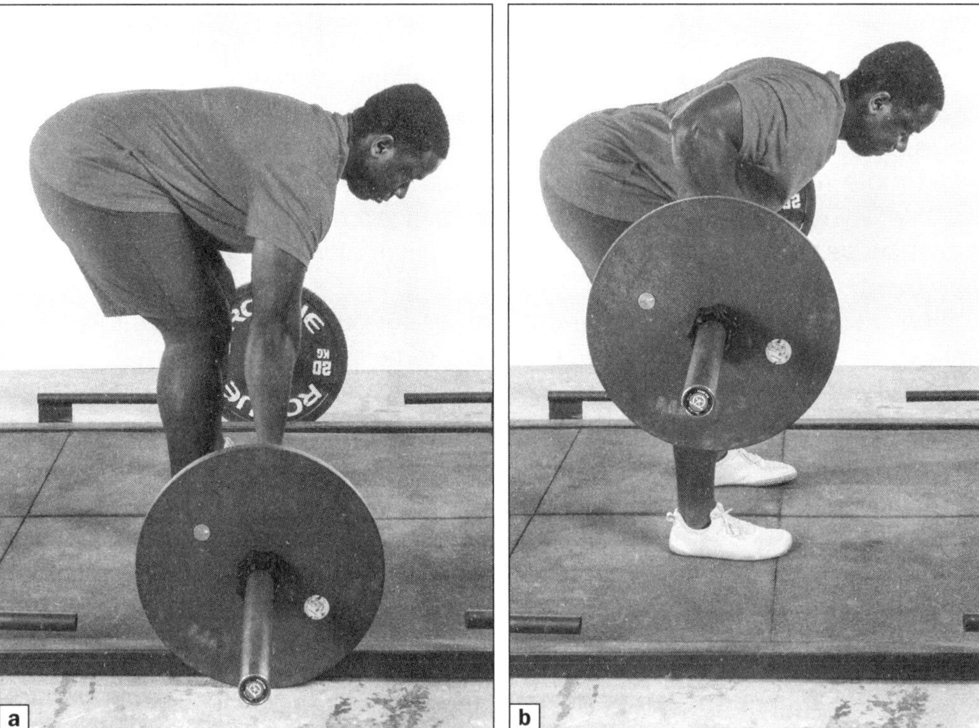

FIGURE 7.8 With the Pendlay row, *(a)* start with the bar on the floor at around mid-shin height, then *(b)* pull it directly off the ground and up to the sternum, and hold for a one- to two-second pause before bringing the bar back to the ground.

Squat Accessory Lifts

If I could squat every day in training, I would. There are actual programs out there that do, but I don't suggest them because they can be very difficult to recover from. Instead, use squat-focused accessories to help build the musculature that will support a big squat: the quads, the glutes, and the adductors, as well as some other hip and leg muscles. In a well-rounded program, these exercises happen on squat days and are sometimes sprinkled into deadlift days as well.

Lunges

I know you don't like lunges. Nobody really likes lunges. But they are one of the greatest unilateral leg builders of all time, so they cannot be ignored. There are endless variations of lunges: from stationary lunges to walking lunges to reverse lunges to lateral lunges. The type of lunge we are going to cover is the stationary lunge. One of the main reasons I want to cover this variation is that it requires less real estate. If you don't have a lot of space to train or you operate in a very busy gym, this is a workable option.

Why use a unilateral movement to build a bilateral movement? The answer is a simple concept related to handedness. Most people have a dominant hand or side, and that carries over into your lifts. You may feel like one leg is stronger than the other, but aside from just squatting all the time, what can you do for this? Lunges allow you to load one side at a time to address this. Additionally, because it's a unilateral movement, you can use less load than with the squat.

This allows you to better manage the load throughout the entire training program while still getting great stimulus on the legs.

With my athletes, I start lunges unloaded. Then I progress to a dumbbell on one side, then to a dumbbell in each hand, and then to a barbell on their back. The setup for all of these is the same. Start in a rack with your feet parallel and shoulder width apart. Take a small step forward with the leg you're going to start with, and step your other foot back so that it's close to double the distance from your front foot. Your feet should still be shoulder width apart in this position. Interestingly enough, you should feel more weight on the front foot than the back foot, but the back foot should have some weight on it. I like to think of the weight in the lunge starting position as being a 70/30 or a 60/40 split between the back foot and front foot, respectively. So your front foot should feel like it has 60 to 70 percent of the weight on it, and the back foot should feel like it has 30 to 40 percent of the weight on it (see figure 7.9*a*).

Keep your torso tall and drop your back knee to the floor. You may be thinking to yourself that because this is a lunge, the front foot should be doing all the work. Why am I focusing on where the back knee goes? Because with lunges, the body should move straight up and down, not forward and backward, and the easiest way to accomplish this is to take the back knee and drop it straight to the floor (see figure 7.9*b*). It does not always have to touch the floor, but the intent of bringing that knee directly to the floor helps keep this lunge in the best position possible. Once your knee is down to the floor, or as close to it as you can tolerate, push through both feet and come back to the start position.

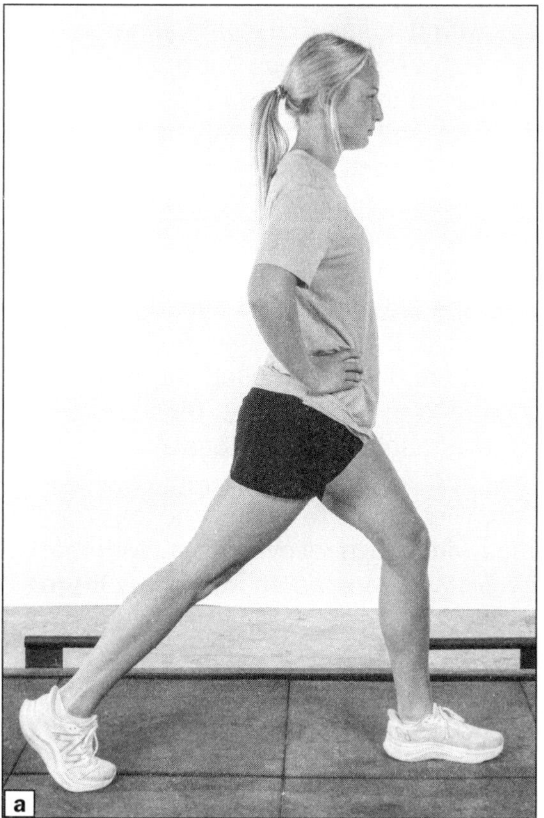

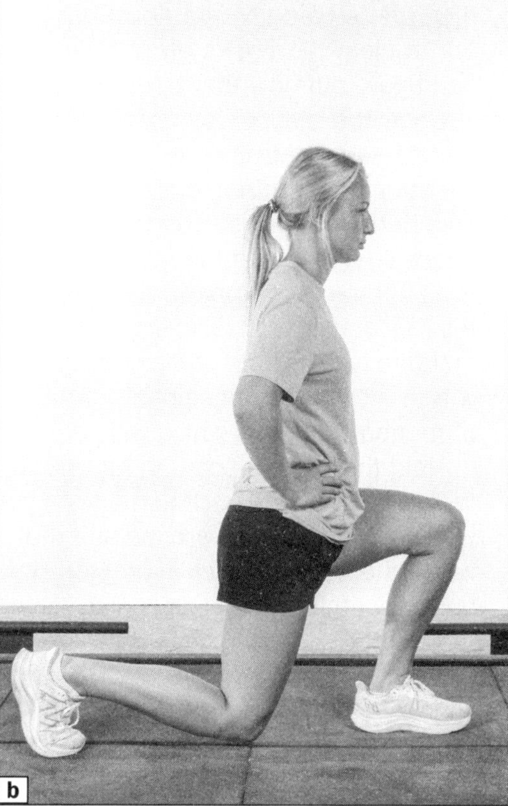

FIGURE 7.9 The start position of the lunge *(a)* with the front foot slightly forward and the back foot about twice that distance back, and *(b)* the bottom position of the lunge with the knee going directly down to the floor and either touching or nearly touching the floor.

You can hold on to the rack or a dowel rod for balance if you need to, and you can also use your hands for a little bit of assistance to come up during the movement. One of the reasons I love lunges so much even though everyone hates them is that they are infinitely scalable from an assistance and load standpoint.

Lunges work larger muscle groups than some of the other accessory movements we've talked about. With that being the case, I typically program these for 8 to 12 reps on each side—and not much more than that—because they have a higher recovery cost. If I'm doing some sort of walking lunge, I typically prescribe a distance rather than a number of reps for each side (50 feet of walking lunges instead of 8 to 12 reps on each side, for example).

Leg Press

Outside of the lat pull-down, the leg press is the only exercise that I have in this book that requires a specialty piece of equipment. Leg presses are very popular and easy to find in most gyms though, and they come in all shapes and sizes and with different functions of operation, If you have a leg press in your gym, it can be one of the best tools for building your squat.

The leg press is a massive piece of equipment, but its operation is relatively simple. The first thing to do once you're seated in the leg press is to find your foot position. There are many different ways you can set your feet, but start by putting them in the middle of the plate with the same stance width and toe-out angle that you squat with. Now you push into the plate to get it off the safeties (see figure 7.10*a*). Many leg presses have similar ways to release the safeties, and typically the safeties are straight down at your sides with handles that rotate either in or out to clear the hooks off of the platform. I suggest you check out the safeties and figure out how they operate before you hop on this machine.

Once the sled is unlocked, bend your knees and allow the weight to come toward you, controlling it all the way until your knees are either touching your chest or slightly outside of your body touching your shoulders (see figure 7.10*b*). This is the bottom position of the leg press and one thing that many people cut short. Just like with the lat pull-down and the pull-up, you want to use as much available range of motion as possible during the leg press. This can help if you feel uncomfortable reaching depth in the squat or if there are certain ranges of motions with certain stances in the squat that are difficult. The leg press allows you to sit in those positions a little bit longer and to work through these ranges of motion with load, which will help you achieve them when you squat.

Hold the bottom position for one to two seconds, and then push through your feet to get the sled back to the start position. Very similar to lunges, the leg press works a lot of muscle groups and that comes with a high recovery cost. With that being the case, I typically program this for 8 to 12 reps as an accessory lift to build my athletes' squats.

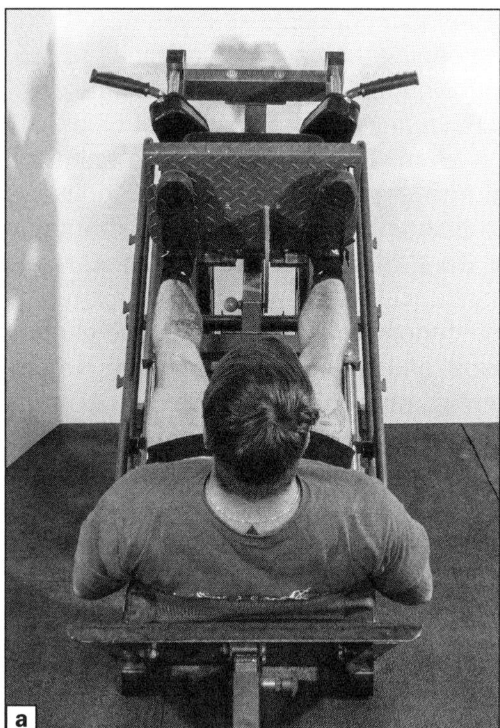
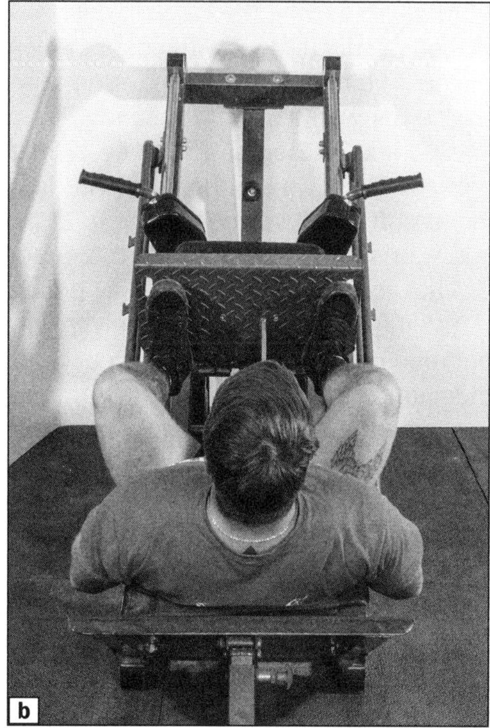

FIGURE 7.10 The start position *(a)* with the knees locked in the leg press, followed by *(b)* the bottom position with the knees at the chest or outside the shoulders to get a full stretch and range of motion on the desired muscle groups.

Hinge Accessory Lifts

We could also call these deadlift accessory lifts, but the movement we are focusing on is the hinge portion of the deadlift. This helps to build up the glutes, the lower back, the hamstrings, and other muscles of the posterior chain. This benefits not only the deadlift but also the squat by helping you maintain position to move big weights. For that reason, you will see hinge-related accessory movements on both squat and deadlift days.

Romanian Deadlift

One of the beautiful things about the Romanian deadlift is that not only does it help build your deadlift but I've seen a massive carryover into my athletes squats as well. Strengthening the posterior chain is paramount to your strength levels in both the squat and the deadlift. This is where the Romanian deadlift shines.

To execute the Romanian deadlift, start with a barbell in the rack at a height that is just below waist level. This may take a little bit of trial and error, but you want it at that level so that you can start the Romanian deadlift from the top. Grasp the barbell using a double overhand grip with your hands just outside shoulder width apart. Bend over slightly with your knees slightly flexed, lift the bar until you are in a fully standing position, and then take two steps back away from the rack. Brace tightly and make your arms long, pinning your elbows to your sides (see figure 7.11*a*). This is the start position for the Romanian deadlift.

To begin moving the barbell, push your hips straight back, as if you were trying to close your car door with your butt, while keeping the bar nice and close to your thighs. The bottom of the movement is when you feel a stretch in the hamstrings as the bar works its way past your knees. For many people, this is just below the knees, and for some, it may be a little bit lower. There is no need to bring the barbell all the way to the floor. The lowest I have my athletes go is to about two inches off the floor (see figure 7.11*b*). To lift the bar up, think about the same cue we use in the lock-out of the deadlift: Bring the hips to the barbell. This will elevate the bar back to the start position, and you'll be ready for the next rep.

You'll feel a challenge not only in your posterior chain (hamstrings and glutes), but also in your upper body in your lats, traps, and upper back. Because so much musculature is used in the Romanian deadlift, I typically prescribe 8 to 10 reps in a program, similar to lunges and the leg press.

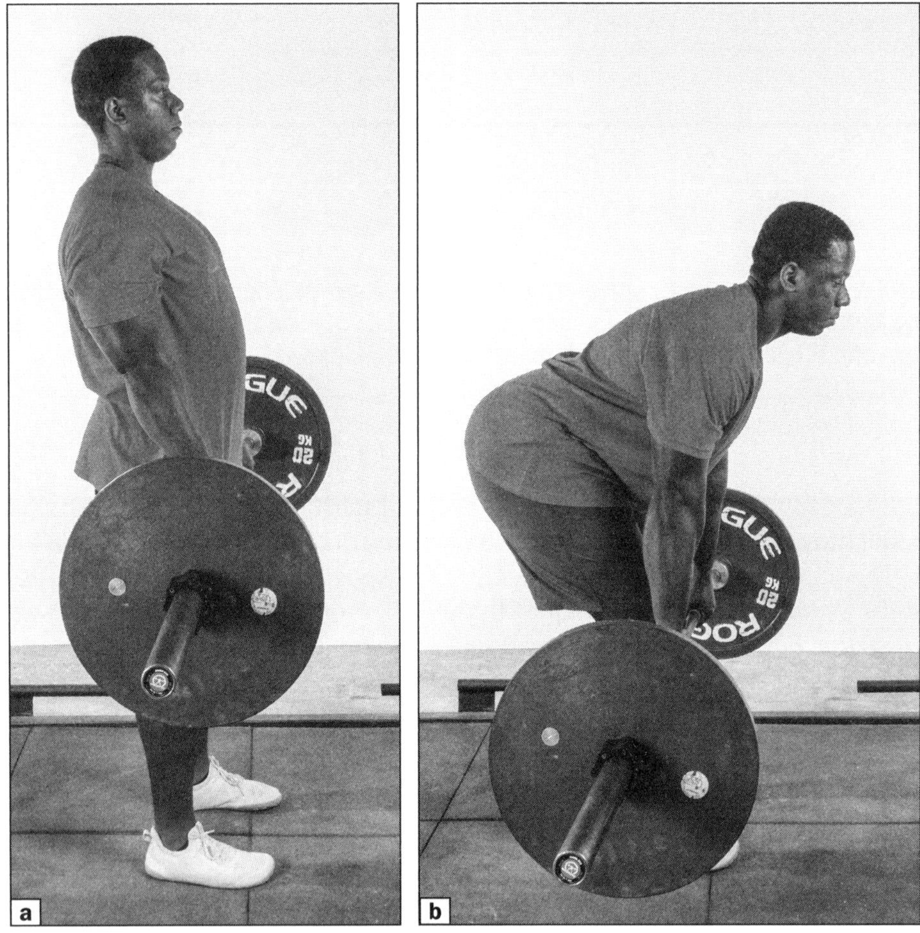

FIGURE 7.11 The start position and the bottom position of the Romanian deadlift. Note that movement essentially starts at the lock-out of the deadlift and moves from the top down. Also note that at the bottom position, the bar doesn't need to go excessively past the knees and that the back stays flat.

Barbell Good Morning

That's right—one of the warm-up variations that I use very frequently is also an accessory exercise that I use to build up the hinge. There were many exercises I could have chosen here, but because this book is based around the barbell, the barbell good morning is an obvious choice. Just like the Romanian deadlift, the barbell good morning helps build not only your deadlift but also your squat.

To set up for the good morning, get under the barbell in the same manner that you would for a barbell back squat. The unrack will be the same as the barbell back squat as well, where you elevate the bar out of the hooks and take your three-step walk out to get to the start position of your squat (see figure 7.12*a*). The difference with the good morning is that you're not going to bend your knees to initiate the movement. Instead, use the same approach as with the Romanian deadlift except with the bar being across your shoulders and in the back squat position. To initiate the movement, push your hips back just like you're closing that car door again. Keep your knees slightly flexed and in a consistent position throughout the movement. Come down far enough to where you feel a stretch in your hamstrings or until your torso is parallel to the ground (see figure 7.12*b*). To reverse this, think about driving your head, neck, and shoulders as a unit back into the barbell while driving your hips forward all the way back to the start position.

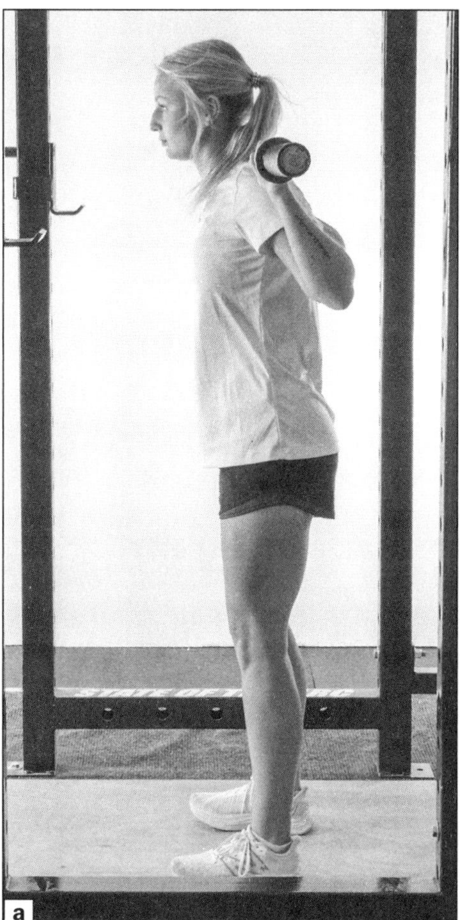

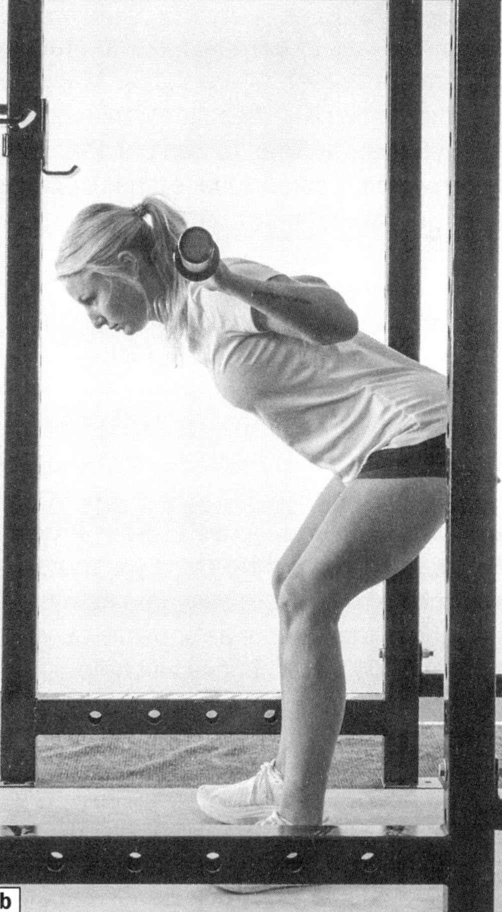

FIGURE 7.12 *(a)* The start position of the good morning looks identical to a squat. *(b)* To initiate the movement, push the hips back while keeping the shins vertical until there's a good stretch in the hamstrings.

You can use lower loads for good mornings than for Romanian deadlifts. Even though it works similar muscle groups, I have used a range of sets and reps with good mornings depending on an athlete's particular weakness and where they are in their training during the year. When first starting out with good mornings, however, I program two to three sets of 8 to 12 reps with a weight that corresponds with about RPE 6 or 7.

Carry Accessory Lifts

Carries are a vastly underutilized accessory movement. They can be done on any day of training, but I like to start doing them twice a week and build to doing them every day of training. Carries help build grip strength and core stability, and I especially like them to get in some cardiovascular work with strength training. The key here is to keep them heavy. They should challenge your grip considerably. I'm not a fan of doing these for minutes on end; sets of 30 seconds to a minute or distances of 50 to 100 feet tend to be a sweet spot. If you mix that with short rest periods for three to four sets, you can increase your heart rate and breathing rate considerably.

Bilateral Carry

When it comes to carries, I like to start with a bilateral carry (see figure 7.13). Many people use dumbbells or kettlebells for this movement, but if you have access to trap bar, that's a great option since it can be loaded heavier. The key is to use something that you can hold while keeping your hands at your sides. This tends to be the easiest position for people to maintain when they first start out doing carries like this.

The execution is simple: Set a timer or select a distance, and start walking. Just because the execution is simple does not mean that this is easy. One of the cues from the deadlift is good for the carry too: Keep your arms long and pinned at your sides. This will decrease the sway of the weights, giving you more control over them. You want to eliminate as much sway or swing of the weights as possible as you carry them around, and this cue will help.

You should also pay close attention to your breathing during carries. Many people brace so hard in their lifts that they don't allow them-

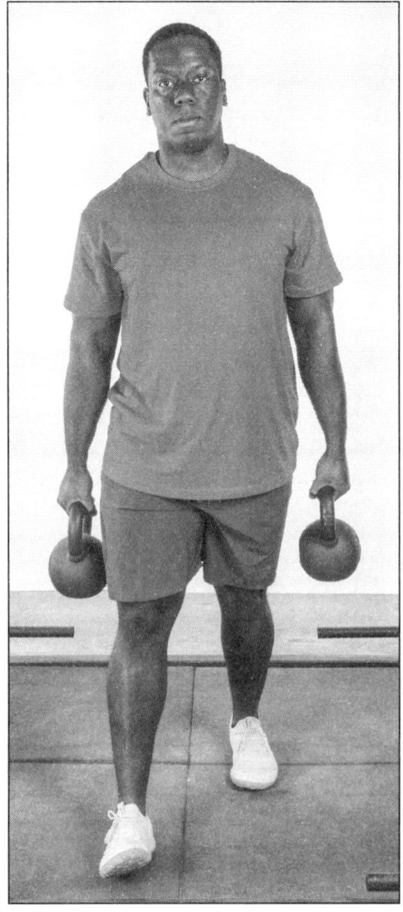

FIGURE 7.13 A well-executed carry builds a strong grip and core. Note that the athlete isn't shrugging up with the shoulders but keeping them back and down.

selves to breathe at a normal rate. One of the greatest gifts that carries can give you is the ability to not always maximally brace. As we discussed earlier in the book, bracing is a reflexive mechanism of the body and you can voluntarily increase your intra-abdominal pressure by bearing down harder. Carries don't require this level of brace, so they can teach you to breathe into your brace better while keeping your breathing regular throughout the exercise.

Front-Rack Carry

The progression of the carry that I like to use next is a front-rack carry where we use a barbell in the front-rack position (see figure 7.14). This is a more challenging position because it's harder to maintain that upright position with the weights at shoulder height as opposed to having the weights hanging down at your sides. I don't start with this variation of carries because the upper-back strength required to maintain this position typically isn't developed enough yet to carry for the distances that I like to carry. During these carries, I tell athletes to think about keeping their chest tall and keeping their eyes on where they are going. "Eyes on target," is the way I like to say it.

When it comes to prescribing carries, I like to use either time or distance but tend to favor time. My most frequently used times are one- to two-minute carries for three to four sets. That can scale up or down depending on the weight being used. The shortest time frame I use is 30 seconds, and that's typically with very heavy loads.

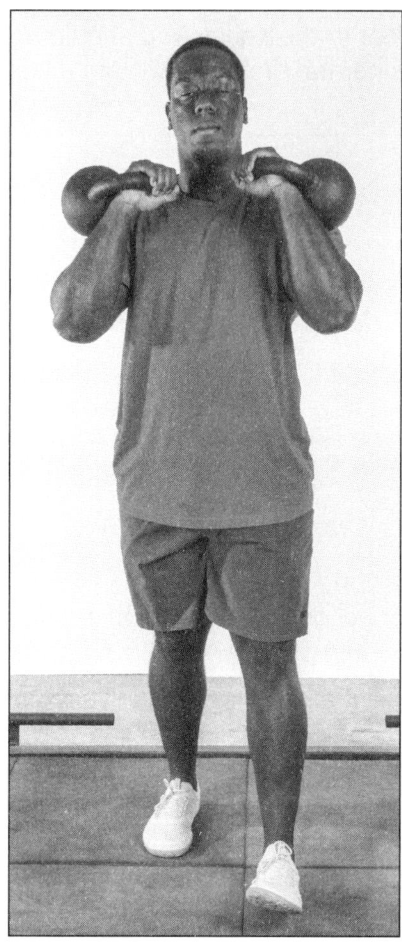

FIGURE 7.14 Front-rack position for a front-rack carry. Note that the athlete keeps their chest tall and their "eyes on target."

Core Accessory Lifts

Last but not least are the core accessory lifts. You may be tempted to skip these, but don't. Because these tend to be at the end of the session in programs, you will hear people say they aren't needed. Don't listen to those people. Make sure to do them, even when you are tired. These help to strengthen the musculature around the trunk like the rectus abdominus, the obliques, and the lower back. These muscles are small and tend to recover quickly, so you'll find these accessories programmed every day. The following are my go-to core accessories.

Plank

The plank is the simplest and most brutal core exercise ever devised. It's a wonderful exercise because it's infinitely scalable in terms of position and load. I like to start off using a basic push-up position, as opposed to up on the elbows, simply because I've found that when people start off on their elbows, they report a lot of discomfort in their shoulders. (see figure 7.15). Set your feet shoulder width apart with your toes on the floor. Your hands should be just underneath your shoulders and set slightly wider than shoulder width apart. If there is any discomfort with your hands on the floor, you can turn them out slightly, just like you would your feet in the squat. You should be braced tightly while also being able to maintain a normal breathing rhythm (like with the carries).

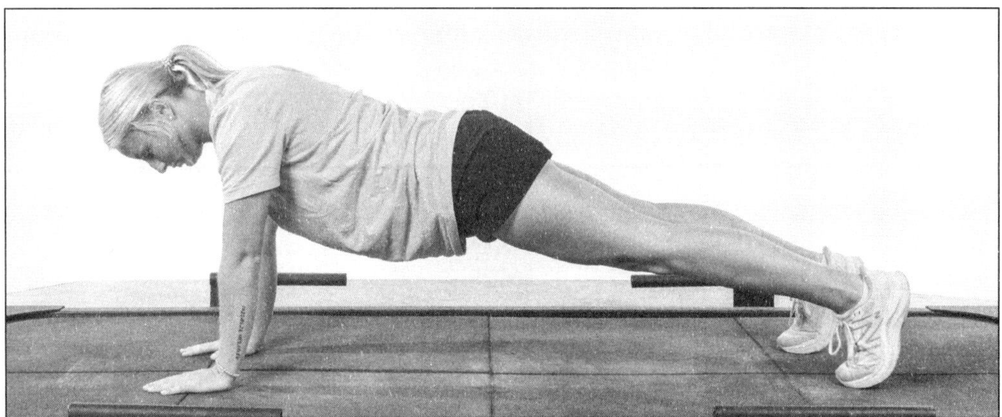

FIGURE 7.15 This is the plank position I like people to start with. It's stable, and it's easier on the shoulders than planking on the elbows.

What makes the plank infinitely scalable is that you can elevate the upper body to make it easier, you can elevate the legs while the hands are on the ground to make it harder, or you can add load with plates stacked on your upper back to make it even more difficult. The additional benefit of the plank is that it can be done multiple times a week because the muscle groups being used are smaller and typically more endurance biased. With that being said, I typically program planks for multiple sets of 30 seconds, three to four times a week depending on training frequency. Which plank position to use is determined by the ability to hold a 30-second plank in the normal push-up position. If you cannot hold a plank for 30 seconds in that position, then raise your hands by using a bench or putting a barbell in a rack and elevating it incrementally until you find the height that challenges you for that entire 30 seconds (see figure 7.16).

If you are able to do a full 30 seconds in the base push-up position, then elevate your feet until your body is parallel to the ground. If you continue to be successful in this position, return to the base push-up position and start adding weight on your middle back (see figure 7.17). I have seen elite-level Olympic weightlifters plank with loads upward of 300 pounds (136 kg). This doesn't mean that you have to work up to 300-pound (136 kg) planks, but it is a good indication that having planks in your program on a regular basis is of high value.

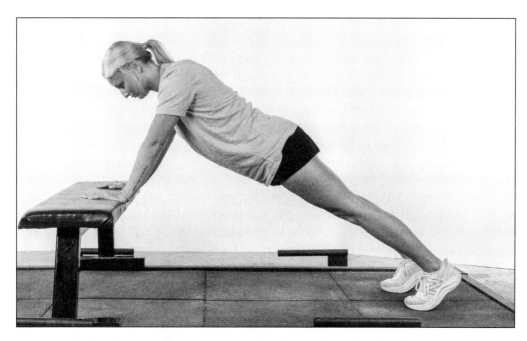

FIGURE 7.16 Many people will regress the plank by bringing their knees to the floor. I prefer to elevate the lifter, using a bar in a rack or box.

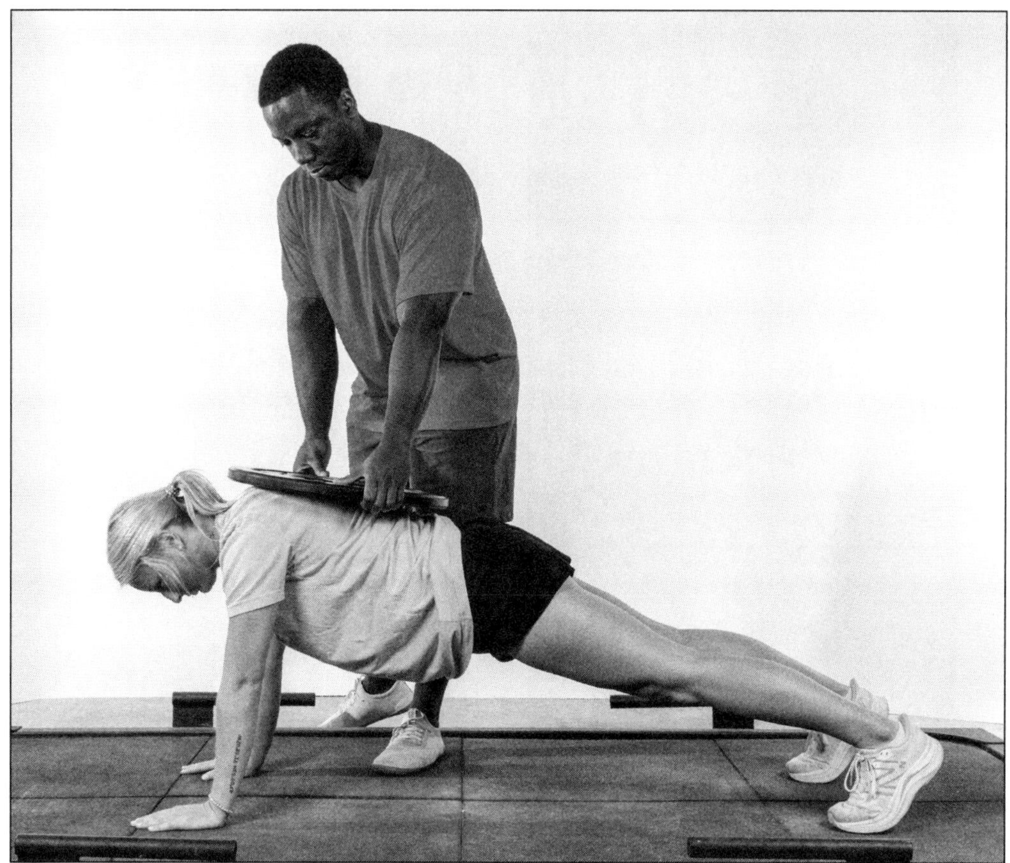

FIGURE 7.17 To progress the base plank position, I prefer to load it by having someone place plates on your back. Make sure to have someone help you to put these plates on and take them off.

Hanging Leg Raise

A very common mistake a lot of trainees make is not having some form of standing or hanging core exercise. Similar to the plank, the hanging leg raise is also very scalable. You can make it easier or harder by changing positions or adding load. It also has the added benefit of helping with grip strength. This makes it a popular accessory movement for strength athletes and other populations.

For the base variation, jump up to a pull-up bar the same way you would to start the pull-up. Keep your feet together and your legs tight while hanging from the pull-up bar. From this position, lift your legs up until they are parallel with the floor (see figure 7.18). If you do this correctly, you should feel your hips push back as you go into this position. This is the top position of the hanging leg raise. To finish, let your legs come back down to the start position, but do not swing into the next rep. The key with the hanging leg raise is to start from a complete stop, move into a complete stop at the top, and then return to a complete stop back in the start position. If this base variation is too difficult, you can bend your knees and do a hanging leg raise with your knees bent (see figure 7.19). This is the starting point for most beginners.

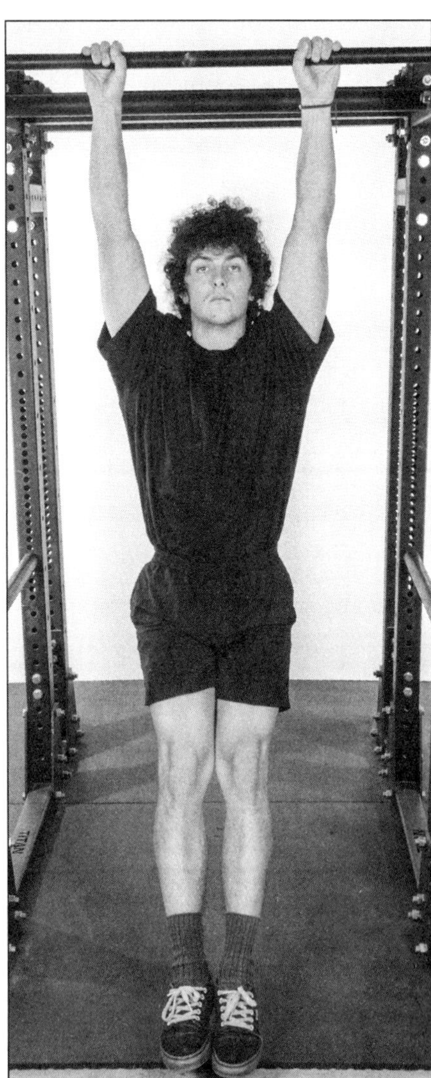

FIGURE 7.18 The base hanging leg raise position should have the legs fully extended, and the body should look like a straight line.

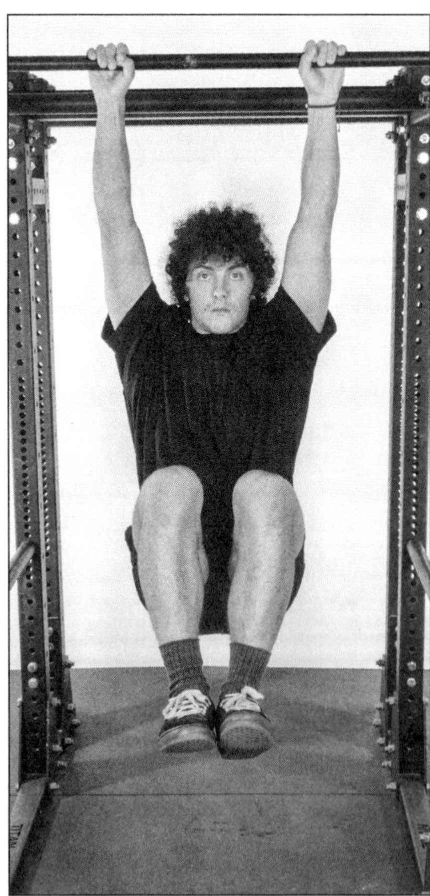

FIGURE 7.19 To modify the leg raise, bend your knees, decreasing the lever arm and therefore the weight of the leg raise.

To progress it beyond the base position, there are two options. The first option is to increase the range of motion until your toes touch the bar (see figure 7.20). This variation is also called a *toes-to-bar*. It became very popular with CrossFit, and it requires much more core strength to pull off. The other option is to add weight by either holding a dumbbell with your feet or using ankle weights to increase the load of the base position (see figure 7.21).

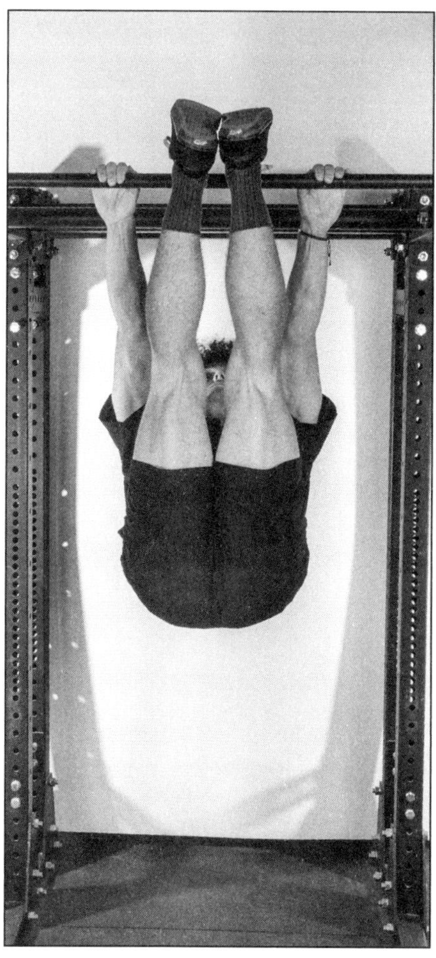

FIGURE 7.20 A toes-to-bar has a much longer range of motion than a normal hanging leg raise. Make sure to return the legs to the starting position in a slow and controlled manner.

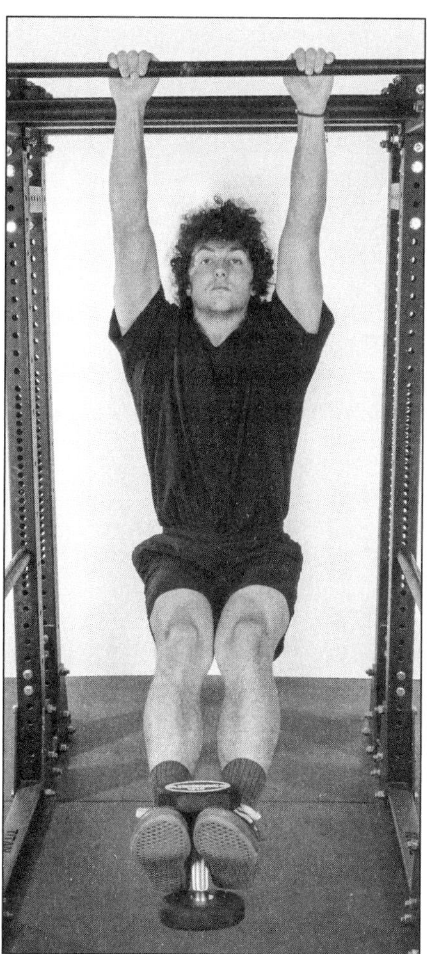

FIGURE 7.21 Adding weight to the leg raise by holding a dumbbell or using ankle weights is another great way to progress the hanging leg raise.

When it comes to dosing for the hanging leg raise, I lean on the same concept that I use in the plank. I prefer sets of 15 to 20 reps, and if those reps aren't able to be maintained in a particular position, I will regress from there.

That's it. At this point we have covered the execution of all of the four major lifts, how to warm up for each one, and how to round out a program with accessory lifts that will help strengthen each of the big four. There are enough variations and choices here for you to create a sustainable program that will lead to long-term strength progress. In the next chapter, you will learn how to do that.

Chapter 8

The Foundations of Programming

Ahhhhh, programming. The Holy Grail. It's the thing that everyone thinks they need to get better at while simultaneously searching for free programs on Google. First of all, if you skipped the entire book and just flipped to this section to find your next program, then go back to the beginning and read the book. For everyone else, the entire book culminates in this chapter. We have laid the foundation of each movement, the terms you need to understand, and the concepts and training principles that can guide you from being a beginner to being an elite lifter. Now you'll learn how to put it all together into a program that you can execute in the gym.

Before we get into the "how," I want to take a second to bust some myths. Whether you use this information to create your own programs or to evaluate programs that you find elsewhere (please, do both), there are a few guidelines I'd like to point out.

Just Because It's Complicated Doesn't Mean It's Effective.

Simple is beautiful, and some of the most effective programming I've used, seen, and experienced is brutally simple. There are always going to be ways to enhance programming and spark progress, but complicating a simple procedure is a great way to get lost. If you are going to add new concepts to your training, do so one at a time. That way, you can evaluate them. If you add too much too quickly, you won't know where the results are coming from. This leads us to the next guideline.

More Is Not Always Better.

Adding for the sake of adding is one of the most common errors I see. While you do want to progress what you're doing and make it progressively harder, adding a mobility program, three new exercises to your warm-up, 15 exercises to the main session, and a post-workout TikTok dance to round it out isn't going to get you to your goal faster. You have been given the tools to use exercise selection as the cornerstone of your program. Be careful when adding things. If you don't have a very good reason for adding something, then don't.

If It Doesn't Work, Save It for Later.

A common philosophy is that if something doesn't work, you should get rid of it. I've seen many long-term trainees box themselves into a corner with this. For instance, they'll say that they tried box squats once and didn't get stronger, so they never used them again. I can understand that. It seems logical. What happens when your knee hurts in a certain range of motion though? What happens when you lose tension in the bottom of a squat? Could that variation help then? You bet. Leave your options open to go back to something if the situation calls for it.

Basic Programming Terminology

Let's start with common programming terms. Many of them have been sprinkled throughout the book, but I want to make sure that everyone is starting on the same page. Here is a quick review of the most important terms we will cover.

Set. A set is a group of repetitions of a particular exercise performed consecutively without rest.

Rep. Rep is short for *repetition*, which is one complete movement of a particular exercise.

Frequency. Frequency refers to the number of times per week a particular exercise or workout is performed.

Intensity. Intensity refers to the amount of weight or resistance used in an exercise. It can also be expressed as a percentage of a person's one-rep maximum (1RM).

Volume: Volume refers to the total amount of work performed in a particular workout, which is calculated by multiplying the number of sets times reps times weight lifted.

Macrocycle. A macrocycle is the complete duration of a training period. It can span several months or even years, and it usually contains several mesocycles.

Microcycle. A microcycle is a shorter training period that typically lasts for one week and contains several training sessions.

Mesocycle. A mesocycle is a mid-length training period that typically lasts for several weeks and is usually focused on a specific training goal.

Overload. Overload refers to the principle of progressively increasing the demands placed on the body during exercise in order to continue making progress.

Hypertrophy. Hypertrophy is the increase in muscle size and strength due to repeated exposure to resistance training.

1RM. 1RM stands for one-rep maximum, which is the maximum amount of weight that can be lifted for a single repetition of a particular exercise.

Relative Intensity. Relative intensity refers to the amount of weight lifted as a percentage of a person's 1RM. It is commonly used to prescribe training loads based on an individual's strength level.

Training Cycle

The best way to learn programming is by doing it. We will start with how to organize your training from a big-picture perspective. Then we will gradually zoom in all the way to the sets and reps for each day.

Macrocycle

The macrocycle is the largest block of training to consider. It can last months, and in some cases (think Olympics prep), even years. For strength sports and barbell training, it's typically divided into off-season training and meet-prep training. If competition isn't on the horizon for you, that's perfectly fine. Think of the macrocycle as the total length of time that you spend pursuing a particular goal before evaluating your progress and updating your plan. Some common lengths of time for a macrocycle are 16 weeks, 12 weeks, and 8 weeks.

Mesocycle

The mesocycle is made up of the consecutive training weeks before you deload. I presented some more advanced deload concepts earlier in the book, but for now let's go with the most common. For reference: "Up" refers to a normal training week, and "down" refers to a deload week. Here are some common lengths of time for a mesocycle:

Three weeks up with one week down

Four weeks up with one week down

Five weeks up with one week down

One word of caution: The more intense the training, the more often deloads need to be planned. If your intention is to build a program that pushes you hard each day in the gym, start with the three-up-one-down setup. The five-up-one-down timeline typically requires lower volume during the mesocycle to keep you from feeling like you've been hit by a truck by the end. It's a great option for when your life is busy and you need to shorten your training sessions, but it can drag out with very intense training.

Microcycle

The microcycle is what each individual week looks like. Let's break this down layer by layer. First, how many days a week can you train? Typically, I recommend training two to five days a week. Very rarely do I suggest people train only once a week or more than five days per week. Even the twice-a-week and the five-days-a-week formats push the limits of minimum viable and maximum recoverable, respectively. Most people train three to four days a week. Be sure to take work, life, kids, hobbies, and anything else into account when you're deciding how often to train each week; when in doubt, round down. Create the habit first, and then you can expand on it later.

Frequency

Now that we have determined the length of your program in weeks and the number of training days in the week, it's time to plan out the frequency of the main lifts. We'll cover this in more detail in the next chapter, but it is important to note here that different lifts require different recoveries. The overhead press has the fastest recovery, followed by the bench press and then the squat. The deadlift has the slowest recovery. The number of days per week that you're training will also affect how frequently you do each lift, and it's best to have no more than two of the four main lifts on the same day. Doing more than two has become more popular in powerlifting circles as preparation for meet days, but outside of specific-use cases like this, keeping it to two main lifts a day is ideal. This is because fatigue is very high by the time you get to the third main lift in a session, which can affect your performance and how much intensity you can handle. For many, the cost of that fatigue and the decreased stimulus from the intensity isn't worth the reward of being able to train the lift more frequently.

Lastly, there is a minimum number of days per week for each movement. For the squat, the bench press, and the overhead press that minimum is one day a week. For the deadlift, I have seen one day every other week be effective in some cases, but for the beginner to intermediate lifter, this is not ideal. Here are some options for how many days per week to train each lift based on the number of days per week you're training:

Minimum of two training days: one bench press, one overhead press, one squat, and one deadlift

Minimum of three training days: two bench press, one overhead press, one squat, and one deadlift

Minimum of three training days: two bench press, two overhead press, two squat, and one deadlift

Minimum of four training days: two bench press, two overhead press, two squat, and one deadlift

Minimum of four training days: three bench press, two overhead press, two squat, and one deadlift

Minimum of five training days: three bench press, two overhead press, two squat, and two deadlift

Minimum of five training days: two bench press, three overhead press, three squat, and one deadlift

There is a maximum number of exposures during the week that we try not to exceed. This threshold for upper body being 5 total exposures during the week and 4 for lower body respectively. The options can be endless here but, a few more things to note. Just as before, be ok with rounding down and remember that more doesn't always mean better and that it's better to err on the side of being conservative.

With these setups, you choose one upper-body main movement and one lower-body main movement each day if the frequency is high enough. To see what I mean, take a look at the following table.

Minimum 2 training days	1 bench press, 1 overhead press, 1 squat, 1 deadlift	*Day 1*: squat, bench press *Day 2*: deadlift, overhead press
Minimum 3 training days	2 bench press, 1 overhead press, 1 squat, 1 deadlift	*Day 1*: squat, bench press *Day 2*: bench press *Day 3*: deadlift, overhead press
	2 bench press, 1 overhead press, 2 squat, 1 deadlift	*Day 1*: squat, bench press *Day 2*: deadlift, overhead press *Day 3*: squat, bench press
Minimum 4 training days	2 bench press, 2 overhead press, 2 squat, 2 deadlift	*Day 1*: squat, bench press *Day 2*: deadlift, overhead press *Day 3*: squat, bench press *Day 4*: deadlift, overhead press
	3 bench press, 2 overhead press, 2 squat, 1 deadlift	*Day 1*: squat, bench press *Day 2*: bench press *Day 3*: deadlift, overhead press *Day 4*: bench press *Day 5*: squat, overhead press
Minimum 5 training days	3 bench press, 2 overhead press, 2 squat, 2 deadlift	*Day 1*: squat, bench press *Day 2*: bench press *Day 3*: deadlift, overhead press *Day 4*: squat, bench press *Day 5*: deadlift, overhead press
	2 bench press, 3 overhead press, 3 squat, 1 deadlift	*Day 1:* squat, overhead press *Day 2:* deadlift, overhead press *Day 3:* squat, bench press *Day 4:* bench press *Day 5:* squat, overhead press

A four-day program that is not listed here—but is one of my personal favorites—is three bench presses, one overhead press, two squats, and one deadlift. It's a starting point for many.

Minimum 4 training days	3 bench press, 1 overhead press, 2 squat, 1 deadlift	*Day 1*: squat, bench press *Day 2*: bench press *Day 3*: deadlift, overhead press *Day 4*: squat, bench press

Why do I like this setup as a starting point? It's great for data collection. There are enough exposures of the squat to learn the movement well. There is enough time between the first day of squat and the first deadlift day to allow ample recovery. The high frequency of pressing takes advantage of those lifts' rapid recovery rates and provides a lot of volume and skill development. Spreading all of that out over four days, enables you to get a good amount of work in while keeping the workouts shorter—and still have three full days of recovery. Is it perfect? Nothing is perfect. However, it's a great starting point from which to begin tracking your recovery so you can find your own sweet spot.

Now you can put together the entire skeleton of the training block. To recap: You have established the total number of weeks in the training block, the number of days per week that you are going to train, and the frequency of each lift during each week. Now it's time to get into the weeds.

Exercise Selection

The details of exercise selection, sets, reps, and the rest are what will complete the program. This is where people overcomplicate things and get lost in the options. Let's break it down. Remember that simple is effective.

The first order of business is to create order. Now that you have selected how many days you are going to do a particular movement, it's time to introduce some new terms to help with organization and exercise selection.

- *Primary movement.* In many cases, this is the baseline main lift—the squat to normal standard or the bench press with your most comfortable grip. Most people want to grow those lifts the most, so having one of them as the primary movement that gets the most work makes sense. However, you have read all about variations and skill development, so let's expand a little more here. If you have identified a particular weakness in a lift, your primary-movement selection can be a variation that addresses that weakness. The key here is to select the movement that is going to move the needle the most based on your needs.
- *Secondary movement.* If you are training a lift two times a week, the second day you train it is a secondary-exercise selection day. This is going to be a variation that directly addresses a weakness to help build your primary movement. This lift tends to be higher volume with less intensity than the primary-day lift in order to help with recovery as well.
- *Tertiary movement.* If you are training a lift three times in a week, this is the movement selected for the third day of training. A tertiary movement continues to attack a weakness but in a less specific way. A great example of this for the powerlifters I work with is a front squat. The bar isn't in the same position as their normal competition squat or closer variations but it's still a squat, and it can help build the leg and upper-back strength needed to move heavier weights in the back squat.

This creates a hierarchy of specificity. You should select movements tactically so that you can address weaknesses and build strengths in a more predictable way. To see this in action, let's look at how two different kinds of athletes might approach the squat. One of them is a beginner who has only squatted a couple of times before, while the other one squats regularly but struggles with good morning squats (where the hips rise too soon).

In this example, the beginner would select an exercise that closely mimics doing the squat itself. The pause squat and box squat allow for plenty of practice while learning the squat movement. However, the lifter who struggles with a good morning error in the squat, where their hips rise early, would select an exercise like the high-bar wide-stance squat to help address that specific issue more directly. One lifter tactically selects a movement in order to address an error, while the other one selects a movement that will allow them to practice the movement they are struggling with.

BEGINNER LIFTER TO SQUATTING	
Primary	Barbell back squat
Secondary	Pause back squat
Tertiary	Box squat
LIFTER'S HIPS RISE EARLY (GOOD MORNING SQUAT)	
Primary	High-bar wide-stance squat
Secondary	Box squat
Tertiary	Front squat

Let's look at an example week with a minimum of four training days, with two squat, three bench, one press, and two deadlift. For this example, let's use a beginner lifter who has no specific weaknesses and who wants to pull sumo in the deadlift. For the setup we outlined earlier, they need a primary-focus main lift for all of the big four, along with a secondary-focus main lift for squat, bench, and deadlift. With the three-times-a-week frequency for the bench, they need to select one more tertiary exercise for the bench. Since this lifter has no known weaknesses, it's good practice to select a very specific exercise as the primary and choose close variations as the secondary and tertiary selections, as shown here:

	Squat	Bench	Deadlift	Press
Primary	Back squat	Pause bench	Sumo deadlift	Overhead press
Secondary	Box squat	Close-grip bench	Sumo deadlift off two-inch blocks	X
Tertiary	X	Dumbbell Bench	X	X

Then they can organize the selected exercises through the week as shown here:

Day 1	Day 2	Day 3	Day 4
Back squat	Sumo deadlift	Box squat	Sumo deadlift off two-inch blocks
Pause bench	Close-grip bench	Overhead press	Dumbbell Bench

Once you have the exercise selections for the main lifts mapped out for a week, you can repeat that for the entire training mesocycle. After your mesocycle ends, you can go through and pick all new exercises or, if you saw very good progress, you can repeat those exercises for the next block. Now it's time to decide how to fill out the rest of the program with your accessory lifts. When selecting accessory lifts, there are three main factors to consider:

1. They should build the main lifts of the day by working similar muscle groups. For example, on a squat day you should select accessory movements that will work the lower body, especially the quads, hamstrings, and glutes.

2. Consider how much time you want to spend in the gym. The more accessory exercises you add, the longer you have to spend in the gym to complete them. Generally, each accessory exercise can add 10 to 15 minutes to a training session.
3. Through the course of the week, you should have at least one of each accessory-lift movement pattern: push, pull, hinge, squat or lunge, and carry or core.

A common mistake is selecting accessory movements that hit muscles and structures that should be recovering from previous training sessions. An example of this would be if your day one was heavy squats, and then day two was heavy leg press and leg extensions as accessory movements. The leg press and leg extensions should be on day one with the squats. This allows for recovery between sessions. Instead of hitting the same muscle groups multiple days in a row, do the accessory movements related to the main lifts on the same day you're doing that lift.

Time management is also important. Nothing feels worse than selecting six different exercises for each day—on top of the main lifts—and then never being able to complete a full workout due to time. For many of us, the main movement—or the two main movements of the day, depending on your frequency—can take 30 to 45 minutes alone. Here are the general time ranges I've seen in my years of coaching:

- Three exercises (the main lift and two accessories) plus warm-up: 30 to 45 minutes.
- Four exercises (the main lift and three accessories) plus warm-up: 45 to 60 minutes.
- Five exercises (the main lift and three to four accessories) plus warm-up: 60 to 75 minutes.
- Six or more exercises (one to two main lifts and four to five accessories) plus warm-up: 75 minutes or longer.

Last but not least: Make sure to get in at least one accessory for each movement pattern. Push, pull, hinge, and squat are pretty much handled by the lifts. In a very minimalist program, I have seen people use a main lift and core exercise alone and see progress. With that said, I still like to include at least one accessory movement for each main lift during the week.

For an example of this, let's return to the four-days-a-week program from earlier. Remember that each accessory lift should match the structures being worked by the main lift that day. Then the number of exercises selected should be based on how long you want to be at the gym. Lastly, make sure each pattern is covered. For a minimum of four training days of two squat, three bench, one overhead press, and two deadlift, and with 60 to 75 minutes as your goal gym time, here's an example of what your training week might look like:

Day 1	Day 2	Day 3	Day 4
Back squat	Sumo deadlift	Box squat	Sumo deadlift off two-inch blocks
Pause bench	Close-grip bench	Overhead press	Incline bench
Leg press	Dumbbell RDL	Walking lunge	Lat pull-down
Lateral arm raise	Hamstring curl	Arnold press	Pendlay row
Tricep push-down	Kettlebell carry	Plank	45-degree back extension

In reality, the options for this are limitless. That's why this framework is needed to make sure we cover all our bases. Let's take a close look at day one to make sure we are on the same page. Squat and bench are the main movements. To build those, you should have accessories that will strengthen the hips and quads for squats, and the chest, shoulders, and triceps for the bench. I selected the leg press to hit a squat-type pattern and to strengthen the quads and hips for the squat. Lateral arm raises strengthen the shoulders and are an isolation exercise that I wouldn't really put in a movement-pattern box, but that's okay because I still have them all covered through the week. Triceps extensions will help strengthen the triceps, and I *do* count this as a push since the triceps are a primary mover and a common limiter of pressing strength. That covers a lot of bases and gets you out of the gym in a manageable amount of time.

Volume and Intensity

We are almost home. Exercise selection is done, but now you have to decide how much volume and intensity you are going to use for each lift. The first thing to do here is to pick a main goal: hypertrophy or strength gain. Is there a right or wrong here? Not at all. But the goal you select determines the bias of your training program.

The Hypertrophy Path

If you want to look like you lift weights, the fastest way to get there is to add size and fill out your shirts a bit more. You won't get stronger at exactly the same rate as you would with a strength focus, but you will grow. The bias of progression with the hypertrophy path is volume. The goal is to gradually increase the total volume of each exercise each week until the completion of the program. For strength athletes, this is a great approach to use during the off-season to build some muscle and create the potential for increased strength. It is also a great starting point for beginners to learn the lifts and to start developing frames of reference with regard to performance. At the end of this kind of block, I do not suggest a one-rep maximum test because you aren't acclimated to that type of lifting. However, I do like to end it in a testing week of repetition maximums.

The Strength Path

In this path, the weight on the bar is the measure of progress. You may not grow at the same rate as you would by focusing on hypertrophy, but you will get noticeably stronger with this focus. The bias of this progression is intensity. The goal is to make the training weights progressively heavier each week while keeping volume relatively stable. For my strength athletes, this is more of an in-season approach. If you are a beginner, I would suggest running a hypertrophy block first to create a routine and a frame of reference for performance. With the strength bias, the block ends in a one-rep-maximum testing week focused on the main lifts.

It's almost time to put it all together, but first you need to incorporate three more principles: acclimatization, accumulation, and realization. These are the mesocycles that you go through as you progress your program, and they help inform the sets, reps, and deloads that you do.

- *Acclimatization.* This is the first mesocycle and the initial phase of the macrocycle. Imagine moving from Florida to Alaska. You would think every single day is extremely cold. It's the same concept here. There is a period of time in your training during which you have to acclimate to the lifts, the volume, and the intensity so that training can stabilize. This is also the time that most athletes complain of the most soreness, especially after the first few sessions. This will subside in the following weeks as you acclimate to the training. This phase can last anywhere from two to four weeks, and it ends in a deload that leads to the next phase.
- *Accumulation.* This is the middle block of the macrocycle, and it's when you start to pile on more volume or more intensity depending on whether you are biased toward hypotrophy or strength. It's where you start to accumulate the most fatigue but also the most stimulus toward your goals. Anecdotally, it's during this phase that I see most lifters become impatient and jump to testing too early. This is the hard-training phase that creates the adaptation needed to build muscle and to get stronger. This training phase can be between three and six weeks long and ends in a deload, leading to the next phase.

  A note here on accumulation: You don't have to move to the next phase of training after this. You can run another round of accumulation with another deload at the end. Some of my athletes never move to the last phase because testing isn't of interest to them. They stay in long phases of accumulation, and they get stronger and stronger. My suggestion, however, is that you restart in the acclimatization phase anytime you deload, and then overhaul your exercise selection. You'll need to acclimate to the new exercises, so give yourself that time.
- *Realization.* This is where you get to see the results of all of your hard work. The goal of the realization phase is to decrease fatigue and to prepare the body for testing (either a new 1RM or a repetition maximum). You can't express the strength that you have built if you're overfatigued. This phase can last between two and four weeks and is characterized by a sharp increase in volume or intensity, followed by a sharp decline in both to decrease fatigue. This is when most people complain about feeling a little beat up. This is normal since fatigue is very high. It's something to monitor though, and it may help determine the number of weeks you spend in this phase prior to testing.

Soreness Does Not Equal Results

Soreness is a commonly used subjective measurement of a good workout. It's not a reliable one though, and you should avoid falling into the trap of using it in this manner. It is, however, a good metric for how new something is. Are you brand new to training? You will be sore. Have you selected a movement that you haven't done before or that you haven't done for a while? You will be sore. Did you decide to run sprints for the first time since high school? That's why your hamstrings are so crushed. It's the novelty and the lack of acclimation to the training that lead to soreness. As you become better trained and your fitness levels improve, you'll experience less soreness. It's not a measure of a great session.

These phases help organize and dictate the sets, the reps, and the intensity that you select. Without them, there wouldn't be any guardrails on progression, and it would be easy to run a portion of the program for too long, for not long enough, or to skip over deloads completely. The following table will help you determine the length in weeks, including a deload at the end of each phase, so that you can stack each of these mesocycles together to create the entire macrocycle. Use the table to select the length of each phase of your training. The first number is the number of weeks in a phase, and the second number represents the deload week. So "2:1" would indicate two weeks in that phase followed by one week of deload.

Acclimatization	Accumulation	Realization
2:1	3:1	2:1
3:1	4:1	3:1
	5:1	4:1
	6:1	

This table shows a training block that is at most 16 weeks long. Does that mean that if you are doing a 16-week block that you have to select all the highest ones? The answer is no, and this is a very important note. As mentioned previously, you can always run more than one accumulation phase. So if you chose 16 weeks, you could easily run two three-to-one or four-to-one phases in the middle of it. There is no right or wrong way do it as long as you make sure to include those deloads and listen to your body.

Now it's time to get the numbers down. Let's return to the different paths—strength and hypertrophy—and outline how to select sets and reps for each exercise. Remember that these are all starting points and commonly used set-and-rep combinations. After these initial selections, you'll select how you'll progress from week to week. One other concept of note here: Select the rep scheme for each individual exercise. Doing eight reps on each exercise across the board is simple—and I don't want to steer you away from that simplicity—but I've found that selecting lower-volume main lifts and higher-volume accessory lifts keeps training fresher and more enjoyable. Also, hypertrophy is driven by volume, and strength is driven by intensity. You can modify accordingly later on down the road as long as you follow those principles.

Hypertrophy Path: Reps, Sets, and RPE

If you are at this point in the book, you more than likely have one of two goals: to get bigger or to get stronger. It's possible that you want to do both, but there always needs to be a bias toward one or the other from a programming standpoint. With that, let's get into the specifics of hypertrophy programming.

Hypertrophy-Path Reps

When it comes to rep selections for hypertrophy, there are quite a few options. This is by no means an exhaustive list of the options that work. I have seen countless combinations of reps, but these are a great place to begin for the first week of the training block. Take a look:

	Option 1: low volume	**Option 2: moderate volume**	**Option 3: high volume**	**Option 4: highest volume**
Main lift 1	5	8	10	12
Main lift 2	5	8	10	12
Accessory 1	8	12	15	20
Accessory 2	8	12	15	20
Accessory 3	8	12	15	20
Accessory 4	8	12	15	20
Accessory 5	8	12	15	20

Hypertrophy-Path Sets

To select the number of sets for week one of each phase of training, use the following chart to select the number of sets per exercise during each mesocycle of your training:

	Acclimatization	**Accumulation**	**Realization**
Week 1	2	3	4
Week 2	3	4	5
Week 3 onward		5	

The acclimatization phase tends to be lower volume by nature, so there are fewer total sets in that portion of the table. For realization, two sets of an exercise won't be adequate to maintain the fitness you are looking for in that phase, so there are more total sets in that phase.

Hypertrophy-Path RPE

RPE should also increase throughout the macrocycle, and training should get more intense from mesocycle to mesocycle. I like to think of each phase as having a top-limit RPE and a bottom-limit RPE, restricting acclimatization to two RPEs that are relatively easy but that will still create some hypertrophy. Use the chart below to help set the RPE selections for week one of your program:

	Acclimatization	Accumulation	Realization
Week 1	5	6	7
Week 2	6	7	8
Week 3 onward		8	9

You now have the sets, reps, and intensity for week one of each phase of the program. There are three ways we can increase the volume of each lift, and one of these you may not think of. The first is to increase the number of reps per set. This is typically done in two-rep increments: If you started with eight reps in week one you would do 10 reps in week two, 12 reps in week three, and so on. This is the smallest incremental increase in volume, and it is easier to recover from.

Another way is to add sets each week to each exercise. If week one starts at three sets, then week two is four sets, and so on. People tend to cap this at six sets because it can become very time consuming; adding sets means adding recovery time between sets as well. The last way to increase volume is to increase the weight, or add intensity. By doing this, you increase a metric known as *tonnage*, which is the total amount of weight lifted in a session expressed as a volume metric. With the intensity of high-rep training being noticeably lower than high-intensity training, it's the accumulation of the weight over reps that makes the difference. Some people suggest adding 5 pounds (2 kg) a week to each lift, but if you bench under 100 pounds (45 kg) that 5 pounds (2 kg) is a lot of weight. Instead, I suggest using an increase in RPE or a percentage increase based on the previous week. Increasing one point in RPE per week or by 5 percent of the weight lifted the week before is reasonable.

Also, it is important to note that you *should not* select all three of these to progress your program. This creates too many variables. The progression moves too fast and can outpace even the best recovery. Pick one, and run the whole program with it. Then select another one for your next program.

To recap, you can progress volume in the hypertrophy path in one of three ways:

- Increase reps in one- to two-rep increments per exercise per week.
- Increase one set per exercise per week.
- Increase the weight used by one point in RPE per week or by 5 percent of the weight lifted the prior week.

The Strength Path: Reps, Sets, and RPE

If strength is your goal, the focus shifts to lower volume and higher intensity. Let's dive in.

Strength-Path Reps

Volume in the strength path will inherently be lower through the entire macrocycle than it is with the hypertrophy path. Here are examples of rep-selection options that will build strength. Again, I have seen numerous combinations of these, but each of these is a great starting point for the first week of the training block. Take a look:

	Option 1: low volume	Option 2: low-moderate volume	Option 3: moderate volume	Option 4: moderate-high volume	Option 5: high volume
Main lift 1	2	3	4	5	6
Main lift 2	2	3	4	5	6
Accessory 1	5	6	8	10	12
Accessory 2	5	6	8	10	12
Accessory 3	6	8	10	12	15
Accessory 4	6	8	10	12	15
Accessory 5	6	8	10	12	15

Strength-Path Sets

Sets per exercise in the strength path actually doesn't look much different than it does in the hypertrophy path. The total volume of an exercise is more controlled here due to the lower reps, meaning the total number of sets is similar to what it is in the hypertrophy path. Again, you shouldn't have too many sets in the acclimatization phase, and you shouldn't have too few during realization or you could lose fitness or adaptation. That's why the sets per exercise are lower for the first week of training as shown here:

	Acclimatization	Accumulation	Realization
Week 1	2	2	3
Week 2	3	3	4
Week 3 onward		4	5

Strength-Path RPE

RPE prescriptions for the strength path will also not look much different from those in the hypertrophy path. A key distinction here is that with lower reps and lower total volume, the weight on the bar during the strength path is going to be higher than it is in the hypertrophy path, even at the same RPE. This makes the strength path higher intensity. It's intensity that builds high levels of strength. Take a look at the following chart to see some common options used during each mesocycle.

	Acclimatization	Accumulation	Realization
Week 1	5	6	7
Week 2	6	7	8
Week 3 onward		8	9

It looks pretty similar to the starting point of the hypertrophy path except for the reps, doesn't it? The reps make a difference here when coupled with the RPE ratings. Lower-rep sets at the same RPE as in hypertrophy training will inherently be heavier because there are just fewer reps to do. This increase in intensity, however, is what makes the difference when it comes to strength.

There is one noticeable difference that needs to be pointed out. As discussed earlier in the book, accessory movements are to build muscle and tissue capacity. Their utility is limited if you are trying to do 1RMs with them. We can still bias them with sets of five or six reps, but the more isolated the movement, the more appropriate higher-rep hypertrophy-type training is. For example, a rope triceps push-down, which is an isolated movement for the triceps, doesn't need to be maxed out and is commonly programmed in the 12- to 20-rep range.

Now how do we progress this? This is where the two paths really differ. The methods used may look similar, but the reasoning behind them is different. Remember that for the hypertrophy path, the goal is to increase volume through higher total volume and tonnage. Here, the focus is on increasing intensity, so the weight gets progressively heavier.

The first option is to do the exact opposite of what's done in hypertrophy: Decrease the number of reps each week. With the same RPE rating from week to week but with fewer reps in each set, the weight on the bar should increase in-line with those two things. Let's say that you start off your week-one accumulation phase with five sets of five reps each in the squat. The next week it would be five sets of four reps each at the same RPE but with more weight.

The next option is to add a set. It's true that you can always add sets anywhere, but I really prefer to do it with very low-rep sets like doubles and triples. This provides more exposure to those heavier weights, increasing not only strength but confidence. At times, I have selected 12 sets of two reps each for the athletes I work with.

Lastly, you can add weight. There are two ways to do this: You can increase RPE or you can increase the weight by 2.5 to 5 percent each week. Increasing RPE will inherently increase the weight on the bar since the sets and the reps are unchanged. However, adding 2.5 to 5 percent more weight to the bar each week means the sets, the reps, and RPE are *all* unchanged. That's how you know you're getting stronger week to week. The weight on the bar increases, but the RPE stays level. That's progress right there.

Again, *do not* select all three of these to progress your program. This creates too many variables. The progression moves too quickly and can outpace even the best recovery. Pick one, and run the whole program with it. Then select another one for your next program.

To recap, you can progress volume and intensity in the strength path in one of three ways:

- Decrease by one or two reps per exercise per week.
- Increase by one set per exercise per week.
- Increase one RPE or increase the weight by 2.5 percent to 5 percent per week.

When you are first starting out, you can apply these suggestions across the entire week of exercises, from week to week. Later on, you can start to run each training day through these selections to get even more granular.

How to Plan a Deload Week

Deloads are the same in the hypertrophy and the strength paths. This is a week when you reduce the fatigue from training while still getting movement in. I like to decrease the volume and the intensity of the last week of training by 50 percent. It's that simple. Cut everything in the last training week in half. For example, if your day-one squat was four sets of six reps with your RPE at eight and you were able to squat 225 pounds (102 kg) for that set, then for the deload week, plan for two sets of six reps with RPE at four to five and with around 115 to135 pounds. (52 to 61 kg).

These weeks are supposed to feel easy. Don't let that feeling trick you into trying to push them harder. Think of these weeks as deposits into the bank, ensuring that you don't go broke in three weeks. Resist the urge, and keep them easy.

Testing

Now that all the work is done, it's time to see how you did. Testing your new maximums allows you to measure progress, to gather information on what worked and what didn't, and to readjust your weights for the next training block now that you've gotten stronger. Testing is typically done after the end of the realization block and after a deload week so that the body is fully rested and ready for peak performance. There is one very important thing to understand though. Testing doesn't make you better. The work before the test does. It's just like in school. The test is the feedback on what you've done, not the driver of progress. This is me trying to deter you from maxing out every single week. Don't do it. Train hard, and then test. You can't skip the train-hard part.

A testing week can be done one of two ways. If you took the hypertrophy path, a repetition-maximum test is ideal because you have accumulated a lot of volume. For the strength path, it's time to find another 1RM or estimated 1RM for each main lift. Before you test, though, you must deload. The realization phase is very high-fatigue. Set yourself up for success by taking a deload week and coming into test week fresh.

For a rep-maximum test, don't select an arbitrary number to test with. A recent frame of reference here is important, and then you can use it as a baseline moving forward. If this is your first time doing this, select the weight you were able to complete for your main lift in week one of your realization phase. Let's say you were able to bench three sets of eight reps at 265 pounds (120 kg) on that day. On test day, you should do as many reps as you can with 265 pounds (120 kg). Go in, do your warm-up, work up to 265 pounds (120 kg), *grab a spotter*, and go for it. Do not sacrifice technique just to get one more rep either. There is no need to go flailing around for this kind of test. When you hit technical failure, note the result. Then use that information to inform your next block, using the exercise-selection concepts that you learned earlier in the book.

The next time you get around to test week, you can use this same method—hopefully with more weight on the bar. You can also use the 265 pounds (120 kg) again and try to get more reps. That choice is yours.

For 1RM or estimated 1RM testing, work up to a maximum lift in each main lift throughout the week. You can work up to a true maximum, which is your 1RM, or you can use a 2RM or 3RM as a proxy. I really like using 2RM and 3RM tests for beginners because they provide a relatively accurate number with a lower chance of failure in a lift. For reference, your 3RM is roughly 87.5 to 90 percent of your 1RM, and your 2RM is between 90 and 92.5 percent of your 1RM.

To test this this way, head into the gym, complete your warm-up, and get started working up the weight in the main lift. When first starting out, I like people to take smaller jumps from set to set so that they can get a better feel for the RPE it's taking to complete the rep. Start out doing five reps per set until the RPE gets to about a six. At that point, cut it to three reps per set until the RPE gets to between seven and eight. Then you can keep increasing RPE using singles. It might look something like this:

Bar × 5 RPE 4

135 pounds (61 kg) × 5 RPE 5

185 pounds (84 kg) × 5 RPE 6

225 pounds (102 kg) × 3 RPE 7.5

245 pounds (111 kg) × 1 RPE 8

265 pounds (120 kg) × 1 RPE 9

275 pounds (125 kg) × 1 Max RPE 9.5

For a 2RM or 3RM set, I would do the exact same workup but instead, take the 3RM at 245 pounds (111 kg) or RPE 8 if it were a single and the 2RM at 265 pounds (120 kg) or RPE 9 as a single.

Missing Lifts

Safety is important. At the same time, missed lifts happen. They just do. At some point, everyone misses a lift. Make good decisions, and if you are unsure, be conservative. A missed lift isn't a guaranteed injury waiting to happen, but it is a missed opportunity. Missed lifts cause more fatigue than successful lifts, and they take a lot of resources to recover from. Don't be reckless with them. We all have goals, but if it's not there on test day, be smart and walk away until the next one. If you do this more often than you miss, you'll achieve every goal you set.

What to do with this information from testing? Use it to reset your goals on new numbers, and go back through this process again. You now have all the tools you need to start barbell training effectively for years to come. You can choose your own warm-ups, create your own program with exercises selected specifically for you, and organize all of it in a way that fits your life.

This is cause for celebration, honestly. Most people never make it to this point, and I thank you from the bottom of my heart for sticking with me through this whole book. You are now part of the 1 percent of lifters who can walk into the gym and know exactly what to do to build a true foundation of strength.

Chapter 9

The Foundations of Long-Term Success

So far, we have spent this entire book talking about how to lift. In order to train successfully and over a long period time, however, you've got to be able to recover between sessions. You can only improve with training that you can recover from. That means the time outside the gym is just as important as the time in the gym. If you can learn this lesson now, it's going to save you massive amounts of time and frustration. I'm a firm believer that people can and should lift for their entire lifetime, and this is how to do it.

We all know that we need to sleep better, eat more vegetables, and manage stress better. Change happens when we know how. With that said, here are the subjects of this chapter so you know what you are getting into.

- *Recovery.* You will gain a deeper understanding of fatigue, rest, and other factors that affect recovery.
- *Quality sleep.* You will learn strategies to improve your sleep in both the short term and the long term.
- *Nutrition.* You will learn about calories and their function, and the baseline of what your body needs. You will also learn how nutrition can help you recover better.
- *Stress management.* You will learn how to tell the difference between different kinds of stressors (since your body can't), how to manage them, and when to find someone that can help you like a counselor or a therapist. I'm a big fan of taking care of your mental health by all means possible. I understand the stigma around it, but I cannot emphasize strongly enough how beneficial getting help can be.

The goal is to be able to manage training and recovery well enough to maintain progress without experiencing long periods of plateau. It's important to note that plateaus happen to all of us at some point. When they do, the first things to look at are how well you are recovering and how well you are managing these factors. Most people just try to train more or train harder to break through plateaus, but more isn't always better, and it has its limits. Look at recovery before pushing harder so you can avoid pushing too hard and burning out or worse, sustaining an injury, which can shorten your lifting career.

Recovery

Training (and life in general) creates fatigue in several forms—central fatigue, peripheral fatigue, and muscular damage. Their specific definitions are as follows:

- *Central fatigue* results from an overactivity-induced decline in muscle function that originates from the central nervous system. A good example of this can be seen in athletes after a powerlifting competition. They have just finished lifting maximal weight. They may not feel tired at all, but everything "just feels heavy," and their performance is heavily diminished after they compete. This can last for days at a time. Without enough recovery, or rest time, it could last for weeks or longer.
- *Peripheral fatigue* results from an overactivity-induced decline in muscle function that originates from non–central nervous system mechanisms such as the motor units within the muscles themselves. This kind of fatigue drops off relatively quickly. Think of the heavy and tired feeling you have after doing a tough workout, or even after something like yard work or moving a friend into their new house. Typically, some food and a good night's rest returns you to 100 percent the next day, even if you have a little soreness. Overall though, your performance isn't affected as much as it is with central fatigue. This is the kind of fatigue that most training creates.
- *Muscular damage* is the result of overload activities that create micro tears in the muscle fibers. Muscular damage is the goal of all resistance training. In cases where an exercise is new, this is a factor that contributes to soreness, but muscular damage can occur without soreness as well. This is a normal response to training, and it's what stimulates hypertrophy and adaptation.

In other words, fatigue leads to a decrease in performance if you don't recover from session to session. This is called *overreaching*. The conundrum many face, however, is that overload and overreaching are required to create adaptation and to get stronger. This is where the fitness–fatigue model comes in (see figure 9.1).

Let's take this graph one line at a time. We'll start with fatigue. As a training program goes on, fatigue accumulates and reaches levels that are difficult to recover from without a change in the program. This is the overreaching phase of training. When you see the decrease in fatigue, this is where a deload, or decrease in training occurs. This is designed to decrease fatigue and to allow the athlete to recover fully. If you do this well, you can drastically decrease fatigue. This drop in fatigue triggers what we see next with performance. Early in training, performance starts high and then starts to decline as fatigue adds up. However, when fatigue decreases again, it creates a phase of super compensation where performance exceeds that of previous bests. It's this repeated cycle—performance increase, fatigue increase, performance decline, fatigue increase, and then super compensation—that creates long-term change and progress.

The next line on the graph to look at is the one for fitness. This shows the capacity for adaptation over time. As you can see, fitness increases as fatigue increases, and it continues increasing for a period of time even when fatigue starts to decrease. Here is the key point of the fitness–fatigue model though: Eventually, both fitness and fatigue drop to low levels, which means that the opportunity for adaptation at that point is low. In the short term, performance is high. This could be viewed as a peak for current performance. Over time however, if fatigue and fitness aren't brought back up, performance declines along with other metrics. This is one of the reasons I like to avoid complete rest during deloads or during periods of injury. Long-term rest can have a negative impact on performance. You should take the opportunity to accumulate fatigue and fitness whenever you can by modifying training appropriately.

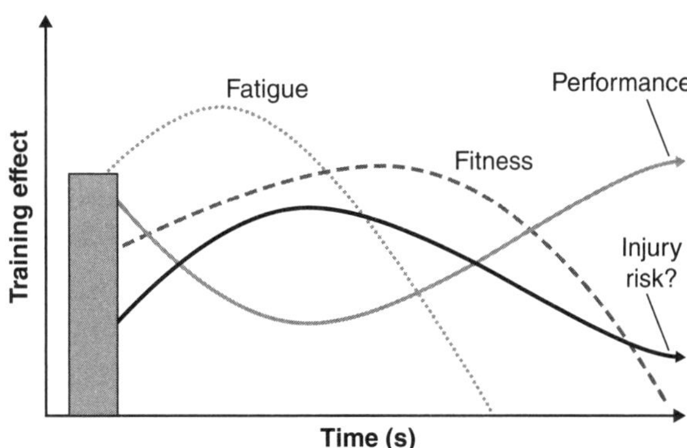

FIGURE 9.1 The fitness–fatigue model illustrates how training can affect fitness and fatigue and why overreaching and recovery are both important.

Reprinted by permission from T. Sawczuk, "Training Loads and Player Wellness in Youth Sport: Implications for Illness," PhD diss., (Leeds Beckett University, 2019), adapted from J.R. Fitz-Clarke et al., "Optimizing Athletic Performance by Influence Curves," *Journal of Applied Physiology* 71, no. 3 (1991): 1151-1158.

Age and Fitness

It's easy to see the benefits of long-term training on fitness levels. The longer you train consistently and follow the guidance in this book, the greater fitness level you will achieve. But what about when the natural aging process starts to affect your general fitness levels?

Here's the scoop: As you age, training becomes even more important. The fitness–fatigue model, as shown in figure 9.1, shows pretty clearly that with limited or no training, all metrics begin to decline. The cessation of training coupled with the natural decline in performance brought about by aging has a compounding effect and creates a rapid loss of fitness and function.

Training regularly as you age won't completely reverse the effects of aging, but it can stop performance declines during the middle-aged years, and it can slow those declines to a crawl during your later years. It's about as close as you can get to a fountain of youth.

There are two additional factors that contribute to fatigue in training, and you should keep them in mind when considering a training plan and your ability to recover from it. These are the athlete qualities and the recovery time for each lift.

Athlete Qualities

"Athlete qualities" sounds nebulous, so let's add some clarity. Each athlete has individual qualities that influence how quickly they can recover. We are going to look at three of them: size, cardiovascular health (or work capacity), and skill level.

Muscular damage is something that happens with all training. It's a desired effect that leads to hypertrophy and strength increases. The rate at which muscle recovers, also called *muscle protein synthesis*, is pretty standard across the board at 0.02 to 0.13 percent per hour after exercise (McGlory et al. 2017). What accounts for that range? The size of the muscle itself, which means that larger athletes (with larger muscles) take longer to recover than smaller athletes. This helps to explain the anecdotal observation that smaller athletes can handle more volume and more frequency than larger athletes.

Another factor to consider is that a larger muscle also has the potential to create more force and lift more weight, thereby creating more damage. To be clear: That doesn't mean that smaller athletes can't lift big weights. I've seen a 155-pound man (70 kg) deadlift well over 800 pounds (363 kg). What some people can do is amazing. What is important about this is the effect that absolute load has on recovery. As your skills improve and you progress to lifting heavier weights, the fatigue you accumulate from that load and activity makes recovery more difficult. Absolute load and skill level matter, and as you climb the ladder, recovery becomes even more important.

Recovery Time of Each Lift

There is a consistent hierarchy with regard to recovery with the main lifts. In order from the fastest recovery to the slowest:

1. Overhead press
2. Bench Press
3. Squat
4. Deadlift

Why is it this way? The overhead press tends to be the lightest of the four lifts and also uses a smaller total amount of musculature. The bench press comes in second. I've seen athletes handle unreal amounts of pressing volume and frequency, especially lighter lifters. It's not uncommon to see some of these people pressing six times in a week. That's more extreme than what I typically suggest, which is to have a pressing movement two to three times a week with a bias to what you want to build the fastest. If you want a bigger overhead press, go with overhead press, bench, overhead press when you lay out your programming for the week. If you want a bigger bench, go with bench, overhead press, bench for the week. If you're a powerlifter and you don't need to overhead press, you can bench three days in the week. (I still advocate for some level of overhead pressing until you begin meet preparation.) From a competition standpoint, it's typical to have a last heavy session on bench or on the overhead press four to seven days ahead of competition, which goes to show how fast the recovery can be.

The next fastest to recover is the squat. It's typical to see people squat two times a week and be okay from a recovery standpoint. I do see some start to struggle when a third day is added, but this is more dependent on the load they are using and on their personal size. When it comes to competing, most athletes take a last heavy set between 10 and 17 days out.

Last to recover is the deadlift. The most I recommend for the athletes I work with is a once-a-week pull with the possibility of a second variation day. It tends to take close to 14 days to fully recover after a heavy session. Leading up to competition, a range of 17 to 21 days to recover is the sweet spot. So why does the deadlift take so much longer? I don't think there is a definitive answer, but there are some theories. First and foremost, it uses a massive amount of musculature.

I've had athletes report that their pecs cramp during heavy attempts on the deadlift. The deadlift uses a lot of muscles to move the weight and to stabilize the rest of the body.

Additionally, with the deadlift being more about force development, it's more like a plyometric or explosive activity. The idea behind this is that since plyometrics demand more from the central nervous system, a deadlift creates more central fatigue than the other lifts. There is conflicting evidence on this subject: Some papers have concluded that it can take days to recover from central fatigue, and other papers have concluded that it can take minutes. This is when I lean on what I've experienced and observed while I wait for further research to emerge.

What I can tell you is this: With the 100 athletes I work with on my team, the average recovery time for the squat is 13 days, and for the deadlift, it is 20 days. That's a big difference, and it can't be ignored. Remember this when you move your training around and then find yourself wondering why you feel so tired.

What About Cardiovascular Health, or Work Capacity?

Cardio is highly underrated in the lifting community. Can cardio training have a negative impact on your lifting? Yes. This is known as the *interference effect.* Because of the SAID principle (specific adaptations to imposed demand), the body adapts to whatever you ask it to do. So if you are hitting the weights hard, your body will make your muscles larger to be more capable of doing what you're asking those big type-two fibers to do. More endurance training will stimulate those smaller, more efficient type-one fibers. However, the impact of the interference effect seems to be a little overblown, and we can create a few goals around baseline cardiovascular performance to help improve performance in the lifts.

How does cardiovascular performance affect performance in strength training? This comes down to energy systems, a subject that could fill an entire book on its own. Basically, heavy resistance training is typically categorized as being in the anaerobic energy system. Anaerobic activity doesn't require oxygen to create the energy needed to complete the activity. The sustainable duration for anaerobic activity tends to be short (less than one minute), and it's less efficient overall. Aerobic activity, such as running or cycling, is more efficient. Oxygen helps to create the energy needed for aerobic activity, so it can be sustained much longer. Here's the deal though: While each resistance exercise you do is an anaerobic activity, as the exercises add up during the session, the demand on the aerobic systems increases. If the aerobic systems aren't performing at some level of baseline, it will affect your recovery between sets and decrease the total amount of work in the session. That's a negative impact on performance.

So what's the baseline you should shoot for? A resting heart rate of 50 bpm is a good reference point. If yours is higher than this, don't panic. Start slowly (i.e., no hill sprints). You don't want the incorporation of cardio to dip into your recovery. Something as simple as an easy 20- to 30-minute walk twice a week can get the ball rolling. I'm also an advocate of purchasing a step-counting device to track your step count during the day. Setting a goal of 10,000 steps a day during your day-to-day activities can be a good starting point. If you are starting out and only getting 3,000 to 4,000 steps in a day, don't worry about getting right to 10,000. Creating a goal of 6,000 to 7,000 steps and hitting that consistently is where I would start. The point is: Don't be afraid to add light cardio work to your program. Not only is it not going to kill your gains, it's going to help them.

So how do you incorporate recovery into training? The most common way is through planned deloads. This is the easiest way to reduce fatigue in a controlled manner, and it's what I most often suggest to people starting out. A deload is a planned decrease in volume and intensity, typically over an entire week of training. The frequency of these deloads can vary, but it's typical to drop them into a plan around the four- to six-week mark. You may hear people refer to their program as being "three up and one down." This means that they train hard and progressively overload over three weeks, and then they insert a back-off, or deload week in the fourth week to allow recovery. Additionally, it's best practice to insert a deload week after competitions or testing weeks to allow for recovery ahead of the next training cycle. If you are just starting out, plan out your deloads and stick to them.

Sleep

Everything slows down during sleep, and the body shifts into repair mode. We've all heard the recommendation that you should get seven to eight hours of sleep per night and even more than that if you're more active. I have seen upward of 11 to 12 hours of sleep recommended for professional athletes with a high training demand. Many of us know we need to improve our sleep. The question is how to do it. Here are some of my top suggestions to get more quality shut eye.

Set Two Bedtime Alarms

Just like you set an alarm to wake up, you should set an alarm to go to bed. In fact, set two of them. The first should be 30 minutes before your planned bedtime. This is when you disconnect from your phone: Stop scrolling on TikTok, plug it in for the night, and turn it over. Doing this 30 minutes before bed allows your normal rhythms to take over and prepares you for sleep. The second alarm is your wrap-up-what-you're-doing-and-go-to-bed alarm. That means putting down this awesome book and going to sleep. This habit alone has helped me to add an hour of sleep a night and also to sleep through the night more consistently.

If you have kids, adding this to their routines can been amazing (I speak from experience here). It's a task at first, but once they get used to it and know what to expect, the pushback becomes less and less. They may still gripe about it every now and then, but it's worth it. It will help them to get better sleep so that you can too.

Have a Nighttime Routine

What should you do during the 30 minutes between the two alarms? This is the time for your bedtime ritual. Get changed, brush your teeth, listen to calming music, read a book, or do whatever it is that calms you down and gets you ready for sleep. The only rule is that your routine should be consistent. Do the same things in the same order and with the same start and end times. If you find that something in the routine isn't working for you, swap it out for something different, but keep it to one variable at a time.

When to Talk to Your Doctor

If I have learned one thing, it's that asking for help pays off. If you experience any of the following, you should talk to your doctor or a sleep specialist.

- Frequent waking up for urination.
- Restless sleep and periods where you stop breathing.
- Pain or numbness that is worsened by sleep.
- Regularly waking up fatigued, even after the recommended eight hours.

This is not an exhaustive list, but if any of these apply to you, talk to your doctor about a sleep study or linking up with a sleep specialist. Your lifting—and your life—will be better for it.

Nutrition

There are so many plans you can follow for consuming food: vegan, paleo, carnivore, South Beach, Atkins, and dozens more. As with training, however, the basics rule. This section will teach you how to look at your nutrition and how to determine whether it's setting you up for success.

The first thing to establish is that food is fuel. Training, lifting, and getting stronger all require fuel. That fuel comes in the form of calories. What is a calorie, and why is it important? A calorie is simply a unit of measurement. Specifically, it's the amount of energy needed to increase the temperature of water by a single degree. That's it. When you process energy, it creates heat. A calorie is how we measure that value in the food you consume. It's like gasoline in a car. As a bigger guy, I like to think of myself as an old diesel truck that has plenty of torque and power but requires 100 gallons of fuel a day to keep running.

This is where *basal metabolic rate*, or BMR, comes in. This is your baseline: The number of calories your body needs in order to perform basic life functions like day-to-day tissue breakdown and recovery, brain function, digestion, and the various processes of all your organs. All of this requires energy. We can calculate how much energy by using the following formulas.

Men

$$\text{BMR} = 88.362 + (13.397 \times \text{your body weight in kg}) + (4.799 \times \text{your height in cm}) - (5.677 \times \text{your age in years})$$

Women

$$\text{BMR} = 447.593 + (9.247 \times \text{your body weight in kg}) + (3.098 \times \text{your height in cm}) - (4.330 \times \text{your age in years})$$

This will tell you how many calories per day you need to survive. The next piece of the puzzle is your activity level, which needs to be factored into the equation. To do this, plug your calculated BMR into one of the following equations based on your activity level, and do the math.

- *Sedentary* (little or no exercise): calories = BMR × 1.2
- *Lightly active* (light exercise or sports 1 to 3 days/week): calories = BMR × 1.375

- *Moderately active* (moderate exercise or sports 3 to 5 days/week): calories = BMR × 1.55
- *Very active* (hard exercise or sports 6 to 7 days a week): calories = BMR × 1.725
- *Extra active* (very hard exercise or sports and a physical job 2x a day for 6 to 7 days a week): calories = BMR × 1.9

Now you know the total amount of daily calories, or the total daily energy expenditure (TDEE), that you need to support your activity level, maintain stable body weight, and be able to recover adequately from workout to workout. It's important to know this number so that you can have a target and take control of your nutrition. In my experience, eating too little has a more negative effect on a lifter's performance than overeating does. When creating or evaluating a diet plan, the calorie intake should be determined using these equations.

Another important part of nutrition is hydration. You have to drink more water. The general guideline is to drink half your bodyweight in ounces per day. Why? Water is critical for most of the processes and environments in your body such as blood volume, brain function, hormonal balance, and digestion. Even a 3 percent decrease in hydration can have a noticeable negative effect on training and performance. So drink up. You may have to go to the bathroom more often, but you'll feel better and rack up more PRs.

Stress Management

When it comes to stress, there are two types: *eustress* and *distress.* Eustress is defined as stress that has a beneficial effect. I like to think of training as a source of eustress. Distress, however, causes a negative effect or emotion. This is the stress from terrible traffic, an argument with your partner, or a bad day at work. The problem is that the body doesn't know how to distinguish between the two. Everything gets lumped together to produce a level of general stress that is either under or over your individual capacity.

The analogy that I have always liked is to imagine that your capacity for stress is a cup. As you train and as life stressors appear, water is added to the cup. When you go to bed at night, you pour all that water out, and you start the next day with an empty cup. There are two possible scenarios that can result in your stress level exceeding your capacity, or your cup overflowing. The first: Some major life event happens and rapidly fills your cup to the point where it overflows and has a negative impact on your life and training.

The second: Chronic stress prevents you from being able to fully empty the cup each night, leaving you with less capacity. This type of ongoing day-to-day stress—whether due to a toxic work environment, a difficult relationship, or a patch of bad training days—compounds until eventually, your cup overflows. Be mindful of stress; it creates fatigue. Control the things you can, like sleep, nutrition, and the way you respond to stressors.

The Mindset Key to Lifting for a Lifetime: Having a "Why."

I'm going to be honest here: You aren't going to feel great every day. The gym won't call to you every session. Some days you will want to curl up on the couch and binge-watch something instead. Not only that, but the longer you lift, the smaller and further apart the jumps in progress become. The experience is not a straight line up. It's a mountain range of ups and downs that all of us have to go through. The idea that your lifting journey is going to be easy, simple, and predictable is completely true, and I've seen many people quit when progress slowed down or things got hard.

That's when it's important to remember your personal "why." If this sounds kind of selfish, that's because it is. Selfishness is not always a negative characteristic though. Everyone needs their own time and space to take care of themselves. Through this, you can be more present in your relationships, work, and life. It is the moments of selfishness that put you in a position to be selfless.

Your "why" is yours alone, whether it's to lose weight, to get stronger, to get bigger, or anything else. To find your deepest "why," ask yourself three follow-ups "whys." Here's what I mean: I work with a young high school wrestler who also competes in powerlifting. When I asked him why he started training, he said it was because he wanted to get stronger. I asked him why. He said, "I want it to carry over to wrestling." I asked him why again. He said, "So I can win more matches." I asked him why one more time. He said, "I want to get to 100 wins before I graduate. There's a short list of people who have been able to do that, and I want to be one of them." He accomplished that goal during his senior year, putting himself in the school's history book. His "why" was way deeper than just to get stronger. It was a mission that had likely been years in the making. That's the stuff that gets you out of bed in the morning. Go through the "three whys" and connect with what is going to keep you going when times get tough.

My goal is for everyone to experience the benefits of strength training and the ways it can affect their lives. More than that, I'd like to make a life-long lifter out of each person who reads this book. We have covered a lot of ground together including:

- The correct execution for the squat, the bench, the deadlift, and the press, and how to modify them for the most progress.
- The proper way to warm up for each lift.
- The incorporation of the right accessory exercises with your main lifts to continue to get stronger and to stay healthy.
- The key elements of effective programming and how to create long-term training plans on your own.
- The importance of understanding what fatigue is and how to manage it, the affect stress has on performance, and how to recover better from session to session.

These are the tools you need to create your own roadmap to lifting success as well as to analyze other programs and determine whether they are effective. More importantly, you now have a framework on the optionality of training. You can make this your own and use it to lift forever. My last challenge to you, as we wrap up this final chapter, is to keep that end in mind. Enjoy each session as much as you can. Have fun with it, and surround yourself with people you can laugh and joke around with while getting stronger. Turn the music up loud and dance a little between sets. Turn off your phone and create your own space for self-improvement. It's not about tomorrow, next week, or even next month. Have fun in the moment, and remember that this lifting journey can go on for as long as you want.

If you've made it this far, thank you. I appreciate the time and energy you have put into reading this book, and my hope is that you implement what it offers and that you find tremendous value in it. Now it's time for me to chase my lifting goals alongside you. And, if we meet in real life in a gym somewhere and you want to lift together, you'll always get a "hell, yes" from me.

APPENDIX: FOUNDATIONAL STRENGTH PROGRAMMING WORKSHEET

1. Pick a length of time for the macrocycle or the length of time that the program you are evaluating lasts.

   16-week macrocycle

   12-week macrocycle

   8-week macrocycle

   Other: ________________

2. Pick your base deload cadence.

   3 up 1 down

   4 up 1 down

   5 up 1 down

   Other: ________________

3. How many days a week will you train?

   5 times a week

   4 times a week

   3 times a week

   2 times a week

4. Select main-lift frequency.

   1 bench, 1 press, 1 squat, 1 deadlift: minimum 2 training days

   2 bench, 1 press, 1 squat, 1 deadlift: minimum 3 training days.

   2 bench, 2 press, 2 squat, 1 deadlift: 3 training days

   2 bench, 2 press, 2 squat, 2 deadlift: 4 training days

   3 bench, 2 press, 2 squat, 1 deadlift: 4 training days

   3 bench, 2 press, 2 squat, 2 deadlift: 5 training days

   2 bench, 3 press, 3 squat, 1 deadlift: 5 training days

   Other: ____

5. Fill in your layout up to this point for a single week.

	Day 1	Day 2	Day 3	Day 4	Day 5
Main lift 1					
Main lift 2					

Input exercise selection for the main lifts.

	Squat	Bench Press	Deadlift	Overhead Press
Primary				
Secondary				
Tertiary				

Now lay out your week based off your previous selections.

Day 1	Day 2	Day 3	Day 4	Day 5

6. Select the time you want to be in the gym.
   3 exercises plus warm up: 30-45 minutes
   4 exercises plus warm up: 45-60 minutes
   5 exercises plus warm up: 60-75 minutes
   6+ exercises plus warm up: 75 minutes plus (also known as *forever*)

Fill out the grid with your accessories:

	Day 1	Day 2	Day 3	Day 4	Day 5
Main Lift 1					
Main Lift 2					
Accessory					
Accessory					
Accessory					
Accessory					
Accessory					

7. Choose your path.
   Hypertrophy
   Strength

Hypertrophy Path

1. Get granular with your training phases and deload cadence.

Total number of weeks for this training block: ________________

Acclimatization	Accumulation	Realization
2:1	3:1	2:1
3:1	4:1	3:1
	5:1	4:1
	6:1	

2. Select reps for hypertrophy path.

Main Lift 1	8	12	15	20
Main Lift 2	8	12	15	20
Accessory 1	8	12	15	20
Accessory 2	8	12	15	20
Accessory 3	8	12	15	20
Accessory 4	8	12	15	20
Accessory 5	8	12	15	20

3. Select sets for week one of each phase for hypertrophy path.

Acclimatization	Accumulation	Realization
2	2	3
3	3	4
	4	

4. Select RPE for week one of each phase of hypertrophy path.

Acclimatization	Accumulation	Realization
5	6	7
6	7	8
	8	9

5. Select a progression method.

   Increase reps by ________ per exercise/per week.

   Increase one set per exercise per week.

   Increase 1 RPE or 5 percent weight lifted per week.

Stop! Now fill out the blank programs at the end of this worksheet with everything you have completed at this point. That is now your program!

The Strength Path

1. Get granular with your training phases and deload cadence.

Total number of weeks for this training block: ________________

Acclimatization	Accumulation	Realization
2:1	3:1	2:1
3:1	4:1	3:1
	5:1	4:1
	6:1	

2. Select reps for strength path.

Main Lift 1	2	3	4	5	6
Main Lift 2	2	3	4	5	6
Accessory 1	5	6	8	10	12
Accessory 2	5	6	8	10	12
Accessory 3	6	8	10	12	15
Accessory 4	6	8	10	12	15
Accessory 5	6	8	10	12	15

3. Select sets for week one of each phase for strength path.

Acclimatization	Accumulation	Realization
2	2	3
3	3	4
	4	

4. Select RPE for week one of each phase of hypertrophy path.

Acclimatization	Accumulation	Realization
5	6	7
6	7	8
	8	9

5. Select a progression method.

   Increase reps by _________ per exercise/per week.

   Increase one set per exercise per week.

   Increase 1 RPE or 5 percent weight lifted per week.

   Stop!! Now fill out the blank programs at the end of this worksheet with everything you have completed at this point. That is now your program!

Week 1 _______________ Phase

	Day 1	Day 2	Day 3	Day 4	Day 5
Main Lift 1					
Main Lift 2					
Accessory					
Accessory					
Accessory					
Accessory					
Accessory					

Week 2_______________ Phase

	Day 1	Day 2	Day 3	Day 4	Day 5
Main Lift 1					
Main Lift 2					
Accessory					
Accessory					
Accessory					
Accessory					
Accessory					

Week 3_______________ Phase

	Day 1	Day 2	Day 3	Day 4	Day 5
Main Lift 1					
Main Lift 2					
Accessory					
Accessory					
Accessory					
Accessory					
Accessory					

Week 4_______________ Phase

	Day 1	Day 2	Day 3	Day 4	Day 5
Main Lift 1					
Main Lift 2					
Accessory					
Accessory					
Accessory					
Accessory					
Accessory					

Week 5_______________ **Phase**

	Day 1	Day 2	Day 3	Day 4	Day 5
Main Lift 1					
Main Lift 2					
Accessory					
Accessory					
Accessory					
Accessory					
Accessory					

Week 6_______________ **Phase**

	Day 1	Day 2	Day 3	Day 4	Day 5
Main Lift 1					
Main Lift 2					
Accessory					
Accessory					
Accessory					
Accessory					
Accessory					

Week 7_______________ **Phase**

	Day 1	Day 2	Day 3	Day 4	Day 5
Main Lift 1					
Main Lift 2					
Accessory					
Accessory					
Accessory					
Accessory					
Accessory					

Week 8_______________ Phase

	Day 1	Day 2	Day 3	Day 4	Day 5
Main Lift 1					
Main Lift 2					
Accessory					
Accessory					
Accessory					
Accessory					
Accessory					

Week 9_______________ Phase

	Day 1	Day 2	Day 3	Day 4	Day 5
Main Lift 1					
Main Lift 2					
Accessory					
Accessory					
Accessory					
Accessory					
Accessory					

Week 10_______________ Phase

	Day 1	Day 2	Day 3	Day 4	Day 5
Main Lift 1					
Main Lift 2					
Accessory					
Accessory					
Accessory					
Accessory					
Accessory					

Week 11_______________ Phase

	Day 1	Day 2	Day 3	Day 4	Day 5
Main Lift 1					
Main Lift 2					
Accessory					
Accessory					
Accessory					
Accessory					
Accessory					

Week 12_______________ Phase

	Day 1	Day 2	Day 3	Day 4	Day 5
Main Lift 1					
Main Lift 2					
Accessory					
Accessory					
Accessory					
Accessory					
Accessory					

Week 13_______________ Phase

	Day 1	Day 2	Day 3	Day 4	Day 5
Main Lift 1					
Main Lift 2					
Accessory					
Accessory					
Accessory					
Accessory					
Accessory					

Week 14_______________ Phase

	Day 1	Day 2	Day 3	Day 4	Day 5
Main Lift 1					
Main Lift 2					
Accessory					
Accessory					
Accessory					
Accessory					
Accessory					

Week 15 _______________ Phase

	Day 1	Day 2	Day 3	Day 4	Day 5
Main Lift 1					
Main Lift 2					
Accessory					
Accessory					
Accessory					
Accessory					
Accessory					

Week 16 _______________ Phase

	Day 1	Day 2	Day 3	Day 4	Day 5
Main Lift 1					
Main Lift 2					
Accessory					
Accessory					
Accessory					
Accessory					
Accessory					

Testing Week Results

	Day 1	Day 2	Day 3	Day 4	Day 5
Main Lift 1					
Main Lift 2					

REFERENCES

Chapter 1

Aasa, U., I. Svartholm, F. Andersson, and L. Berglund. 2017. "Injuries Among Weightlifters and Powerlifters: A Systematic Review." *British Journal of Sports Medicine* 51: 211-219.

National Council on Aging. 2023. "Get the Facts on Falls Prevention." https://ncoa.org/article/get-the-facts-on-falls-prevention.

Prieto-González, P., J.L. Martínez-Castillo, L.M. Fernández-Galván, A. Casado, S. Soporki, and J. Sánchez-Infante. 2021. "Epidemiology of Sports-Related Injuries and Associated Risk Factors in Adolescent Athletes: An Injury Surveillance." *International Journal of Environmental Research and Public Health* 18(9): 4857. https://doi.org/10.3390/ijerph18094857.

Chapter 2

Hammer, S., A. Alexander, K. Didier, T. Barstow. 2020. "Influence of Blood Flow Occlusion on Muscular Recruitment and Fatigue During Maximal-Effort Small Muscle-Mass Exercise." *The Journal of Physiology* 598(19): 4293-306. https://doi.org/10.1113/JP279925.

Chapter 3

Blazek, D., P. Stastny, A. Maszczyk, M. Krawczyk, P. Matykiewicz, and M. Petr. 2019. "Systematic Review of Intra-Abdominal and Intrathoracic Pressures Initiated by the Valsalva Manoeuvre During High-Intensity Resistance Exercises." *Biology of Sport* 36(4): 373-86. https://doi.org/10.5114/biolsport.2019.88759.

Glassbrook, D.J., E.R. Helms, S.R. Brown, and A.G. Storey. 2017. "A Review of the Biomechanical Differences Between the High-Bar and Low-Bar Back-Squat." *Journal of Strength and Conditioning Research* 31(9): 2618-34. https//doi.org/10.1519/JSC.0000000000002007.

Liu-Ambrose, T., K.M. Khan, J.J. Eng, P.A. Janssen, S.R. Lord, and H.A. McKay. 2004. "Resistance and Agility Training Reduce Fall Risk in Women Aged 75 to 85 With Low Bone Mass: A 6-Month Randomized, Controlled Trial." *Journal of the American Geriatrics Society* 52(5): 657-65. https://doi.org/10.1111/j.1532-5415.2004.52200.x.

Miletello, W.M., J.R. Beam, and Z.C. Cooper. 2009. "A Biomechanical Analysis of the Squat Between Competitive Collegiate, Competitive High School, and Novice Powerlifters." *Journal of Strength and Conditioning Research* 23(5): 1611-7. https://doi.org/10.1519/JSC.0b013e3181a3c6ef.

Chapter 4

Cudlip, A.C., J.M. Maciukiewicz, B.L. Pinto, and C.R. Dickerson. 2022. "Upper Extremity Muscle Activity and Joint Loading Changes Between the Standard and Powerlifting Bench Press Techniques. Journal of Sports Sciences 40(9): 1055-1063. https://doi.org/10.1080/02640414.2022.2046937.

Ferland, P.-M., and A.S. Comtois. 2019. "Classic Powerlifting Performance: A Systematic Review." *Journal of Strength and Conditioning Research* 33:S194-S201. https//doi.org/10.1519/JSC.0000000000003099

Saeterbakken, A.H., D.A. Mo, S. Scott, and V. Andersen. 2017. "The Effects of Bench Press Variations in Competitive Athletes on Muscle Activity and Performance." *Journal of Human Kinetics* 57:61-71. http//doi.org/10.1515/hukin-2017-0047.

Tungate, P. 2019. "The Bench Press: A Comparison Between Flat-Back and Arched-Back Techniques." *Strength and Conditioning Journal* 41(5): 86-89. https//doi.org/10.1519/SSC.0000000000000494.

Chapter 5

Bengtsson, V., L. Berglund, and U. Aasa. 2018. "Narrative Review of Injuries in Powerlifting With Special Reference to Their Association to the Squat, Bench Press and Deadlift." *BMJ Open Sport & Exercise Medicine* 4: e000382. https//:doi.org/10.1136/bmjsem-2018-000382.

Blazek, D., P. Stastny, A. Maszczyk, M. Krawczyk, P. Matykiewicz, and M. Petr. 2019. "Systematic Review of Intra-Abdominal and Intrathoracic Pressures Initiated by the Valsalva Manoeuvre During High-Intensity Resistance Exercises." *Biology of Sport* 36(4): 373-86. https://doi.org/10.5114/biolsport.2019.88759.

Escamilla et al. (2000). A three-dimensional biomechanical analysis of sumo and conventional style deadlifts. *Medicine and science in sports and exercise.* https://pubmed.ncbi.nlm.nih.gov/10912892/

Fischer, S.C., D.Q. Calley, and J.H. Hollman. 2021. "Effect of an Exercise Program That Includes Deadlifts on Low Back Pain." *Journal of Sport Rehabilitation* 30(4): 672-5. https://doi.org/10.1123/jsr.2020-0324.

Holmberg, D., H. Crantz, and P. Michaelson. 2012. "Treating Persistent Low Back Pain With Deadlift Training – A Single Subject Experimental Design With a 15-Month Follow-Up." *Advances in Physiotherapy* 14(2): 61-70. https://doi.org/10.3109/14038196.2012.674973.

Nogueira, A., A. Resende-Neto, J. Aragão-Santos, L. da Silva Chaves, L. Azevêdo, C. La Scala Teixeira, G. Senna, and M. Da Silva-Grigoletto. 2017. "Effects of a Multicomponent Training Protocol on Functional Fitness and Quality of Life of Physically Active Older Women." *Motricidade* 13.

Soriano-Maldonado, A., Á. Carrera-Ruiz, D.M. Díez-Fernández, A. Esteban-Simón, M. Maldonado-Quesada, N. Moreno-Poza, M.D.M. García-Martínez, et al. 2019. "Effects of a 12-Week Resistance and Aerobic Exercise Program on Muscular Strength and Quality of Life in Breast Cancer Survivors: Study Protocol for the EFICAN Randomized Controlled Trial." *Medicine* 98(44): e17625. https://doi.org/10.1097/MD.0000000000017625.

Chapter 9

McGlory, C., M.C. Devries, and S.M. Phillips. 2017. "Skeletal Muscle and Resistance Exercise Training; the Role of Protein Synthesis in Recovery and Remodeling." *Journal of Applied Physiology* 122(3): 541-8.

INDEX

J

K

L

M

N

O

P

ABOUT THE AUTHOR

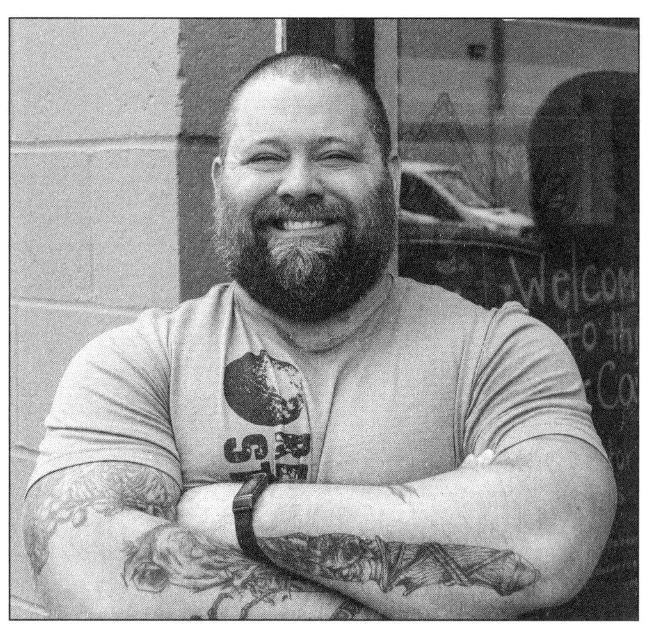

John Flagg is a strength coach, athletic trainer, and competitive powerlifter. He is the owner of Rebuild Stronger, an online coaching company that helps powerlifting, weightlifting, and strongman athletes return from injury and overcome training plateaus. He has helped thousands of athletes recover from injuries while also developing elite athletes preparing for national and international levels of competition. He currently coaches nearly 100 athletes, both online and in person. He is also the cohost of the *Rebuild Stronger* podcast, covering all things related to strength training and health.

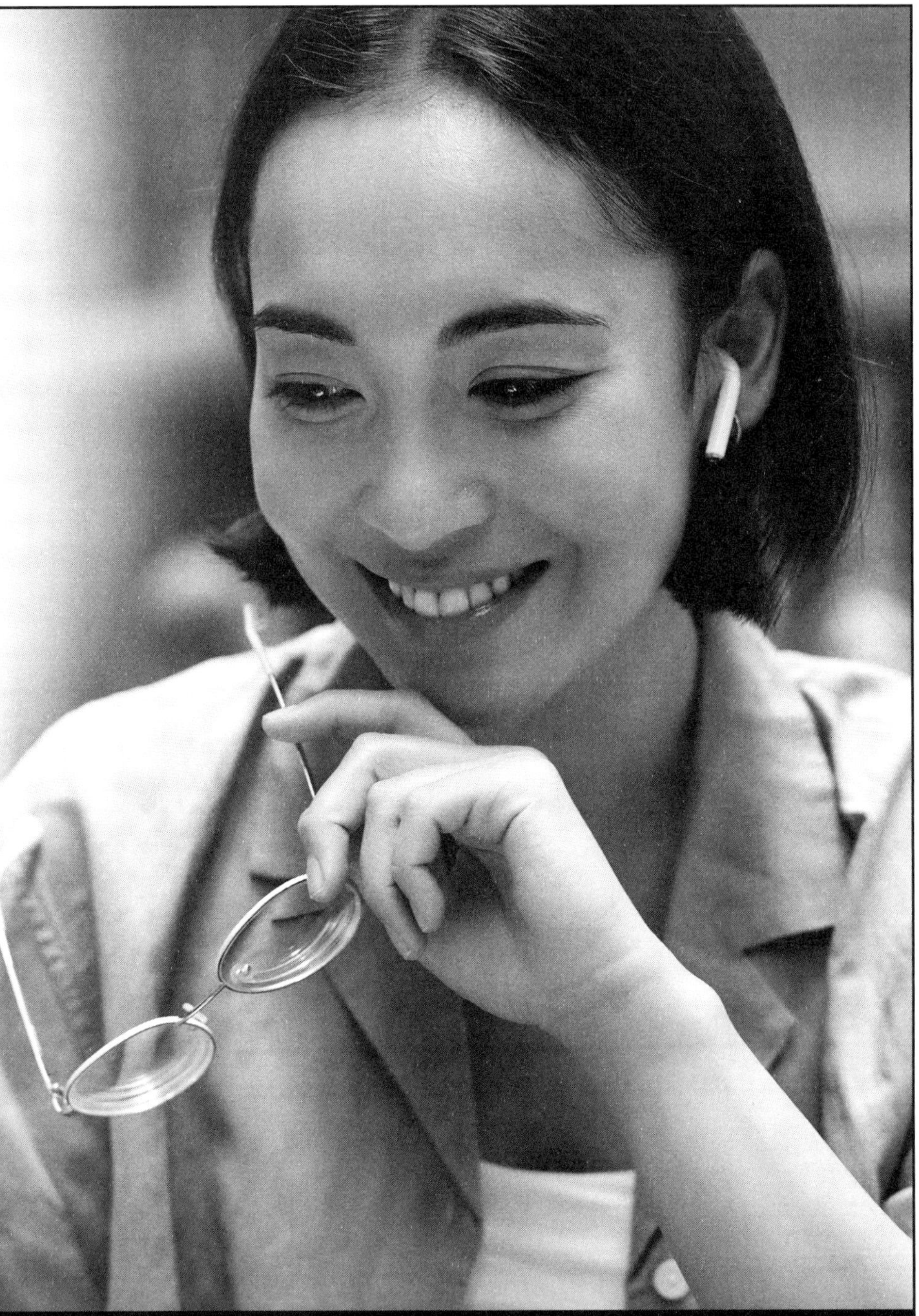

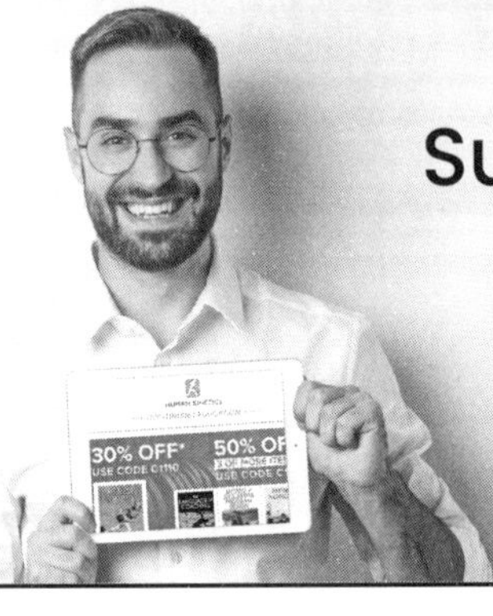